GENETICS OF HYPERTENSION

PUBLISHED VOLUMES IN THE SERIES

SERIES EDITORS: W. H. BIRKENHÄGER AND J. L. REID

Volume 24

GENETICS OF HYPERTENSION

Editors

Anna F. Dominiczak
British Heart Foundation Professor of
Cardiovascular Medicine; Director,
BHF Glasgow Cardiovascular
Research Centre, University of Glasgow,
Glasgow, UK

John M. C. Connell
Professor of Endocrinology,
BHF Glasgow Cardiovascular
Research Centre, University of Glasgow,
Glasgow, UK

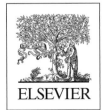

ELSEVIER

EDINBURGH   LONDON   NEW YORK   OXFORD
PHILADELPHIA   ST LOUIS   SYDNEY   TORONTO   2007

Elsevier B.V.
Radarweg 29, 1043 NX, Amerstam, The Netherlands

© 2007, Elsevier B.V. All rights reserved.

First published 2007

ISBN-13: 978 0 444 51456 1 (Vol 24)
ISBN-10: 0 444 51456 2 (Vol 24)

ISBN-13: 978 0 444 90341 9
ISBN-10: 0 444 90341 0 (Series)

British Library Cataloguing in Publication Data
A catalogue record for this book is available from the British Library

Library of Congress Cataloging in Publication Data
A catalog record for this book is available from the Library of Congress

Notice
Knowledge and best practice in this field are constantly changing. As new research and experience broaden our knowledge, changes in practice, treatment and drug therapy may become necessary or appropriate. Readers are advised to check the most current information provided (i) on procedures featured or (ii) by the manufacturer of each product to be administered, to verify the recommended dose or formula, the method and duration of administration, and contraindications. It is the responsibility of the practitioner, relying on their own experience and knowledge of the patient, to make diagnoses, to determine dosages and the best treatment for each individual patient, and to take all appropriate safety precautions. To the fullest extent of the law, neither the Publisher nor the Editors assume any liability for any injury and/or damage to persons or property arising out or related to any use of the material contained in this book.

The Publisher

Printed in China

Contributors

G. Bianchi
Chair and School of Nephrology
Division of Nephrology, Dialysis and
   Hypertension,
University Vita-Salute,
San Raffaele Hospital,
Milan, Italy

F. Broughton Pipkin
Professor of Perinatal Physiology
University Department of Obstetrics &
   Gynaecology
Maternity Unit
City Hospital
Nottingham, UK

P. R. Burton
Professor of Genetic Epidemiology
Departments of Health Sciences
   and Genetics,
University of Leicester,
Leicester, UK

M. Caulfield
Professor of Clinical Pharmacology
   and Director of The William Harvey
   Research Institute,
Bart's and The London School of
   Medicine and Dentistry,
London, UK

L. Citterio
Senior Scientist
Division of Nephrology, Dialysis and
   Hypertension,
University Vita-Salute,
San Raffaele Hospital,
Milan, Italy

Tara Collidge
Specialist Registrar in Renal Medicine,
Renal Unit, Glasgow Royal Infirmary,
Glasgow, UK

J. M. C. Connell
Professor of Endocrinology,
BHF Glasgow Cardiovascular
   Research Centre,
University of Glasgow,
Glasgow, UK

A. W. Cowley Jr
Chair
Department of Physiology,
Medical College of Wisconsin,
Milwaukee, Wisconsin,
USA

W. J. de Lange
Postdoctoral research scholar
Ray J. and Lucille A. Carver College of
   Medicine
University of Iowa,
Iowa City, Iowa,
USA

A. F. Dominiczak
British Heart Foundation Professor of
   Cardiovascular Medicine; Director,
BHF Glasgow Cardiovascular
   Research Centre,
University of Glasgow,
Glasgow, UK

M. R. Garrett
Assistant Professor
University of Toledo
Health Science Campus
Toledo, Ohio,
USA

D. S. Geller
Section of Nephrology,
Yale University School of Medicine,
New Haven, Connecticut,
USA

J. E. Goodwin
Section of Pediatric Nephrology,
Yale University School of Medicine,
New Haven, Connecticut,
USA

H. J. Jacob
Director, Human and Molecular
   Genetics Center, Professor,
   Department of Physiology
Medical College of Wisconsin,
Milwaukee, Wisconsin,
USA

B. Joe
Assistant Professor
Physiological Genomics Laboratory
University of Toledo
Health Science Campus
Toledo, Ohio,
USA

B. Keavney
Professor of Cardiology
Institute of Human Genetics,
University of Newcastle
Newcastle-upon-Tyne, UK

K. Lindpaintner
Roche Distinguished Scientist and VP
   Research,
Head, Roche Genetics & Roche Center
   for Medical Genomics,
Basel, Switzerland

C. Moreno
Assistant Professor
Department of Physiology
Medical College of Wisconsin,
Milwaukee, Wisconsin,
USA

L. Morgan
Senior lecturer and honorary consultant
   in clinical chemistry
Clinical Chemistry Department,
Queen's Medical Centre,
Nottingham, UK

J. J. Mullins
Professor,
Centre for Cardiovascular Science,
Queen's Medical Research Centre,
The University of Edinburgh,
Edinburgh, UK

P. B. Munroe
Reader in Molecular Genetics
Clinical Pharmacology, The William
   Harvey Research Institute,
Bart's and The London School of
   Medicine and Dentistry,
London, UK

M. I. Phillips
Research Professor
Keck Graduate Institute
Claremont, California,
USA

N. J. Samani
British Heart Foundation Professor of
   Cardiology
Department of Cardiovascular Sciences,
University of Leicester,
Glenfield Hospital
Leicester, UK

P. Sharma
Reader in Cerebrovascular Biology &
   Consultant Neurologist
Department of Clinical Neuroscience,
Imperial College and Hammersmith
   Hospitals,
London, UK

N. A. Sheehan
Senior Lecturer in Statistical Genetics
Departments of Health Sciences and
   Genetics,
University of Leicester,
Leicester, UK

C. D. Sigmund
Director, Carver Research Program
  of Excellence on the Functional
  Genomics of Cardiovascular
  Disease
Roy J. and Lucille A. Carver College
  of Medicine
University of Iowa
Iowa City, Iowa,
USA

M. D. Tobin
Clinical Senior Lecturer in Genetic
  Epidemiology
Departments of Health Sciences and
  Genetics,
University of Leicester,
Leicester, UK

G. Tripodi
Group Leader Molecular Biology
Prassis-Sigma Tau Research Institute
Milan, Italy

C. Wallace
Research Fellow
Department of Clinical Pharmacology,
The William Harvey Research
  Institute,
Bart's and The London School of
  Medicine and Dentistry,
London, UK

MZ. Xue
Senior Research Officer
Disease Mechanisms and
  Therapeutics Group
Department of Biological Sciences
University of Essex
Colchester, UK

Y. C. Zhang
Assistant Professor of Pediatrics
Children's Research Institute
University of South Florida
St. Petersburg, Florida,
USA

Foreword

In the late 1970s basic and clinical research in hypertension and related cardiovascular diseases was rapidly expanding. Physicians and researchers had difficulty keeping up with the quantity and range of research publications of relevance. The Handbook of Hypertension was conceived as a series of freestanding volumes which would provide a series of authoritative reviews and update of aspects of hypertension and cardiovascular disease. Some 30 years on 24 volumes have been published reviewing, analyzing and setting in context discoveries in a wide range of clinical and experimental areas in hypertension.

Early in the Series, volume 4, on Experimental and Genetic Models of Hypertension was commissioned, edited by Professor Wybren de Jong. The volume provided a valuable update on experimental models of hypertension including the recently developed inbred strains of hypertensive rats which have provided key information on pathogenesis of hypertension and the pathological implications of high blood pressure in humans.

10 years later in 1994 a further volume updated experimental and genetic models of hypertension (volume 16) with Professor Detlev Ganten joining Wybren de Jong as Co-Editors. There had been further elucidation of genetic mechanisms of experimental hypertension and the implications for human disease were emerging. However even in the late 1990s the information on genetic influences in man was minimal (volume 19). Over the last 10 years the implications of genetics on human disease have been expanded greatly. Extensive research studies performed in humans have characterized not only the genetics of rare forms of inherited hypertension but also polygenic influences in essential hypertension in different populations.

Volume 24 provides a timely review of our present understanding of the genetics of hypertension based on experimental studies and now extended to man. The volume is edited by Professors Anna Dominiczak and John Connell and includes contributions from a range of distinguished colleagues working in clinics and laboratories around the world on genetic aspects of hypertension.

We as Series Editors are delighted that our original concept continues to develop and provide a useful information resource for researchers and clinicians in hypertension. The Handbook of Hypertension series will provide updates and new titles are in preparation. An update volume in clinical pharmacology and therapeutics of hypertension is in an advanced stage of preparation and other new titles are in the pipeline. We are grateful to the Volume Editors and all contributors for their creative input and to our publishers for their continuing support and encouragement.

WILLEM H BIRKENHÄGER, Rotterdam

JOHN L REID, Glasgow

Series Editors

Preface

Classic and modern tools of genetics have been applied to hypertension research for some 20 years. The current volume aims to go beyond a simple summary of discoveries and provides a critical commentary on many controversial issues. The editors believe that this volume will be particularly useful for clinician scientists at all stages of their careers, graduate students and post-doctoral scientists as well as all those interested in cardiovascular medicine and research throughout the entire spectrum from bench to bedside.

As in every relatively young area of research, the initial excitement over the early positive observations has not always been confirmed by subsequent larger studies with greater statistical power. Issues related to current recommendations on design of studies and their analysis are included in Chapters 2, 4 and 7. Pharmacogenetics and pharmacogenomics have been the subjects of many debates in recent years and are of particular importance in hypertension as life-long treatments, frequently with multiple drugs are given to millions of people worldwide. A critical appraisal of this controversial topic is provided in chapter 8. We have also included several chapters on experimental genetics of hypertension with a special focus on physiological genomics.

This book is dedicated to our past, current and future students, coworkers and collaborators at the BHF Glasgow Cardiovascular Research Centre where genetics and genomics of hypertension and cardiovascular disease have been a major strength and focus for several years.

ANNA F. DOMINICZAK
JOHN M. C. CONNELL

Contents

1 | Overview

Anna F. Dominiczak and John M. C. Connell

Human essential or primary hypertension is a substantial public health problem, with more than 25% of the adult population being affected in industrial societies. Moreover, the cardiovascular disease epidemic has now moved to the developing countries, with the projected increase in the proportion of all death attributable to cardiovascular causes expected to go from approximately 25% in 1990 to more than 40% in 2020.[1] The cardiovascular continuum runs from risk factors such as hypertension, insulin resistance, type 2 diabetes, obesity and hyperlipidemias through traits such as metabolic syndrome and atherosclerosis to disease phenotypes including myocardial infarction, heart failure, stroke, peripheral vascular disease and renal failure (Fig. 1.1) The modifiable cardiovascular risk factors listed above are best described as complex, polygenic or at least oligogenic traits with significant environmental influences.[2] It is therefore unsurprising that genetic dissection of these complex phenotypes has been less than straightforward.

The chapters presented in this volume of the *Handbook of Hypertension* summarize the current status of knowledge on the genetics of hypertension together with suggestions of future developments and directions. It should be acknowledged that understanding the genetics of hypertension in parallel with other common complex traits is best described as work in progress. Over the last decade we have moved from studying single markers in candidate genes in small-family, case-control studies to multiple single nucleotide polymorphisms (SNPs) and haplotypes in large (thousands of subjects) samples; this is described in detail in Chapter 2. Major international initiatives such as the human genome project[3,4] and the HapMap[5,6] have played an important role in facilitating new and better strategic approaches to cardiovascular genetics. Moreover, significant advances in rat and mouse programs on cardiovascular genetics, described in detail in Chapters 10–13, have resulted in several important candidate genes and pathways for human genetic studies. Major examples here include novel genetical genomic strategies utilized by Hübner et al[7] in a genome-wide gene expression study in rat recombinant inbred strains, which resulted in the identification of 50 or more putative candidate regions for human hypertension. It is expected that the combined forces of new 'omics' (genomics, proteomics and metabonomics), together with increasing technological advances of bioinformatics and comparative genome analysis, will make it feasible to translate individual discoveries between species.[8]

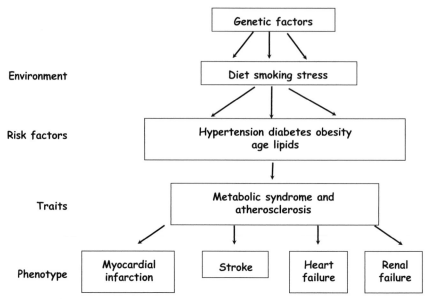

Fig. 1.1 Multiple interactions between genetic and environmental factors that can lead to cardio-vascular target organ damage. (Modified from ref. 2.)

Equally important are the new therapeutic approaches, including pharmacogenetics and pharmacogenomics (which are summarized in Chapter 8) and gene therapy strategies (summarized in Chapter 14). The major challenge for the next decade is to introduce some of our genetic – and particularly the pharmacogenetic – tools into clinical practice. Will this be achieved, and if so when? Many clinical scientists, including the authors of this overview, have debated this extensively in front of clinical and genetic audiences. The optimists cite major diagnostic and therapeutic advances that have resulted from our thorough understanding of monogenic forms of hypertension (see Chapter 3); the pessimists tell us about a major role of environmental influences (50% or more) and small effects of the individual polymorphisms in any complex polygenic trait. The real answer for the current debate will only come from well-designed studies and clinical protocols of the future. However, let us finish this overview by quoting from Sydney Brenner:[9]

> . . . Many people base their lives on the proposition that they can do what they like to their bodies because medical science will come and save them with a pill. Perhaps the prime value of our work to society will be the creation of a new public health paradigm in which we are all taught how to look after our somatic selves; those who have a genetic background that makes them especially liable to one of the diseases of our civilization will have to learn how to take extra care.

References

1. Reddy KS. Cardiovascular disease in non-Western countries. *N Engl J Med* 2004; 350:2438–2440.
2. Dominiczak AF, Graham D, McBride MW, et al. Arthur Corcoran Lecture 2004. Cardiovascular genomics and oxidative stress. *Hypertension* 2005; 45:636–642.
3. International Human Genome Sequencing Consortium. Initial sequencing and analysis of the human genome. *Nature* 2001; 409:860–921.

4. Venter CJ, Adams MD, Myres EW, et al. The sequence of the human genome. *Science* 2001; 291:1304–1351.
5. The International HapMap Consortium. A haplotype map of the human genome. *Nature* 2005; 437:1299–1320.
6. Goldstein DB, Cavalleri GL. Understanding human diversity. *Nature* 2005; 437:1241–1242.
7. Hübner A, Wallace CA, Zimdahl H, et al. Integrated transcriptional profiling and linkage analysis for identification of genes underlying disease. *Nat Genet* 2005; 37:243–253.
8. McBride MW, Graham D, Delles C, Dominiczak AF. Functional genomics in hypertension. *Current Opinion in Nephrology and Hypertension* 2006; 15(2):145–151.
9. Brenner S. Humanity as the model system. *Science* 2003; 302:533.

2 | The genetic epidemiology of hypertension

Martin D. Tobin, Nuala A. Sheehan, Nilesh J. Samani and Paul R. Burton

INTRODUCTION

Hypertension is a major public health burden, affecting around 1 billion people worldwide.[1] It increases the risk of several common cardiovascular diseases including stroke, myocardial infarction and congestive heart failure.[2,3] Furthermore, changes in blood pressure within the 'normal' range affect the risk of these cardiovascular endpoints. Even from a systolic blood pressure as low as 115 mmHg, a 2 mmHg higher usual systolic blood pressure in middle age is associated with an approximate 10% higher mortality from stroke and a 7% higher mortality from ischemic heart disease or other vascular causes[4] (see Chapter 1). The genomics revolution has provided new opportunities for improving the understanding of the molecular mechanisms underlying Mendelian and complex hypertensive disorders in human populations. Improvements in the understanding of the mechanisms that underlie human hypertension, and indeed of those that regulate blood pressure throughout its range, should facilitate advances in the prevention and treatment of hypertension (Fig. 2.1).

In this chapter we outline some of the ways that genetic epidemiology studies could contribute towards a better understanding of the relevant molecular mechanisms of blood pressure regulation and hypertension and we review, from a genetic epidemiology perspective, the progress of these studies and consider some promising approaches that may benefit this area of research in the near future. This chapter specifically focuses on genetic epidemiology approaches aimed at improving the understanding of human hypertension as a complex trait, but we note that many advances in the understanding of the etiology of hypertension have also come through the study of animal models (see Chapters 12–14) and of monogenic disorders[5] (see Chapter 3).

Essential hypertension and blood pressure as complex traits

Across a wide range of disease areas, genetic epidemiology studies are increasingly focusing on the investigation of so-called complex disorders, and the field of

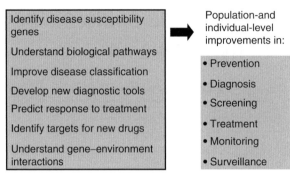

Fig. 2.1 Potential benefits of genetic epidemiology studies.

hypertension research is no exception. Complex disorders are characteristically caused by multiple genetic and environmental determinants that interact in complex ways.[6] Blood pressure and essential hypertension might therefore be described as complex traits or complex phenotypes. A range of genetic epidemiology approaches has been employed to dissect the genetic determinants of these traits (see Fig. 2.2, below). All these studies are constrained by the small effect sizes of the individual genetic variants they seek to detect and by the complexity of the phenotype under study. Accordingly, various practical problems are encountered in the design, conduct, analysis and interpretation of genetic epidemiology studies of these phenotypes. The strengths and weaknesses of such studies are not unique to these traits. They are also encountered in genetic epidemiology studies of a wide range of complex disorders.[7] Just as the molecular techniques employed in any genetic study draw from advances in other disease areas, optimal approaches to study design, conduct, analysis and interpretation in genetic studies of essential hypertension and blood pressure depend on a sound application of the advances in, and lessons learned from, genetic epidemiology studies of other complex disorders.

In this chapter we review the genetic epidemiology approaches that have been used to study essential hypertension and blood pressure. The practical problems encountered in studying these complex phenotypes are considered throughout the chapter.

AN OVERVIEW OF GENETIC EPIDEMIOLOGY APPROACHES TO STUDY ESSENTIAL HYPERTENSION AND BLOOD PRESSURE

Fig. 2.2 provides a schematic representation of how the investigation of the genetic etiology of essential hypertension and blood pressure can be viewed as a series of manageable steps, from the descriptive studies shown in steps (i)–(iii) to the analytical studies that search for specific etiological determinants, i.e. steps (iv) and (v). Early researchers in this field, although limited to the descriptive studies shown in steps (i)–(iii), clearly showed that genes were important determinants of blood pressure and essential hypertension risk (see 'Evidence for genetic determinants of blood pressure and essential hypertension', below). Research is actually proceeding simultaneously in all the areas shown in Fig. 2.2 rather than in any prescriptive order. However, a logical framework for appraising existing evidence and for planning studies can be helpful and we therefore structure our chapter around this framework.

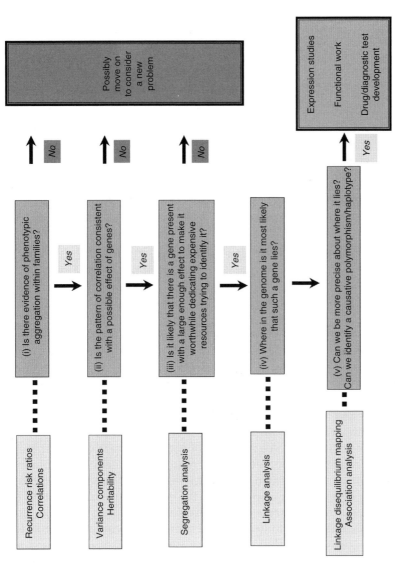

Fig. 2.2 Schematic framework outlining a systematic approach to the identification and characterization of the genetic determinants of a complex disease. Note that the failure of a segregation analysis to find a major gene would no longer be considered an absolute barrier to proceeding with steps (iv) and (v). (Adapted, with permission, from ref. 32.)

PHENOTYPE CHARACTERIZATION

In any genetic epidemiology study of a complex disorder, the way in which one characterizes the phenotype under study has profound implications for the ability to detect genetic etiological determinants of that phenotype. This is particularly evident in studies of the genetics of essential hypertension and blood pressure, and we therefore outline some of the principal dilemmas below.

First, there is the fundamental question of whether blood pressure should be considered as a quantitative trait or as a binary trait (hypertension) in the context of its genetic causation. This was the subject of the controversial debate between Platt and Pickering in the 1950s. The observation of a bimodal blood pressure distribution among members of a small number of families with hypertension was interpreted by Platt as support for the traditional view that hypertension was a qualitative abnormality, and thus likely to be subject to Mendelian patterns of inheritance. However, the aggregation in quantitative blood pressure that Pickering and colleagues observed between family members persuaded them of the rationale for the study of blood pressure as a quantitative trait, particularly when investigating its genetic influences. Pickering stated:[8]

> The new idea that blood pressure was inherited as a graded character dawned, and steadily became convincing, when it became apparent that there was a quantitative relationship between the deviations from the norm of arterial pressures of our patients and those of their first-degree relatives.

We now know that there are rare monogenic syndromes that underlie hypertension in a small proportion of the population so that Platt was at least partially correct. However, the weight of evidence relating to the etiology and the sequelae of raised blood pressure now supports the Pickering concept.[9] Even clinical hypertension has been 'operationally defined as the blood pressure level above which therapeutic intervention has continued to demonstrate benefit'.[5] This supports the following theories: (1) that essential hypertension represents the dichotomization of quantitative blood pressure; and (2) that the risk of essential hypertension is primarily influenced by multiple genetic and environmental determinants that, through their individual actions and interactions, increase quantitative blood pressure.

Second, there are pragmatic considerations that might influence the choice of phenotype in genetic epidemiology studies of essential hypertension or blood pressure. These relate to the power to detect modest genetic determinants, attempts to minimize measurement error and to avoid bias due to the effects of antihypertensive therapy, and also relate to the convenience of recruiting the sample. If the genetic determinants of interest affect blood pressure throughout its range, the statistical power to detect a determinant of a continuous trait will be considerably greater than that of a binary trait,[6] whether the context is a genetic linkage study[10] or an association study.[11] This will particularly be the case if the binary trait represents a dichotomization of the quantitative trait.

However, there are a number of reasons why researchers have chosen to study essential hypertension rather than quantitative blood pressure: (1) conventional blood pressure measurement can be subject to substantial measurement error[12] in epidemiological studies, whereas a diagnosis of hypertension is usually made after a series of blood pressure measurements; (2) to avoid bias where a proportion of the study population take antihypertensive medication, quantitative blood pressure may have been translated into a binary trait by defining as 'hypertensive' those subjects who are treated or have an observed blood pressure in excess of a stated quantitative threshold;[13-17] (3) etiological hetero-geneity should be minimized in studies of more extreme phenotypes,[7] such as early-onset hypertension;[18] (4) for case-control studies, convenience samples of subjects with hypertension may be recruited with relative ease, although the choice of control subjects warrants careful consideration.[19]

Box 2.1 (p 17) shows a practical illustration of some choices related to pheno-type characterization and their impact on the power of a study. It also shows the potential impact of the effects of antihypertensive therapy on the power to detect genes that affect quantitative blood pressure and the consequences of some methods that aim to avoid, or to adjust for, the effects of antihypertensive treat-ment. These methods have been described in more detail elsewhere.[11,20]

EVIDENCE FOR GENETIC DETERMINANTS OF BLOOD PRESSURE AND ESSENTIAL HYPERTENSION

Is there evidence of aggregation of blood pressure and essential hypertension risk within families?

Familial aggregation of quantitative blood pressure [Fig. 2.2, step (i)] can be described in terms of correlation coefficients within a correlation structure.[21-23] Pickering reported a correlation coefficient of around 0.2 between the blood pres-sures of hypertensives and their first-degree relatives[8] and noted that this correla-tion applied to blood pressure observations throughout the range. Although the estimates of the correlation coefficients for blood pressure between first-degree rel-atives have varied due to differing study populations, differing relationship types and random error, these correlation coefficients have typically been between 0.1 and 0.3. The aggregation of binary hypertension has been described in terms of the ratio of incidence rates of hypertension in families of hypertensive subjects and in the general population (referred to as 'relative risk'). Hunt and colleagues showed that the relative risk of developing hypertension was around 2.0 in first-degree rel-atives of hypertensive subjects using family data in a cohort study of 94 000 sub-jects. However, the relative risk increased markedly with a younger age of onset of hypertension and with the number of first-degree relatives affected. For example, for subjects aged 20–39 with at least two first-degree relatives affected by hyper-tension before 55 years, the relative risks of developing hypertension were 4.1 in men and 5.0 in women.[24,25] The collection of such detailed incidence data is expen-sive. If only prevalence data are available, the recurrence risk ratio in relatives (lambda R)[26] can be used to describe the aggregation of hypertension within fami-lies. This is defined as the ratio of prevalences in particular relatives (e.g. sibs) of an affected individual and in the general population.

Is the pattern of aggregation of blood pressure within families consistent with the effect of genes?

Researchers have addressed this question primarily by comparing the correla-tion coefficients of adoptive and nonadoptive siblings, and those of monozy-gotic and dizygotic twins. For systolic blood pressure, the Montreal adoption study demonstrated correlation coefficients of 0.27 between mother and biologi-cal child, 0.08 between mother and adoptive child and correlation coefficients of 0.38 and 0.16 between biological sibs and adoptive sibs, respectively.[27] Providing that one is prepared to assume that environmental sharing is similar between the comparison groups, this provides support for a genetic influence on blood pressure. The Victorian Family Heart Study estimated correlation coefficients for systolic blood pressure of 0.12 for spouse–spouse pairs, 0.22 for parent–offspring pairs, 0.44 for nontwin siblings, 0.50 for dizygous twins and 0.78 for monozygous twins.[28] The correlation patterns in other twin studies have been broadly consistent with these findings.[29]

A more sophisticated approach for family data explicitly models the components of variance that may be attributed to shared genes and those that may be attributed to shared and unshared environment. These types of models are termed variance components models.[30] A key aim of this approach is to understand how blood pressure might be modulated by the additive effect of one or more genes, i.e. additive polygenic effects or 'S^2_A'.[31,32] Such models incorporate the different probabilities with which different classes may share alleles that are identical by descent (IBD). Note that two alleles are described as IBD when it is *known* that they have been inherited from a common ancestor, and that while all alleles with the same 'call' at a particular locus may be described as identical by state (IBS), not all of these will be IBD.

If the total variance of the phenotype is denoted 'S^2_T' then the narrow sense heritability can be defined as: $H^2_N = S^2_A/S^2_T$. Narrow sense heritability is thus the proportion of the total conditional variance of a phenotype that can be attributed to variation in additive genetic effects. Certain types of study design, such as those including monozygous twin pairs, allow one to estimate 'S^2_G' – the phenotypic variance attributable to *all* genetic effects, including nonadditive effects at individual loci (dominance variance) and between loci (epistatic variance). Broad sense heritability (H^2_B) is then defined as: $H^2_B = S^2_G/S^2_T$.[32]

Before we consider the findings of studies that have investigated the heritability of blood pressure, it is important to clarify what this term actually means given that it is so commonly misunderstood. Heritability is not about cause *per se*, but about the causes of variation in a particular trait in a particular population at a particular point in time.[32,33] Note that the magnitude of S^2_T, the denominator in the estimate of heritability, is determined by measurement error in addition to the variances attributable to genes, shared environment, unshared environment and unmeasured determinants. This means that heritability must be interpreted with caution.[32] That said, the power of a study for discovering genes is positively associated with the heritability of the trait of interest in the population concerned. If the heritability of a trait is known to be low, it forewarns those contemplating doing the study – and those considering its funding – that genetic effects may be difficult to find.

The impact of measurement error on heritability estimates is illustrated by the Framingham Heart Study, which reported narrow sense heritability (H^2_N) for systolic and diastolic blood pressure of 0.42 and 0.39 (respectively) based on measurement at a single follow-up, but H^2_N of 0.57 and 0.56 based on the average blood pressure from all follow-up measures.[34] Another study that used ambulatory monitoring to minimize measurement error reported H^2_N of 0.69 and 0.51 for mean night-time systolic and diastolic blood pressure.[35] In contrast, H^2_N estimates have generally fallen between 0.15 and 0.46 for systolic blood pressure and between 0.15 and 0.31 for diastolic blood pressure in family studies employing a small number of clinic blood pressure measurements.[28,36–38]

Is there evidence of a gene with a substantial enough effect on blood pressure to justify expensive genetic studies?

Using segregation analysis it is possible to assess whether there are one or more genes with variants that have a strong effect on susceptibility and whose Mendelian segregation within families explains all or part of the observed familial aggregation of blood pressure or essential hypertension risk. Such genes are called major genes, even if the variants are rare. Segregation analyses have not only been used to inform the search for major genes[32] but have also been used to generate estimates for parametric linkage analyses.[39] There are many detailed accounts of segregation analysis.[39–41] For most readers, it will be sufficient to be acquainted with the key interpretational caveat of segregation analyses, i.e. that the conclusions of a segregation analysis might be sensitive to a variety of factors. These include the characteristics of the phenotype under study and the way that it is measured; the size and mechanism of ascertainment of the study population; and the modeling assumptions, e.g. the number of loci modeled[42] and the age at onset.[43] That said, major gene effects on blood pressure have now been reported in a variety of populations,[43–47] justifying the search for such genes using linkage and association approaches (see Genetic linkage studies of blood pressure and essential hypertension and Genetic association studies of blood pressure and essential hypertension, below).

GENETIC LINKAGE STUDIES OF BLOOD PRESSURE AND ESSENTIAL HYPERTENSION

The context of linkage analysis

The evidence for a genetic component to the etiology of hypertension (see 'Evidence for genetic determinants of blood pressure and essential hypertension', above) has justified investment in attempts to locate and identify causative genes. If there were only a small number of genes that were obvious candidates for having variants that affected blood pressure and risk of hypertension, an obvious approach would be to study the effect of variants in those genes in association studies (see 'Genetic association studies of blood pressure and essential hypertension', below). In reality, there are so many candidates for hypertension, and so many genes whose usual effects are completely unknown, that the work on such candidate genes might logically be preceded by attempts to localize (or map) regions of the genome that appear to contain one or more genes that are causally relevant.

An introduction to linkage study design

Genetic linkage analysis[39,48–50] relies on the tendency for shorter haplotypes to be passed on to the next generation intact, i.e. without being subject to recombination due to a crossover at meiosis. Put simply, if a genetic marker is passed down through a family such that it consistently accompanies hypertension (i.e. the marker and hypertension 'cosegregate'), this suggests that a gene that influences hypertension risk is located close to the marker. Linkage analysis can be focused on candidate loci or on the whole genome, using evenly spaced markers.

Parametric linkage analysis involves the study of the cosegregation of loci within pedigrees to estimate the probability of recombination (the recombination fraction) between markers and trait loci. A genetic model is specified requiring estimates of the parameters defining the mode of inheritance, allele frequency, penetrance and genetic heterogeneity.[51] However, for complex diseases there is no clear single mode of inheritance, and nonparametric methods have been developed that do not rely on the full specification of a disease model.[49] In general, these methods test whether the degree of IBD sharing at a locus is greater than that expected under the null hypothesis of no linkage. Many different types of pairs of relatives could be used, but a simple and common approach involves the study of sibling pairs. For a binary trait, such as hypertension, linkage would be suggested by the sharing of more alleles at a candidate locus between affected siblings than would be expected by chance. Under the null hypothesis of no linkage one would expect 0, 1 and 2 haplotypes to be shared IBD at any locus with probability 0.25, 0.5 and 0.25, respectively. For a quantitative trait, such as blood pressure, Haseman and Elston[52] suggested regressing the squared difference in the siblings' trait values on the estimated proportion of alleles shared IBD. More recently, modified versions of this test have been suggested and variance components linkage has also been used for quantitative traits.[53] All these methods rely on the principle that siblings sharing more alleles IBD would be expected to have more similar trait values if the gene is related to the trait.[51]

Genetic linkage studies of hypertension have used a variety of different populations. Many studies, although not all, have attempted to limit etiological heterogeneity by sampling from populations that are relatively homogeneous. For example, the BRIGHT study focused on Caucasian families in the UK.[54] A more extreme approach is to recruit families from isolated, inbred populations[55,56] but the real advantage of such populations, which typically exhibit a high degree of linkage disequilibrium (LD), is exploited when they are used for LD mapping (see 'An introduction to genetic association study design', below).[55]

The choice of phenotype in a linkage study of a complex disease is usually driven by attempts to maximize statistical power and to reduce heterogeneity. Studying quantitative traits can increase statistical power and can often avoid problems with difficult or inconsistent diagnostic criteria for complex diseases.[10] However, in an attempt to minimize etiological heterogeneity, researchers might study 'extreme' phenotypes, for example, severe hypertensives[54] or those with early-onset disease.[18] In many linkage studies, the attempts to obtain a sample of families that is as informative as possible leads to a study sample that is unrepresentative of the general population. These studies are then analyzed as if their mode of ascertainment was irrelevant. This form of ascertainment will not bias the estimates obtained from the genetic linkage study provided that the informative individuals/families for the analysis have been identified *either* on the basis of the disease of interest *or* on the basis of the distribution of markers, *but not both*.[57] Under designs where families that have already been recruited are extended in a manner that depends on the distribution of disease status amongst its members this logic can break down and ascertainment bias can distort the findings of the study.[57,58]

As the power of any individual study is usually very limited (see the following two sections) it could be helpful to combine the evidence from different linkage studies. Meta-analysis offers one approach to evidence synthesis and such methods have been developed[59] and applied to linkage studies of essential hypertension.[60] However, meta-analysis of studies that have used different populations, different phenotypes and different study designs is not a trivial problem (see also the interpretational caveats described in the two sections below).

Interpretation of results from linkage studies

In reporting the results of linkage analyses, the magnitude of a linkage peak is typically expressed as a maximum 'log odds' (LOD) score. Although comparable to other likelihood ratio tests, LOD scores are based on logarithms to the base 10. The LOD score is a function of the recombination fraction or of the IBD sharing.[51]

The interpretation of linkage peaks from studies of complex diseases is often not straightforward. First, linkage can extend over tens of centimorgans (cM), with these large regions often including hundreds of genes, and linkage peaks are highly variable.[51,61] Second, the criteria for statistical significance are complex because the LOD score threshold that equates to a genome-wide significance of 5% depends on the analytical approach employed. Traditionally, LOD scores exceeding 3 have generally been considered indicative of statistically significant linkage at a genome-wide level,[62] whereas LOD scores exceeding 2.0 could be considered suggestive of linkage. As different analytical approaches have been employed, different thresholds have been proposed.[63] Recent recommendations for statistical significance include thresholds for LOD scores of greater than 3.3 and 3.6 for parametric linkage analysis and a sibpair nonparametric analysis, respectively.[51] Alternatively, significance can be determined by simulation.

The interpretation of linkage findings, both positive and negative, depends on considerations of statistical power. Linkage studies of complex traits will have adequate power to detect linkage to genes with a large genotype relative risk. However, to detect linkage to a gene with a genotype relative risk of less than 2, which is a likely scenario with essential hypertension (see 'Essential hypertension and blood pressure as complex traits', above), adequate power will only be achieved with unrealistically large sample sizes.[64]

Results of linkage studies of essential hypertension and blood pressure in humans

In contrast to the success in locating the genes for monogenic forms of hypertension using genetic linkage analysis, there have been fewer successes with locating the genes that underlie blood pressure and essential hypertension risk as complex traits. Although loci with suggestive LOD scores have been reported on every chromosome, only a few have been replicated in independent populations. The studies that have reported evidence of linkage that reached genome-wide levels of significance include some of the largest such studies undertaken to date.[34,54,65] This is unsurprising given that most genetic linkage studies have been too small to have the power to detect genes of modest effect. Other reasons, such as the recruitment of heterogeneous populations, misclassification or measurement error in phenotype definition, and genotyping error may also partially explain the lack of positive linkage findings in some linkage studies of blood pressure and essential hypertension as complex traits.

Details of genetic linkage studies of blood pressure and essential hypertension undertaken to date and their findings can be found in Chapter 4.

'Comprehensive' linkage and linkage disequilibrium studies

Some studies have staged their approach so that they progress from genome wide linkage to typing further markers in regions of interest. Even finer mapping can be undertaken using LD mapping (see 'Introduction to genetic association study design'). For example, Angius et al, in their study of an inbred isolated Sardinian population, reported evidence suggestive of linkage on chromosome 2p24-25, but highly significant evidence ($P = 0.00006$) from their LD mapping in this genomic region, with localization of the signal to a 7.57 cM region.[55] The US Family Blood Pressure Program has also undertaken LD mapping of a chromosome 2 region in which evidence suggestive of linkage was found, reporting association between *SLC4A5*, a gene encoding a sodium bicarbonate cotransporter, and hypertension.[66]

GENETIC ASSOCIATION STUDIES OF BLOOD PRESSURE AND ESSENTIAL HYPERTENSION

The context of genetic association studies

Ideally, one might build on the evidence from linkage studies to 'fine map' the genomic regions of interest and to identify the functional genetic variants that predispose to essential hypertension (see Fig. 2.2, p 7). Unfortunately, due to limited statistical power, genetic linkage studies of essential hypertension have provided little in the way of replicable findings to inform such a fine mapping approach. Genetic association studies have therefore been undertaken in parallel to genetic linkage studies, often selecting genes as candidates based on their known or putative role in blood pressure homeostasis, or based on evidence of their involvement in rare monogenic forms of hypertension. This raises challenges for the interpretation of such studies, given the large number of plausible candidate genes.

The design and interpretation of genetic association studies depends on an appreciation of the concept of LD. Put simply, LD occurs between two loci when they are so tightly linked that, even after a large number of ancestral meioses, they still tend to occur on the same haplotype, leading to an association at a population level.[67]

An introduction to genetic association study design

Direct and indirect association studies

There are three main reasons for association between a marker and a phenotypic trait of interest. First, the marker might be a functional variant that has a direct causal role. Second, the marker might be in LD with a causal variant that has a causal role. Third, a noncausal association between the marker and the trait might occur in the presence of ethnic stratification or admixture in the population under study.[68–70] The first two reasons for association are exploited in 'direct' and 'indirect' association studies (respectively). So whereas direct association studies rely on knowledge of candidate variants, indirect association (or 'LD mapping') studies employ one or more markers that act as surrogates for a causal variant.[71–73] The third type of association, attributable to confounding by population stratification or admixture, is generally regarded as a nuisance that should be avoided or controlled for where possible.

Indirect associations based on LD also offer the potential of whole genome scans based on association rather than linkage analysis. The International HapMap Project (see: http://www.hapmap.org) is a major collaborative initiative to map out regions of LD and to 'develop a haplotype map of the human genome'.[74] However, indirect association studies are less powerful than direct association studies and provide additional analytical and interpretational challenges. In particular, it is difficult to exclude the possibility that a causal variant lies in a region in which no indirect association has been shown, because the negative result could simply be attributable to the choice of markers. As current genotyping costs render this type of study relatively inefficient at a genome-wide level, an alternative would be to use selected subsets of the 10 000–15 000 coding single nucleotide polymorphisms (SNPs) identified to date. That said, it is important to note that not all SNPs that affect complex traits will be coding SNPs.

Hinds and colleagues described 'whole-genome' patterns of common DNA variation in individuals of European, African and Asian ancestry using over 1.5 million SNPs.[75] Their findings, particularly those relating to the extent of LD and of the redundancy of SNP information in different genomic regions, will assist the development of more efficient tools to relate common genomic variation to human diseases, such as hypertension. The HapMap project has already advanced our understanding of LD in the human genome and provides a valuable tool for genetic association studies. Genotyping costs continue to fall and commercial platforms have been developed for genome-wide association studies employing hundreds of thousands of SNPs. Genome-wide LD mapping is already being employed in genetic studies of hypertension. For example, in the UK, the Wellcome Trust Case Control Consortium (see: http://www.wtccc.org.uk) has brought together 3000 controls together with 2000 cases for each of seven disorders, including hypertension. It will undertake genome-wide association using over 600 000 SNPs. The rapid developments in this area provide optimism but also fresh challenges for the analysis, the interpretation of the findings and the follow-up of the relevant genomic regions of interest.

Genotype or haplotype as the unit of exposure?

Haplotype blocks exist within the genome as regions of high LD interspersed by recombination hotspots and with limited haplotype diversity within blocks.[76] There has been a growing interest in the use of the haplotype as the unit of exposure in genetic association studies given some of the limitations of testing individual SNPs, particularly when these are in LD with one another. However, for marker regions in which LD is strong, it is questionable whether the use of haplotype information is a 'better' approach, given that this may lead to an increase in the degrees of freedom in the analysis, resulting in loss of power. Haplotype analyses also provide additional challenges. First, laboratories almost always measure genotype, which means that additional information is required to define genetic exposure as a haplotype. In the absence of the knowledge of genetic phase from extensive family data, this usually means that haplotypes must be imputed from genotype information using certain assumptions (such as that of Hardy–Weinberg equilibrium). However, phase uncertainty must be properly taken into account. There is also interest in 'haplotype tagging' SNPs (htSNPs), following the observation that a few SNPs capture most of the polymorphism of a haplotype. The aim of haplotype tagging is to improve the cost-effectiveness of studies by allowing more limited genotyping and yet discarding minimal information. Several different methods of defining haplotype blocks and selecting tag SNPs have been suggested,[76–81] and these approaches are far from standardized at present.

Confounding, population structure and admixture

All association studies attempt to avoid confounding that could obscure causal associations or lead to noncausal association. Traditional epidemiology studies are susceptible to confounding by lifestyle factors, such as smoking or alcohol intake. In contrast, genetic association studies are *not* subject to confounding by lifestyle factors since genotype is assigned at conception by a seemingly random process (see 'Public health benefits of genetic epidemiology and Mendelian randomization', below).[82,83] However, genetic association studies based on unrelated individuals *are* subject to confounding due to population stratification. Two main strategies have evolved to prevent this source of confounding from distorting the findings of genetic association studies. First, one could recruit families rather than unrelated individuals. Second, one could attempt to detect and control for population stratification using large numbers of unlinked markers (genomic control).[84] The former approach is less powerful than a study of an equivalent number of unrelated subjects, whereas the latter might lead to residual confounding if too few markers are used and to substantial loss of power in other settings.[85] There are other reasons why one might want to study related individuals. For example, to study the heritability of a particular trait, or to estimate the likelihood that there is an as yet unobserved major gene having already adjusted for the effects of known candidate gene variants on the trait.[86] In addition, family-based studies can provide extra information about the phase of markers that are in LD to facilitate haplotype analysis.[32] Different family designs are available to suit different research questions. Trios, consisting of an affected individual and genotyped (but not necessarily phenotyped) parents, can be recruited specifically to test for association in the presence of linkage using a transmission disequilibrium test (TDT).[87]

Sample size

Studies involving at least 5000 cases are now regularly recommended.[88,89] Given that the sample size requirements critically depend on the study design and analytical approaches (Box 2.1), researchers should focus on achieving adequate statistical power to detect modest genetic effects. Given the limited power of individual studies to date, methods of evidence synthesis, including meta-analysis, have been developed[90,91] and also used for genetic association studies of essential hypertension and blood pressure (see 'Interpretation of results from genetic association studies', below and also the examples in Chapter 7).

Box 2.1 Considerations of power to detect genetic associations with blood pressure and essential hypertension

Measurement of systolic blood pressure (SBP)	Number of subjects	Statistical power (P < 0.001)				
		(a) Knowing underlying	(b) No adjustment SBP	(c) Normal censored approach	(d) Treatment covariate	(e) Convert SBP to binary trait, essential hypertension
Conventional SBP	5000	77.9%	73.1%	77.3%	51.5%	46.5%
Mean 24-hour ambulatory SBP	1300	81.6%	54.5%	79.5%	53.2%	48.2%

TWO SIMPLE SCENARIOS

Datasets were simulated to estimate the power to detect the effect of a single nucleotide polymorphism that increased systolic blood pressure (SBP) by 2 mmHg per copy of the minor allele (P < 0.001). Each dataset was of size 5000 for conventional SBP, and of size 1300 for ambulatory SBP. In each case, 42.5% of subjects were hypertensive and two-thirds of hypertensives (27.9% of subjects) received antihypertensive treatment. Treatment was assumed to reduce SBP by an average of 15 mmHg. Ignoring for the moment the effects of measurement error, the 'observed' SBP was equal to the underlying SBP in untreated subjects and, in treated subjects was equal to the underlying SBP less the individual treatment effect. The measurement error was greater with conventional SBP measures (assumed to be observed with standard deviation of 21.3 mmHg) than with mean 24-hour ambulatory SBP (observed with a standard deviation of 10.5 mmHg). Empirical power was estimated based on 10 000 simulated datasets. The box above shows the empirical power: (a) supposing that one did know the underlying SBP (this is to illustrate the extent of loss of power but in practice the underlying SBP is not observable) and (b)–(e) based on the 'observed' SBP using some different approaches that attempt to adjust for, or avoid, the effects of antihypertensive treatment. Method (c) assumes that, in treated subjects, the observed SBP is greater than the underlying SBP. Method (d) involves dealing with treatment as one might deal with any confounder (i.e. by including it as a covariate in a regression analysis) and simultaneously models the tendency for underlying SBP to be higher in treated subjects and the tendency for treatment to lower SBP. These methods have been described in more detail elsewhere.[11]

STATISTICAL POWER TO ESTIMATE THE SIMULATED GENETIC EFFECT

What the scenarios illustrate

- The study of precisely measured quantitative blood pressure provides adequate statistical power with realistically achievable sample sizes (*n* = 1300), whereas very large sample sizes (*n* = 5000) are required where an imprecise measure of blood pressure is used (assuming that the minor allele does not contribute to the extra variance in clinic BP compared with ambulatory BP).

- Where a gene has a modest effect on hypertension risk via its effect on quantitative risk throughout the range, then the study of quantitative SBP is more powerful than the study of hypertension as a binary trait.
- Antihypertensive treatment effects reduce the power to detect genetic effects. In an ideal situation one would be able to study the underlying SBP, but this is rarely possible. An appropriate adjustment method needs to be used for the study of the observed SBP where some of the observations are subject to antihypertensive treatment effects.
- A censored normal approach is a useful adjustment for the effects of antihypertensive treatment. Approaches such as making no adjustment or adjusting for treatment as a covariate are commonly used in practice but are incorrect and can result in loss of power.[11] Converting blood pressure to the binary trait, hypertension, is a low power approach.
- For a precisely measured trait such as mean 24-hour ambulatory BP, treatment accounts for a greater proportion of the standard deviation and even greater loss of power and it is therefore particularly important to use an appropriate correction for treatment (assuming here that the treatment has the same quantitative impact on ambulatory BP as on clinic BP).

The study of gene–environment interactions

The study of gene–environment interactions requires even larger sample sizes than would be required for simply testing for overall association between the gene and disease, or between the environmental factor and disease.[71] Two main strategies exist for studying gene–environmental interactions. One approach is to use large case-control studies.[71] However, although more efficient than cohort studies, case-control studies are usually unable to collect accurate data on premorbid characteristics and environmental exposures. The second approach is to undertake very large cohort studies, such as the UK Biobank.[92] Although these studies are very expensive, they do permit the collection of detailed prospective environmental exposure data and some efficiency may be gained by the judicious use of case-control studies nested within the cohort.

Interpretation of results from genetic association studies

A general feature of association studies of hypertension and related phenotypes has been the inability to replicate early findings. In fact, this has generated great concern for genetic association studies of all complex diseases. Recent reviews have discussed the problems of reporting and interpreting genetic association studies.[88,89] In an attempt to improve practice, guidelines have been issued for reporting gene-disease associations.[91] Practical guidance is also available for critically appraising literature related to genetic association studies.[93] We will briefly consider some of the issues here, but we refer readers to other sources for detailed discussion.[89,93]

Statistical significance

Any causal genetic variant is expected to have only a small effect on blood pressure or the risk of essential hypertension. Whereas genetic association studies might be considerably more powerful than genetic linkage studies,[64] most have been underpowered to detect such modest effects and more powerful study designs are needed. The increasing ease with which large numbers of candidate gene variants can be tested means that many hypotheses can be tested in a single study. Thus the most appropriate threshold for statistical significance warrants careful consideration in such studies to maximize the power to detect true positive associations while minimizing false-positive findings. This issue has generated considerable debate, and there is no universal agreement as to the most appropriate approach.[89] Setting a threshold of $0.05/n$ for n independent hypotheses is generally regarded as appropriate in nongenetic applications using a classic statistical approach. In a genetic application, the threshold one adopts depends critically on whether this is a test on a single candidate gene or merely one gene among many that are being tested as part of a whole genome scan and therefore demanding adjustment for extreme multiple testing.[63] It is not unusual for researchers to test a large number of genetic associations in the same dataset, sometimes over a prolonged period of time. An ideal correction for multiple testing in a genetic association study would account for the fact that some hypotheses are not independent (e.g. where the polymorphisms under study are in LD) and would take account of *a priori* evidence. At present such evidence is usually very weak as so little is known about the underlying biology and so few real genetic associations are known,[88] but as more biological information accrues, Bayesian approaches that can incorporate *a priori* evidence should be more widely used.

False-positive findings, reporting and publication bias

As the *a priori* probability of a causal association between essential hypertension and each of the genetic variants tested is probably low, one would expect a high proportion of the positive results of genetic association studies to be false-positive findings.[89] Positive findings also tend to be reported and published in preference to negative findings from studies of an equivalent size. The resulting reporting bias and publication bias mean that researchers attempting to integrate the evidence from many genetic association studies of the same candidate gene need to be very cautious. A simple and safe approach to interpret evidence from individual studies that circumvents many of these problems may be to view small studies (e.g. several hundred cases for a binary trait such as hypertension) as hypothesis generating, but larger studies (e.g. several thousand cases for a binary trait) as hypothesis testing.[94] For meta-analysis, statistical methods can be employed to assist in detecting publication bias.[95]

Replication of true positive findings

As most genetic association studies are underpowered, even true positive findings are likely to be reported with exaggerated effect sizes in the initial report of the association, leading to difficulty in replicating findings. It is therefore recommended that replication studies should be powered to look for an effect size that is more modest than that reported in the original study.[89]

Bias and confounding

Selection and information bias can be minimized in candidate gene association studies by the use of a careful sampling strategy and appropriate laboratory procedures.[89] When utilizing large scale (e.g. genome-wide) genotyping platforms, it is important to be aware of the potential sources of bias. Recent indications are that the extent of bias in the calling of genotypes may be substantial. In particular, some algorithms may only call genotypes where there is a high degree of certainty (separation of the signal clouds on signal intensity plots) and, in this situation, the failure to call is not independent of genotype and this 'informative missingness' can lead to false-positive association.[96]

Genetic association studies of unrelated individuals are susceptible to confounding due to population stratification or admixture (see 'Introduction to genetic association study design', p 14).

Evidence synthesis

In the absence of powerful primary studies it is useful to use a systematic approach to synthesize the available evidence in a qualitative manner (such as a systematic review) or in a quantitative fashion (meta-analysis).[91] However, synthesis of the results of very heterogeneous genetic association studies of hypertension and blood pressure presents several challenges. Studies may differ in their phenotype definition, the genetic variants studied, the genetic models assumed and the statistical methods adopted. Distinct study populations may be exposed to different environmental modifiers of genetic effects, and LD might vary so that a marker that is a good surrogate for a functional allele in one population is a poor surrogate in another population. Moreover, the problems of reporting and publication bias might seriously distort the true pattern of findings so that incorrect inferences may be drawn from the pooled data. Statistical methods to detect publication bias can be used[95] before applying meta-analytical approaches.[97]

Results of genetic association studies of blood pressure and hypertension

Reported associations with hypertension or blood pressure have related to polymorphisms in a number of plausible candidate genes, including the genes coding for angiotensin I converting enzyme (ACE),[98] angiotensinogen,[99] alpha-adducin[100] and the G-protein beta subunit.[101] These initial reports of associations have been followed by many 'replication' studies with mostly negative findings. Given that the replication studies have been generally underpowered, it has been difficult to assess whether the lack of replication is entirely due to low power to replicate a true positive association or due to a false positive initial report. In assessing the 'candidate' status of these genes in the etiology of essential hypertension other information must also be used, such as that from linkage studies[99,102,103] and from studies investigating the effect of the candidate gene variants on intermediate phenotypes.[104,105]

Associations have been reported between variants in over 30 candidate genes and hypertension, but the majority of these findings are far from robust.[9] Genes that are now regarded as strong candidates for blood pressure regulation and essential hypertension risk (not all of which have yet been investigated in genetic association studies) are described throughout this volume. In addition, examples of meta-analyses of association studies relating to some strong candidates for hypertension are considered in Chapter 7. Furthermore, genetic association studies of stroke, a major complication of hypertension, are described in Chapter 5. The results of association studies of hypertension and its complications have also been reviewed comprehensively elsewhere.[2,9,106–109]

EXPRESSION STUDIES AND PHARMACOGENETIC STUDIES

Building on the findings of linkage and association studies considered above, there has been a rapid increase in gene expression studies and in pharmacogenetic studies.[110] Gene expression studies bring fresh methodological challenges, not least the magnitude of multiple-testing usually involved.[111] However, the refinement of microarray approaches and the successful integration of gene expression data with other types of genomic information[112,113] give hope that such studies will provide valuable insight into the mechanisms underlying the development of essential hypertension.

A recent review identified 28 published pharmacogenetic studies of hypertension treatment.[114] Only ten of these studies included more than 100 participants. It is unsurprising, therefore, that the results of these studies have been highly variable. For example, of 11 studies that studied the influence of the *ACE* deletion polymorphism on the blood pressure-lowering effect of angiotensin-converting enzyme (ACE) inhibitors, three studies reported a greater effect, four studies reported a smaller effect and four studies reported no difference.[114] However, larger pharmacogenetic studies are being undertaken and the findings of these studies will be of great interest to clinicians that prescribe antihypertensive drugs. Chapter 8 considers pharmacogenetic studies in detail.

ADMIXTURE MAPPING

Although not a new idea, an alternative approach that is currently gaining favor is termed 'admixture mapping'.[115] This approach specifically makes use of recently admixed populations and depends on assessing the extent to which the population's ancestry proportions at a given locus differ from the average proportions over the genome.[116] Zhu and colleagues recently used admixture mapping to search for hypertension loci using genome-scan markers in an African–American population.[117] At chromosome regions 6q24 and 21q21 they found an excess of African ancestry in hypertensive cases but not in normotensive controls. These findings are consistent with the theory that these particular genomic regions harbor genes conferring susceptibility to hypertension in this admixed population.

In many respects, the admixture mapping approach falls between linkage analysis and association analysis, because it offers improved mapping resolution and greater statistical power than linkage studies (subject to markedly differing frequencies of the disease susceptibility alleles in the ancestral populations)[116] and it requires fewer markers than LD mapping.[118] Furthermore, admixture mapping offers an apparent solution to the dilemma of studying specific populations that are otherwise difficult to analyze using other approaches. Such populations are those that have been subject to recent admixture, where the admixture may actually confound estimates of gene–disease associations.[68] There are parallels with the TDT approach, which was also well suited to the analysis of samples of a particular kind, i.e. trios consisting of affected probands and genotyped parents with missing phenotype information. For a time, the TDT became so 'fashionable' that its use was suggested even for problems where other designs would have been more appropriate.[68,119]

Undoubtedly, more admixture mapping studies of hypertension and its complications will be undertaken in the near future, many of these exploiting existing biomedical collections from admixed populations. However, for the method to offer real advantages over linkage or LD studies, the allele frequencies of the disease susceptibility alleles need to differ substantially between the ancestral populations of the admixed population. As these allele frequencies are usually unknown, it is unclear whether this condition will be satisfied in many realistic settings,[116] although preliminary evidence as to the utility of this approach will be gained by testing whether the phenotypic status is correlated with ancestry within the admixed study population.[120]

Admixture mapping appears to be a promising approach. However, enthusiasm for this approach should be tempered with some caution, given the recent tendency of genetic epidemiology studies of complex diseases (including hypertension) to follow study design 'fashions'[119] and given concerns about the number of settings for which admixture mapping will be effective.[121]

PUBLIC HEALTH BENEFITS OF GENETIC EPIDEMIOLOGY AND 'MENDELIAN RANDOMIZATION'

The emphasis on the utility of genetic epidemiology to inform 'personalized medicine'[110] has generated concern that genetic epidemiology is the antithesis of public health epidemiology,[122] but because genetic epidemiology can help identify biological pathways and intermediates that are amenable to public health intervention, it could inform interventions that act at either a population or an individual level (see Fig. 2.1, p 6). The public health utility of genetic epidemiology studies has been particularly apparent in studies that employ the concept of 'Mendelian randomization'[82] or 'Mendelian deconfounding'[83] to circumvent the confounding and reverse causation that have undermined the findings of traditional epidemiological studies.[123]

In many public health and clinical settings, we wish to assess the evidence for a causal relationship between a quantitative intermediate phenotype, such as circulating homocysteine levels, and a quantitative or binary outcome, for example blood pressure or risk of stroke. Such knowledge can inform public health interventions, such as the fortification of flour with folate, or individual level interventions, such as prescribing folate tablets. Observational epidemiological studies have shown that raised homocysteine levels are associated with a higher risk of stroke.[124,125] However, many lifestyle factors, such as smoking, are associated both with homocysteine levels and the risk of stroke and might therefore confound the relationship. Furthermore, atherosclerosis and stroke might elevate homocysteine levels, leading to an apparent association due to reverse causation. Thus confounding or reverse causation could account for some or all of the association observed between homocysteine levels and stroke risk.

One can attempt to minimize the effect of confounders by measuring such variables and by adjusting for them in any analysis, but residual confounding might still be problematic, as many confounders are not known or easily measurable. Furthermore, this will not control for reverse causation. An alternative approach, based on work of Katan and colleagues,[126] is to generate indirect inferences about the relationship between a phenotype and a disease given direct information about gene-disease and gene-phenotype associations. According to Mendel's laws of segregation and independence,[127] a subject's genotype is determined by an apparently random process at conception, so that gene–disease and gene–phenotype associations cannot be subject to reverse causation or confounded by lifestyle factors. Therefore, the phenotype–disease estimate that is obtained through the use of the genotype as an instrumental variable[128] is 'deconfounded'.[83] Providing that one has sufficient information to account for the uncertainty in the estimates of the genotype–phenotype and genotype–disease associations, e.g. using data from meta-analyses,[129] then this method could have great utility for informing public health interventions. For example, Casas and colleagues investigated the causal link between homocysteine levels and stroke by integrating evidence from meta-analyses of the relationships between the methylenetetrahydrofolate reductase (MTHFR) C677T genotype and homocysteine level and between the MTHFR genotype and stroke risk.[130] They obtained estimates close to those obtained from observation studies, adding to the weight of evidence for a causal relationship between elevated homocysteine and increased stroke risk that may be modifiable by folic acid supplementation at a population level.

Mendelian randomization has been employed to assess the relationship between C-reactive protein (CRP) level, and blood pressure and hypertension by using a polymorphism in the CRP gene as an instrumental variable in a single study.[131] The unconfounded estimates from this study did not support the apparently causal association between elevated circulating CRP levels reported from a number of observational epidemiology studies. Other phenotype disease relationships relevant to cardiovascular epidemiology have been investigated using Mendelian randomization.[82] For example, a polymorphism in the beta-fibrinogen gene has been used as an instrument to assess the unconfounded relationship between circulating fibrinogen levels and the risk of myocardial infarction.[132] These studies have provided a 'proof of concept'. Although skepticism remains about Mendelian randomization studies,[133] and about the validity of their findings in the presence of the genetic heterogeneity and pleiotropy that inevitably accompany complex diseases such as essential hypertension,[83] methodological work is underway that will address some of these issues. In the near future it is likely that Mendelian randomization studies will be applied to test associations between a range of potentially modifiable phenotypes and blood pressure, essential hypertension, and their complications.

CONCLUDING REMARKS

A range of strategies has been used to investigate the genetic architecture of essential hypertension and blood pressure as complex traits. Rapid advances in genomics have provided exciting opportunities but also fresh challenges. Over the next two decades, there are likely to be substantial advances in the understanding of the etiology of these complex traits and resulting improvements in treatment and prevention. The use of Mendelian randomization studies offers the possibility that the benefits of these developments might be realized by whole populations.

References

1. Chobanian AV, Bakris GL, Black HR, et al. The Seventh Report of the Joint National Committee on Prevention, Detection, Evaluation, and Treatment of High Blood Pressure: the JNC 7 report. *JAMA*. 2003; 289:2560–2572.
2. Staessen JA, Wang J, Bianchi G, Birkenhager WH. Essential hypertension. *Lancet* 2003; 361:1629–1641.
3. National Institutes of Health (NIH). JNC 7 express: the seventh report of the Joint National Committee on Prevention, Detection, Evaluation and Treatment of High Blood Pressure. Bethesda, MD: National Institutes of Health; 2003.
4. Lewington S, Clarke R, Qizilbash N, et al. Age-specific relevance of usual blood pressure to vascular mortality: a meta-analysis of individual data for one million adults in 61 prospective studies. *Lancet* 2002; 360:1903–1913.
5. Lifton RP, Gharavi AG, Geller DS. Molecular mechanisms of human hypertension. *Cell* 2001; 104:545–556.
6. Palmer LJ. Complex diseases. In: Elston R, Olson JM, Palmer LJ, eds. *Biostatistical genetics and genetic epidemiology*. Chichester: Wiley; 2002:141–143.
7. Lander ES, Schork NJ. Genetic dissection of complex traits. *Science* 1994; 265:2037–2048.
8. Pickering GW. The nature of essential hypertension. *Lancet* 1959; 5 December:1027–1028.
9. Samani NJ. Genetics of hypertension. In: Warrell DA, Cox TM, Firth JD, Benz EJJ, eds. *Oxford textbook of medicine, 4th edn*. Oxford: Oxford University Press; 2003:1–9.
10. Olson JM, Witte JS, Elston RC. Genetic mapping of complex traits. *Stat Med* 1999; 18:2961–2981.
11. Tobin MD, Sheehan NA, Scurrah K, Burton PR. Adjusting for treatment effects in studies of quantitative traits: antihypertensive therapy and systolic blood pressure. *Stat Med* 2005; 24:2911–2935.
12. Rothman KJ, Greenland S. Validity and generalizability in epidemiologic studies. In: Elston R, Olson JM, Palmer LJ, eds. *Biostatistical genetics and genetic epidemiology*. Chichester: Wiley; 2002:771–777.
13. Sagnella GA, Rothwell MJ, Onipinla AK, et al. A population study of ethnic variations in the angiotensin-converting enzyme I/D polymorphism: relationships with gender, hypertension and impaired glucose metabolism. *J Hypertens* 1999; 17:657–664.
14. Sethi AA, Nordestgaard BG, Agerholm-Larsen B, et al. Angiotensinogen polymorphisms and elevated blood pressure in the general population: the Copenhagen City Heart Study. *Hypertension* 2001; 37:875–881.
15. Zhu X, Chang YP, Yan D, et al. Associations between hypertension and genes in the renin–angiotensin system. *Hypertension* 2003; 41:1027–1034.
16. Iwai N, Baba S, Mannami T, et al. Association of sodium channel gamma-subunit promoter variant with blood pressure. *Hypertension* 2001; 38:86–89.
17. Pereira AC, Mota GF, Cunha RS, et al. Angiotensinogen 235T allele 'dosage' is associated with blood pressure phenotypes. *Hypertension* 2003; 41:25–30.
18. von Wowern F, Bengtsson K, Lindgren CM, et al. A genome wide scan for early onset primary hypertension in Scandinavians. *Hum Mol Genet* 2003; 12:2077–2081.
19. Wacholder S, Hartge P, Palmer LJ. Case-control study. In: Elston R, Olson JM, Palmer LJ, eds. *Biostatistical genetics and genetic epidemiology*. Chichester: Wiley; 2002:95–109.
20. Tobin MD. The genetic epidemiology of blood pressure in human populations. Department of Health Sciences, University of Leicester; Leicester:2004.
21. Galton F. Typical laws of heredity. *Proc Roy Inst* 1877; 8:282–301.
22. Galton F. Family likeness in stature. *Proc Roy Soc* 1886; 40:42–73.
23. Pearson K. Mathematical contributions to the theory of evolution – III. Regression, heredity, and panmixia. *Phil Trans Roy Soc A* 1896; 187:253–318.
24. Hunt SC. Genetics and family history of hypertension. In: Izzo JL, Black HR, eds. *Hypertension primer, 3rd edn*. Dallas, TX: American Heart Association; 2003:218–221.
25. Hunt SC, Williams RR, Barlow GK. A comparison of positive family history definitions for defining risk of future disease. *J Chronic Dis* 1986; 39:809–821.
26. Risch N. Linkage strategies for genetically complex traits. II. The power of affected relative pairs. *Am J Hum Genet* 1990; 46:229–241.
27. Mongeau JG, Biron P, Sing CF. The influence of genetics and household environment upon the variability of normal blood pressure: the Montreal Adoption Survey. *Clin Exp Hypertens A* 1986; 8:653–660.
28. Harrap SB, Stebbing M, Hopper JL, et al. Familial patterns of covariation for cardiovascular risk factors in adults: the Victorian Family Heart Study. *Am J Epidemiol* 2000; 152:704–715.
29. Luft FC. Twins in cardiovascular genetic research. *Hypertension* 2001; 37:350–356.
30. Hopper J. Variance components for statistical genetics: applications in medical research to characteristics related to human diseases and health. *Stat Methods Med Res* 1993; 2:199–223.

31. Khoury MJ, Beaty TH, Cohen BH. Genetic approaches to familial aggregation: I. Analysis of heritability. In: *Fundamentals of genetic epidemiology*. New York: Oxford University Press; 1993:200–232.

32. Burton PR, Tobin MD. Epidemiology and genetic epidemiology. In: Balding DJ, Bishop M, Cannings C, eds. *Handbook of statistical genetics, 2nd edn*. Chichester: Wiley; 2003.

33. Hopper JL. Variance component analysis. In: Elston R, Olson J, Palmer L, eds. *Biostatistical genetics and genetic epidemiology*. Chichester: Wiley; 2002:778–788.

34. Levy D, DeStefano AL, Larson MG, et al. Evidence for a gene influencing blood pressure on chromosome 17. Genome scan linkage results for longitudinal blood pressure phenotypes in subjects from the Framingham Heart Study. *Hypertension* 2000; 36:477–483.

35. Kotchen TA, Kotchen JM, Grim CE, et al. Genetic determinants of hypertension: identification of candidate phenotypes. *Hypertension* 2000; 36:7–13.

36. Gu C, Borecki I, Gagnon J, et al. Familial resemblance for resting blood pressure with particular reference to racial differences: preliminary analyses from the HERITAGE Family Study. *Hum Biol* 1998; 70:77–90.

37. Atwood LD, Samollow PB, Hixson JE, et al. Genome–wide linkage analysis of pulse pressure in Mexican Americans. *Hypertension* 2001; 37:425–428.

38. Skaric-Juric T. Path analysis of familial resemblance in blood pressure in Middle Dalmatia, Croatia. *Collegium Antropologicum* 2003; 27:229–237.

39. Terwilliger JD. Linkage analysis model-based. In: Elston R, Olson JM, Palmer LJ, eds. *Biostatistical genetics and genetic epidemiology*. Chichester: Wiley; 2002:448–460.

40. Blangero J. Segregation analysis, complex. In: Elston R, Olson J, Palmer L, eds. *Biostatistical genetics and genetic epidemiology*. Chichester: Wiley; 2002:696–708.

41. Elston RC. Segregation analysis. *Adv Hum Genet* 1981; 11:63–120, 372–373.

42. Crockford GP, Bishop DT, Barrett JH. Segregation analysis comparing liability and quantitative trait models for hypertension using the Genetic Analysis Workshop 13 simulated data. *BMC Genet* 2003; 4(suppl 1):S79.

43. Kopciuk KA, Briollais L, Demenais F, Bull SB. Using an age-at-onset phenotype with interval censoring to compare methods of segregation and linkage analysis in a candidate region for elevated systolic blood pressure. *BMC Genet* 2003; 4(suppl 1):S84.

44. Rice T, Bouchard C, Borecki IB, Rao DC. Commingling and segregation analysis of blood pressure in a French–Canadian population. *Am J Hum Genet* 1990; 46:37–44.

45. Chien KL, Yang CY, Lee YT. Major gene effects in systolic and diastolic blood pressure in families receiving a health examination in Taiwan. *J Hypertens* 2003; 21:73–79.

46. Cheng LS, Livshits G, Carmelli D, et al. Segregation analysis reveals a major gene effect controlling systolic blood pressure and BMI in an Israeli population. *Hum Biol* 1998; 70:59–75.

47. An P, Rice T, Perusse L, et al. Complex segregation analysis of blood pressure and heart rate measured before and after a 20-week endurance exercise training program: the HERITAGE Family Study. *Am J Hypertens* 2000; 13:488–497.

48. Thompson EA. Linkage analysis. In: Balding DJ, Bishop M, Cannings C, eds. *Handbook of statistical genetics*. Chichester: Wiley; 2001:541–563.

49. Holmans P. Non-parametric linkage. In: Balding DJ, Bishop M, Cannings C, eds. *Handbook of statistical genetics*. Chichester: Wiley; 2001:487–505.

50. Olson J. Linkage analysis model-based. In: Elston R, Olson JM, Palmer LJ, eds. *Biostatistical genetics and genetic epidemiology*. Chichester: Wiley; 2002:461–472.

51. Teare MD, Barrett JH. Genetic linkage studies. *Lancet* 2005; 366:1036–1044.

52. Haseman JK, Elston RC. The investigation of linkage between a quantitative trait and a marker locus. *Behav Genet* 1972; 2:3–19.

53. Amos C. Robust variance-components approach for assessing genetic linkage in pedigrees. *Am J Hum Genet* 1994; 54:535–543.

54. Caulfield M, Munroe P, Pembroke J, et al. Genome-wide mapping of human loci for essential hypertension. *Lancet* 2003; 361:2118–2123.

55. Angius A, Petretto E, Maestrale GB, et al. A new essential hypertension susceptibility locus on chromosome 2p24-p25, detected by genomewide search. *Am J Hum Genet* 2002; 71:893–905.

56. Hsueh WC, Mitchell BD, Schneider JL, et al. QTL influencing blood pressure maps to the region of PPH1 on chromosome 2q31-34 in Old Order Amish. *Circulation* 2000; 101:2810–2816.

57. Hodge SE. Ascertainment. In: Elston R, Olson J, Palmer L, eds. *Biostatistical genetics and genetic epidemiology*. Chichester: Wiley; 2002:20–28.

58. Cannings C, Thompson EA. Ascertainment in the sequential sampling of pedigrees. *Clin Genet* 1977; 12:208–212.

59. Wise LH, Lanchbury JS, Lewis CM. Meta-analysis of genome searches. *Ann Hum Genet* 1999; 63 (Pt 3):263–272.

60. Province MA, Kardia SL, Ranade K, et al. A meta-analysis of genome-wide linkage scans for hypertension: the National Heart, Lung and Blood Institute Family Blood Pressure Program. *Am J Hypertens* 2003; 16:144–147.

61. Roberts SB, MacLean CJ, Neale MC, et al. Replication of linkage studies of complex traits: an examination of variation in location estimates. *Am J Hum Genet* 1999; 65:876–884.
62. Morton NE. Sequential tests for the detection of linkage. *Am J Hum Genet* 1955; 7:277–318.
63. Lander E, Kruglyak L. Genetic dissection of complex traits: guidelines for interpreting and reporting linkage results. *Nat Genet* 1995; 11:241–247.
64. Risch NJ. Searching for genetic determinants in the new millennium. *Nature* 2000; 405:847–856.
65. Kristjansson K, Manolescu A, Kristinsson A, et al. Linkage of essential hypertension to chromosome 18q. *Hypertension* 2002; 39:1044–1049.
66. Barkley RA, Chakravarti A, Cooper RS, et al. Positional identification of hypertension susceptibility genes on chromosome 2. *Hypertension* 2004; 43:477–482.
67. Johnson GC, Esposito L, Barratt BJ, et al. Haplotype tagging for the identification of common disease genes. *Nat Genet* 2001; 29:233–237.
68. Cardon LR, Palmer LJ. Population stratification and spurious allelic association. *Lancet* 2003; 361:598–604.
69. Hoggart CJ, Parra EJ, Shriver MD, et al. Control of confounding of genetic associations in stratified populations. *Am J Hum Genet* 2003; 72:1492–1504.
70. Freedman ML, Reich D, Penney KL, et al. Assessing the impact of population stratification on genetic association studies. *Nat Genet* 2004; 36:388–393.
71. Clayton D, McKeigue PM. Epidemiological methods for studying genes and environmental factors in complex diseases. *Lancet* 2001; 358:1356–1360.
72. Zondervan KT, Cardon LR. The complex interplay among factors that influence allelic association. *Nat Rev Genet* 2004; 5:89–100.
73. Chakravarti A. Linkage disequilibrium. In: Elston R, Olson JM, Palmer LJ, eds. *Biostatistical genetics and genetic epidemiology*. Chichester: Wiley; 2002:472–475.
74. International HapMap Consortium. The International HapMap Project. *Nature* 2003; 426:789–796.
75. Hinds DA, Stuve LL, Nilsen GB, et al. Whole-genome patterns of common DNA variation in three human populations. *Science* 2005; 307:1072–1079.
76. Daly MJ, Rioux JD, Schaffner SF, et al. High-resolution haplotype structure in the human genome. *Nat Genet* 2001; 29:229–232.
77. Anderson EC, Novembre J. Finding haplotype block boundaries by using the minimum-description-length principle. *Am J Hum Genet* 2003; 73:336–354.
78. Gabriel SB, Schaffner SF, Nguyen H, et al. The structure of haplotype blocks in the human genome. *Science* 2002; 296:2225–2229.
79. Mannila H, Koivisto M, Perola M, et al. Minimum description length block finder, a method to identify haplotype blocks and to compare the strength of block boundaries. *Am J Hum Genet* 2003; 73:86–94.
80. Patil N, Berno AJ, Hinds DA, et al. Blocks of limited haplotype diversity revealed by high–resolution scanning of human chromosome 21. *Science* 2001; 294:1719–1723.
81. Phillips MS, Lawrence R, Sachidanandam R, et al. Chromosome-wide distribution of haplotype blocks and the role of recombination hot spots. *Nat Genet* 2003; 33:382–387.
82. Davey Smith G, Ebrahim S. 'Mendelian randomisation': can genetic epidemiology contribute to understanding environmental determinants of disease? *Int J Epidemiol* 2003; 32:1–22.
83. Tobin MD, Minelli C, Burton PR, Thompson JR. The development of Mendelian randomisation: from hypothesis testing to 'Mendelian deconfounding.' *Int J Epidemiol* 2004; 33:26–29.
84. Devlin B, Roeder K. Genomic control for association studies. *Biometrics* 1999; 55:997–1004.
85. Marchini J, Cardon LR, Phillips MS, Donnelly P. The effects of human population structure on large genetic association studies. *Nat Genet* 2004; 36:512–517.
86. Palmer LJ, Cookson WO, James AL, et al. Gibbs sampling-based segregation analysis of asthma-associated quantitative traits in a population-based sample of nuclear families. *Genet Epidemiol* 2001; 20:356–372.
87. Ewens WJ, Spielman RS. The transmission/disequilibrium test: history, subdivision, and admixture. *Am J Hum Genet* 1995; 57:455–464.
88. Cardon LR, Bell JI. Association study designs for complex diseases. *Nat Rev Genet* 2001; 2:91–99.
89. Colhoun HM, McKeigue PM, Davey Smith G. Problems of reporting genetic associations with complex outcomes. *Lancet* 2003; 361:865–872.
90. Attia J, Thakkinstian A, D'Este C. Meta-analyses of molecular association studies: methodologic lessons for genetic epidemiology. *J Clin Epidemiol* 2003; 56:297–303.
91. Little J, Bradley L, Bray MS, et al. Reporting, appraising, and integrating data on genotype prevalence and gene-disease associations. *Am J Epidemiol* 2002; 156:300–310.
92. Wellcome Trust and Medical Research Council. Draft Protocol for BioBank UK: A study of genes, environment and health. London: Medical Research Council; 2002.
93. Little J. Reporting and review of human genome epidemiology studies. In: Khoury MJ, Little J, Burke W, eds. *Human genome epidemiology*. Oxford: Oxford University Press; 2004:168–192.

94. Tobin MD, Braund PS, Burton PR, et al. Genotypes and haplotypes predisposing to myocardial infarction: a multilocus case-control study. *Eur Heart J* 2004; 25:459–467.
95. Sutton AJ, Song F, Gilbody SM, Abrams KR. Modelling publication bias in meta-analysis: a review. *Stat Methods Med Res* 2000; 9:421–445.
96. Clayton DG, Walker NM, Smyth DJ, et al. Population structure, differential bias and genomic control in a large-scale, case-control association study. *Nat Genet* 2005; 37:1243–1246.
97. Thakkinstian A, McElduff P, D'Este C, et al. A method for meta-analysis of molecular association studies. *Stat Med* 2005; 24(9):1291–1306.
98. Fornage M, Amos CI, Kardia S, et al. Variation in the region of the angiotensin-converting enzyme gene influences interindividual differences in blood pressure levels in young white males. *Circulation* 1998; 97:1773–1779.
99. Jeunemaitre X, Soubrier F, Kotelevtsev YV, et al. Molecular basis of human hypertension: role of angiotensinogen. *Cell* 1992; 71:169–180.
100. Casari G, Barlassina C, Cusi D, et al. Association of the alpha-adducin locus with essential hypertension. *Hypertension* 1995; 25:320–326.
101. Siffert W, Rosskopf D, Siffert G, et al. Association of a human G-protein beta3 subunit variant with hypertension. *Nat Genet* 1998; 18:45–48.
102. Cusi D, Barlassina C, Azzani T, et al. Polymorphisms of alpha-adducin and salt sensitivity in patients with essential hypertension. *Lancet* 1997; 349:1353–1357.
103. Wong ZY, Stebbing M, Ellis JA, et al. Genetic linkage of beta and gamma subunits of epithelial sodium channel to systolic blood pressure. *Lancet* 1999; 353:1222–1225.
104. Cox R, Bouzekri N, Martin S, et al. Angiotensin-1-converting enzyme (ACE) plasma concentration is influenced by multiple ACE-linked quantitative trait nucleotides. *Hum Mol Genet* 2002; 11:2969–2977.
105. Soubrier F, Cambien F. The angiotensin I-converting enzyme gene polymorphism: implication in hypertension and myocardial infarction. *Curr Opin Nephrol Hypertens* 1994; 3:25–29.
106. Mein CA, Caulfield MJ, Dobson RJ, Munroe PB. Genetics of essential hypertension. *Hum Mol Genet* 2004; 13(suppl 1):R169–R175.
107. Turner ST, Boerwinkle E. Genetics of blood pressure, hypertensive complications, and antihypertensive drug responses. *Pharmacogenomics* 2003; 4:53–65.
108. Hopkins PN, Hunt SC. Genetics of hypertension. *Genet Med* 2003; 5:413–429.
109. Nabel EG. Cardiovascular disease. *N Engl J Med* 2003; 349:60–72.
110. Goldstein DB, Tate SK, Sisodiya SM. Pharmacogenetics goes genomic. *Nat Rev Genet* 2003; 4:937–947.
111. Pravenec M, Wallace C, Aitman TJ, Kurtz TW. Gene expression profiling in hypertension research: a critical perspective. *Hypertension* 2003; 41:3–8.
112. Yagil C, Hubner N, Monti J, et al. Identification of hypertension–related genes through an integrated genomic-transcriptomic approach. *Circ Res* 2005; 96:617–625.
113. Hubner N, Wallace CA, Zimdahl H, et al. Integrated transcriptional profiling and linkage analysis for identification of genes underlying disease. *Nat Genet* 2005; 37:243–253.
114. Koopmans RP, Insel PA, Michel MC. Pharmacogenetics of hypertension treatment: a structured review. *Pharmacogenetics* 2003; 13:705–713.
115. McKeigue PM. Prospects for admixture mapping of complex traits. *Am J Hum Genet* 2005; 76:1–7.
116. Montana G, Pritchard JK. Statistical tests for admixture mapping with case-control and cases-only data. *Am J Hum Genet* 2004; 75:771–789.
117. Zhu X, Luke A, Cooper RS, et al. Admixture mapping for hypertension loci with genome-scan markers. *Nat Genet* 2005; 37:177–181.
118. Darvasi A, Shifman S. The beauty of admixture. *Nat Genet* 2005; 37:118–119.
119. Spence MA, Greenberg DA, Hodge SE, Vieland VJ. The emperor's new methods. *Am J Hum Genet* 2003; 72:1084–1087.
120. Kittles RA, Chen W, Panguluri RK, et al. CYP3A4-V and prostate cancer in African Americans: causal or confounding association because of population stratification? *Hum Genet* 2002; 110:553–560.
121. Nievergelt CM, Schork NJ. Admixture mapping as a gene discovery approach for complex human traits and diseases. *Curr Hypertens Rep* 2005; 7:31–37.
122. Davey Smith G, Harbord R, Ebrahim S. Fibrinogen, C-reactive protein and coronary heart disease: does Mendelian randomization suggest the associations are non-causal? *Quart J Med*. 2004; 97:163–166.
123. Taubes G. Epidemiology faces its limits. *Science* 1995; 269:164–169.
124. Homocyseine Lowering Trialists' Collaboration. Homocysteine and risk of ischemic heart disease and stroke: a meta-analysis. *JAMA* 2002; 288:2015–2022.
125. Wald DS, Law M, Morris JK. Homocysteine and cardiovascular disease: evidence on causality from a meta-analysis. *Br Med J* 2002; 325:1202.
126. Katan MB. Apolipoprotein E isoforms, serum cholesterol, and cancer. *Lancet* 1986; 1:507–508.
127. Wijsman EM. Mendel's laws. In: Elston R, Olson JM, Palmer LJ, eds. *Biostatistical genetics and genetic epidemiology*. Chichester: Wiley; 2002:527–529.

128. Thomas DC, Conti DV. Commentary: the concept of 'Mendelian randomization'. *Int J Epidemiol* 2004; 33:21–25.
129. Minelli C, Thompson JR, Tobin MD, Abrams KR. An integrated approach to the meta-analysis of genetic association studies using Mendelian randomization. *Am J Epidemiol* 2004; 160:445–452.
130. Casas JP, Bautista LE, Smeeth L, et al. Homocysteine and stroke: evidence on a causal link from mendelian randomisation. *Lancet* 2005; 365:224–232.
131. Smith GD, Lawlor DA, Harbord R, et al. Association of C-reactive protein with blood pressure and hypertension. life course confounding and Mendelian randomization tests of causality. Arterioscler Thromb Vasc Biol 2005; 25(5):1051–1056; erratum in: Arterioscler Thromb Vasc Biol 2005; 25(8):e129; comment in: *Arterioscler Thromb Vasc Biol* 2005; 25(9):e137.
132. Youngman L, Keavney B. Plasma fibrinogen and fibrinogen genotypes in 4685 cases of myocardial infarction and in 6002 controls: test of causality by 'Mendelian randomisation.' *Circulation* 2000; 102:31–32.
133. Little J, Khoury MJ. Mendelian randomisation: a new spin or real progress? *Lancet* 2003; 362:930–931.

3 | Monogenic disorders of blood pressure regulation

Julie E. Goodwin and David S. Geller

INTRODUCTION

Hypertension is among the most common diseases of the industrialized world and is an important risk factor for heart disease, stroke and kidney failure. Nevertheless, the molecular basis of disease remains unknown in the vast majority of hypertensive patients. The study of Mendelian disorders featuring primary effect on blood pressure has yielded great insights into the underlying molecular etiology of hypertension. Here, we will review the various monogenic disorders with primary effect on blood pressure regulation with an emphasis on how the elucidation of the mechanisms of these disorders has enhanced our understanding of the molecular basis of hypertension.

HYPERTENSIVE DISORDERS (Table 3.1)

Liddle syndrome

First described in 1963, Liddle syndrome is an autosomal dominant form of human hypertension characterized by severe, early-onset hypertension, hypokalemia and metabolic alkalosis in the setting of low plasma renin and aldosterone levels. Recent advances in the last decade have demonstrated that the disease can be caused by mutations in either the β or the γ subunit of the epithelial sodium channel (ENaC) gene on chromosome 16p. Both subunits are known to increase channel activity.[1,2] The elucidation of the molecular basis of Liddle syndrome has demonstrated it to be perhaps the most straightforward form of hypertension, developing solely on the basis of excess renal sodium reabsorption in the distal nephron. This notion has been reinforced by the clinical observation that renal transplantation cured hypertension in a patient with Liddle syndrome and end-stage renal disease.[3]

ENaC, located in the distal nephron as well as the colon and lung, plays a crucial role in maintaining fluid and electrolyte homeostasis and represents the final effector molecule of the renin–angiotensin–aldosterone system in the kidney. By mediating aldosterone-sensitive apical Na$^+$ transport in conjunction with the

Table 3.1 Mendelian disorders of hypertension

Syndrome	Gene	Renin	Aldo	K	Treatment
Liddle syndrome*	SCNN1B,G (β, γ ENaC)	Low	Low	Low/ Normal	Amiloride, triamterene, low-sodium diet
HTN exacerbated by pregnancy*	MR	Low	Low	Low/ Normal	Amiloride, triamterene, low-sodium diet
GRA	Aldo S/11 β-OHase chimera	Low	High	Low/ Normal	Dexamethasone
AME**	11βHSD2	Low	Low	Low	Spironolactone, low-sodium diet
PHA 2	WNK1, 4	Low	Normal	High	Thiazide diuretics
HTN with brachydactyly*	Unknown	Normal	Normal	Normal	Multiple antihypertensives
FH II*	Unknown	Low?	High	Low?	Spironolactone?, surgery?

* Autosomal dominant inheritance.
** Autosomal recessive inheritance.
FH II, Familial hyperaldosteronism type II; GRA, Glucocorticoid remediable aldosteronism; HTN, Hypertension; PHA 2, Pseudohypoaldosteronism type 2; AME, Syndrome of apparent mineralocorticoid excess.

basolateral Na/K ATPase, ENaC regulates whole body sodium balance. The channel is composed of three subunits in the following proportion: two α, one β and one γ. Each subunit consists of two transmembrane domains and intracellular NH_2 and COOH termini; the COOH termini all contain highly conserved sequences known as PY motifs, which play a role in the removal of ENaC from the cell surface.[4] Mutations causing Liddle syndrome have in common a disruption of these PY motifs, via frameshift mutations, premature stop codons or site-specific point mutations, resulting in increased ENaC activity via an increase in the number of channels at the apical surface.[5]

As Liddle syndrome is characterized by mineralocorticoid-independent activation of renal sodium reabsorption via ENaC, renin and aldosterone levels are suppressed and spironolactone is not an effective therapy. By contrast, amiloride and triamterene, to which the channel is sensitive, do provide amelioration of symptoms. Amiloride/hydrochlorothiazide combinations are also effective.[6] It is notable that hypokalemia is not necessary to make the diagnosis, nor is it universally present in affected patients.[3] In some older patients, beta-blockers and vasodilators may be needed in addition to diuretics to achieve adequate blood pressure control, and a low-salt diet is an important and synergistic adjunct treatment. Left untreated, patients develop significant sequelae of hypertension including left ventricular hypertrophy (LVH), congestive heart failure (CHF) and cerebrovascular complications.

Hypertension exacerbated by pregnancy

Although blood pressure is usually lower than normal during pregnancy, hypertension is a significant problem in a small percentage of pregnant patients. In the majority of these cases, many of which progress to pre-eclampsia, the cause of the hypertension is unknown. However, in rare cases, a genetic mutation in the mineralocorticoid receptor (MR) can account for this aberrant condition.

As MR binds aldosterone, a primary regulator of blood pressure and sodium homeostasis, and as mutations in MR have been implicated in other genetic conditions involving blood pressure derangements (see adPHA1, p 37), it was a reasonable candidate in the search for genes underlying hereditary predispositions to hypertension. In a screen of 75 patients with early-onset hypertension, we detected a missense mutation in MR in a single patient, which resulted in a substitution of leucine for serine at residue 810 in the hormone-binding domain of the receptor.[7] MR_{S810L} cosegregated in an autosomal dominant fashion with early-onset hypertension and low aldosterone levels in family members of the index case, demonstrating that this allele is causative of the disease. All affected individuals had severe hypertension diagnosed before the age of 20, with suppression of serum aldosterone levels. Although hypokalemia might have been an expected feature of this disease, it was not uniformly present.

Further characterization of the mutant receptor demonstrated two key properties that help to explain the clinical phenotype. First, the receptor has some constitutive activity in the absence of added aldosterone. Second, steroids lacking 21-OH groups, such as progesterone and spironolactone, activate the mutant, but not the wild-type, receptor. As progesterone levels increase markedly during pregnancy, the authors predicted that pregnant women with MR_{S810L} would become severely hypertensive. Two MR_{L810} carriers had a total of five pregnancies. As expected, each was characterized by severe and uncontrollable hypertension and hypokalemia that required premature delivery in the seventh month of pregnancy or premature termination of the pregnancy.

There is still the puzzling question of why carriers of MR_{S810L}, notably men and nonpregnant women, who have much lower levels of progesterone, also develop hypertension. However, Rafestin-Oblin et al have recently shown that cortisone, a metabolite of cortisol in the distal nephron, is a potent activator of the mutant, but not the wild-type, receptor *in vitro*.[8] This finding suggests that cortisone might be responsible for the hypertension found in men and nonpregnant women with the mutant receptor.

Hypertension exacerbated in pregnancy is among the rarest diseases ever described. To date, it has been identified in only the original family, despite screening specifically for this disorder in hypertensive pregnant women.[9] An explanation for this scarcity came in part from substitution mutagenesis studies, which revealed that only methionine and leucine at residue 810 are permissive for progesterone-mediated activation of the receptor. Based on this finding, it appears that only one specific mutation in the entire genome, a substitution of cytosine to thymine in codon 810, can lead to this phenotype. Furthermore, if such a mutation were to arise, the severe hypertension experienced by female carriers during pregnancy would lead to a strong selection bias against propagation of this allele.

Glucocorticoid-remediable aldosteronism

Glucocorticoid-remediable aldosteronism (GRA) is an autosomal dominant form of primary aldosteronism characterized by elevated aldosterone levels and hypertension despite suppressed renin levels. GRA is distinguished by the marked overproduction of the hybrid steroids 18-hydroxycortisol and 18-oxo-cortisol. The pathognomonic feature of the disease, however, is extreme sensitivity of the aldosteronism to glucocorticoids. Physiologic doses of glucocorticoids lead to a prompt regression of aldosterone excess and marked improvement of hypertension.

GRA results from inheritance of a chimeric gene, which is caused by unequal mitotic crossover of the genes coding for 11-hydroxylase (*CYP11B1*), the final step in cortisol biosynthesis, and aldosterone synthase (*CYP11B2*), the final step in aldosterone synthesis.[10] The resulting chimeric gene produces a protein with aldosterone synthase activity under the regulatory control of the adrenocorticotrophic hormone (ACTH)-dependent *CYP11B1* promoter. This explains why glucocorticoids reverse the disease so rapidly. Whereas aldosterone synthase is normally produced exclusively in the zona glomerulosa, the chimeric gene is expressed in all three layers of the adrenal gland.[11] The expression of aldosterone synthase, with its 18-hydroxylase activity in the zona fasciculata, where cortisol is normally produced, accounts for the production of the 'hybrid steroids' 18-hydroxycortisol and 18-oxo-cortisol.[12]

Although the prevalence of GRA remains unknown and the degree of hypertension can be variable, diagnosis of this disorder remains clinically relevant. Diagnosis of GRA has traditionally been made by a positive dexamethasone suppression test. Suppression of aldosterone levels to < 4 ng/dL has been reported to have greater than 90% specificity and sensitivity for diagnosing GRA.[13] However, because false positives have been noted using these criteria,[14] the diagnosis is best confirmed via demonstration of elevated urinary hybrid steroid levels or by identification of the chimeric gene.

The mainstay of treatment for GRA is dexamethasone, although the optimal dose required and the extent to which aldosterone should be suppressed are unclear. Studies have shown that complete normalization of urinary steroid levels and abolition of ACTH-induced aldosterone production is not necessary to control hypertension effectively and, in fact, might result in Cushingoid side effects.[15] Thus, physiologic replacement doses of glucocorticoids appear to be adequate for control of hypertension. A starting dose of 0.125 mg dexamethasone (or 2.5–5 mg prednisolone) once per day in adults has been suggested.[15] Concerns about the adverse effects of high aldosterone levels on cardiac health[16,17] have resulted in the employment of selective mineralocorticoid receptor blockers, including spironolactone, as an adjunctive treatment.

Apparent mineralocorticoid excess

The first reports of what are now known to be cases of apparent mineralocorticoid excess (AME) were described in children in the late 1970s. The phenotype was invariable: severe, early-onset hypertension, hypokalemia, metabolic alkalosis and low renin and aldosterone levels. Additional features included failure to thrive and persistent polyuria/polydipsia. Although AME patients have all the features of mineralocorticoid excess, their levels of aldosterone are nearly undetectable and an exhaustive search for other, as yet unknown, mineralocorticoids proved unsuccessful. It was only when the metabolism of the body's own endogenous glucocorticoid, cortisol, was studied that the molecular basis for this condition was discovered.

Studies noted that AME patients have impaired metabolism of cortisol to cortisone with greatly elevated levels of serum cortisol and prolonged serum half-life of this hormone.[18,19] Furthermore, it was observed that administration of exogenous cortisol (hydrocortisone) or ACTH seemed to worsen the syndrome.[20] Two conclusions were drawn from these clinical observations: (1) 11β-HSD2, the enzyme responsible for conversion of cortisol to cortisone, was deficient or nonfunctional; and (2) cortisol was acting as a mineralocorticoid in these patients. The demonstration that cortisol is a potent mineralocorticoid agonist *in vitro* led to the question of why cortisol didn't function as such in all individuals.[21]

We now recognize that: (1) although cortisol levels are 100 times more abundant than aldosterone levels at steady state, cortisol is prevented from activating MR through the action of 11β-HSD2, which converts cortisol to the inactive cortisone; and (2) patients with AME are deficient in this enzyme.[22] Of note, a similar clinical presentation can be seen with excessive ingestion of black licorice, which contains glycyrrhetinic acid, a competitive inhibitor of 11β-HSD2.[23]

Diagnosis of this disorder is based on clinical presentation as well as measurement of urinary cortisol (compound F) to cortisone (compound E) ratios. A normal F/E ratio is approximately 1.0; AME patients demonstrate significantly elevated ratios. The disease remains exceedingly rare, with only about 40 cases reported worldwide since its recognition over 20 years ago.[24] Most of these patients demonstrate homozygosity for one of ten described mutations affecting enzymatic activity or structure. The disease is inherited in an autosomal recessive manner and most commonly occurs in areas of the world with high rates of consanguinity.[24]

Recent studies have revealed the existence of a milder form of AME. Termed AME type II, this form is characterized by a later age of presentation (> 30 years), a more variable degree of hypertension (sometimes asymptomatic), low renin and aldosterone levels and normal serum electrolytes. The urinary F/E ratio is largely normal.[25] These patients have homozygous alterations in 11β-HSD2 which produce a partial decrease in enzymatic activity and result in mild hypertension in affected individuals.[25,26] It has since been suggested that both types of AME are part of a continuum and that perhaps it is inappropriate to classify them individually.[25]

Treatment of AME is aimed at managing hypertension and hypokalemia. Thus, spironolactone is a mainstay of treatment; a low-salt diet is also important. There is a reported case of AME cured by renal transplantation.[27] Without treatment, patients sustain significant end-organ damage secondary to the hypertension and progress to renal and cardiac failure at an early age.

Pseudohypoaldosteronism type 2

Like most Mendelian disorders, pseudohypoaldosteronism type 2 (PHA 2), also known as familial hypertension with hyperkalemia, was first recognized many years ago[28,29] but current studies continue to elucidate the mechanism of this disorder. The phenotype of PHA 2 consists of hypertension and hyperkalemia despite a normal GFR, with varying degrees of hyperchloremia and metabolic acidosis. A relative hyperaldosteronism is present in response to high potassium levels. Inheritance is autosomal dominant with high penetrance. Clinically, this disorder is a mirror image of Gitelman's syndrome (discussed below) and therefore, as might be suspected, all abnormalities can be corrected with administration of thiazide diuretics. Although the phenotype is suggestive of some sort of defect in renal electrolyte handling, there had not been a readily apparent physiological mechanism to explain these findings until quite recently.

Linkage studies had previously localized genes causing PHA 2 to chromosomes 17q, 1q and 12p.[30–32] Wilson et al showed that each of the two PHA 2 kindreds linked to chromosome 12 had a large deletion in the first intron of *WNK1*, the gene encoding a recently described serine-threonine kinase. It was so named because it lacked a highly conserved lysine (WNK = with no lysine) in the catalytic domain of the protein.[33] This group subsequently identified three paralogs of *WNK1* and demonstrated that one of these, *WNK4*, localized to the same region of chromosome 17 previously implicated in PHA 2. They therefore screened the *WNK4* gene in PHA 2 patients and identified disease-causing mutations in a number of kindreds.[33]

Consistent with their role in producing hypertension and hyperkalemia, both WNK1 and WNK4 localized to the distal nephron, a key site regulating salt and water homeostasis.[33] Specifically, WNK1 is cytoplasmic whereas WNK4 is part of the tight junction complex. However, their role in these tissues was not known.

The association of WNK1 and WNK4 to human hypertension and hyperkalemia was the first clue to the function of these two novel kinases. WNK4 functions as a negative regulator of the thiazide-sensitive cotransporter (TSC) by preventing incorporation into the cell membrane and expression at the apical surface. Interestingly, this activity is lost in a WNK4 protein mutated in the catalytic domain, implicating this function as WNK4 kinase-dependent.[34,35] This activity is also lost in WNK4 protein carrying PHA 2 disease-causing mutations. Whereas loss of this TSC inhibition could explain the hypertensive phenotype in patients carrying WNK4 mutations, it could not explain the coexistent hyperkalemia. Subsequent studies, however, showed that WNK4 also functions as a negative regulator of potassium secretion by ROMK in kinase-independent fashion. In addition, WNK4 protein carrying PHA 2 disease-causing mutations maintains or even increases its ability to inhibit potassium secretion via ROMK, providing a mechanism by which these mutations can cause hypertension and hyperkalemia.[36] WNK4 also increases paracellular chloride transport in the collecting duct, resulting in an increase in salt and water reabsorption and a simultaneous decrease in the electrochemical gradient driving K^+ and H^+ secretion.

Although the role of WNK1 in mediating hypertension and hyperkalemia is not as well understood, it appears that WNK1 might function as a negative regulator of WNK4.[34] The increase in WNK1 expression induced by the intronic deletions in this gene[33] might therefore be expected to relieve WNK4-mediated suppression of TSC, leading to increased renal salt reabsorption and hypertension.[35]

Elucidation of the molecular basis of disease in PHA II has allowed studies of genotype–phenotype correlation in extended kindreds. Consistent with the known effects of TSC on calcium handling in the distal convoluted tubule, PHA 2 patients carrying WNK4 mutations have evidence of hypercalciuria leading to osteopenia, osteoporosis and stone disease. However, hypercalciuria was not observed in a French kindred carrying a WNK1 mutation. The reasons underlying this phenotypic difference are not clear. However, it is important to realize that the metabolic abnormalities precede the development of hypertension; the hyperkalemia can precede the hypertension by as many as 13 years.[37]

It is interesting to note that the molecular basis of PHA 2 might have significant implications for determining the etiology of 'essential hypertension' in the general population. The *WNK4* gene lies in close proximity to the site showing the strongest linkage to hypertension in the Framingham Heart Study.[33,38] Further delineation of the mechanisms of PHA 2 seems to hold great promise for continued advancement of our understanding of more general forms of hypertension.

Hypertension with brachydactyly

Hypertension with brachydactyly, sometimes called Bilginturan's syndrome for the investigator who initially described it, was first identified in a large Turkish kindred in the 1970s.[39] The phenotype consists of hypertension, brachydactyly, cone-shaped epiphyses, short stature with normal intelligence and an autosomal dominant inheritance pattern with complete penetrance. The hypertension typically worsens with age, with blood pressure reaching elevations greater than 50 mmHg above normal by age 50, resulting in premature stroke.[40] Aldosterone and renin levels are normal. No one particular drug class provides optimal therapy; a multidrug regimen is necessary to control the hypertension. Interestingly, an ophthalmologic exam of affected patients showed no evidence of hypertensive retinopathy despite long-standing, severe hypertension.[41]

Two other clinical correlations have emerged that are of unknown significance as of yet. Studies of fibroblast growth in the original kindred showed that it was accelerated compared to controls similar to the phenomenon seen in spontaneously hypertensive rats.[42] In addition, Bähring et al identified bilateral or unilateral looping in the posterior inferior cerebellar artery (PICA) by MR angiography in 15 affected members of the kindred and none of the unaffected members; this looping has also been observed in patients with essential hypertension.[43] The authors speculated that neurovascular compression resulting from the looping might have been a possible mechanism of the hypertension.

In 1996, Schuster et al performed linkage analysis on the original kindred and identified two polymorphisms on chromosome 12p that are specific for the phenotype.[42] A number of candidate genes have been suggested, several of which have since been disproven. Most recently, Gong et al have offered two more genes on chromosome 12p for consideration: *PDE3A*, a cyclic nucleotide phosphodiesterase and *SUR2*, a sulfonyl urea receptor subunit of an ATP-sensitive potassium channel.[44] At present, the molecular basis of this disorder remains unknown.

Familial hyperaldosteronism type II

Familial hyperaldosteronism type II (FH II) is the most recently described genetic hypertensive disorder, first recognized in five families in the early 1990s.[45] By definition, the disorder is present when two or more individuals in a kindred have evidence of primary aldosteronism of any subtype aside from GRA. Although this expansive definition could lead to overdiagnosis of the syndrome, there are a few kindreds in whom there does appear to be Mendelian transmission of the disorder, permitting genetic linkage analysis. The most recent work on this syndrome has re-examined the original pedigree and mapped FH II to a locus on chromosome 7p.[46] However, the underlying basis of this disease remains unknown.

HYPOTENSIVE DISORDERS (Table 3.2)

So far, we have focused on disorders featuring a rise in blood pressure. However, a moment's reflection makes it clear that disorders featuring low blood pressure are equally relevant to our understanding of molecular factors underlying blood pressure regulation.

Pseudohypoaldosteronism type 1

First described in 1958 by Cheek and Perry, pseudohypoaldosteronism type 1 (PHA1) is a rare disorder characterized by neonatal salt wasting, hyponatremia and hyperkalemic metabolic acidosis despite hyperreninemia and hyperaldosteronemia.[47] The clinical picture is thus one of renal aldosterone resistance. Children typically present in the first weeks of life with failure to thrive, volume depletion and vomiting. Two forms of the disease have been described, an autosomal dominant (adPHA1) form and an autosomal recessive form (arPHA1).[48] These will be discussed separately below.

Autosomal recessive PHA1

The autosomal recessive form of PHA1 (arPHA1) is caused by homozygous or compound heterozygous loss-of-function mutations in either the α, β, or γ subunit of the epithelial sodium channel (ENaC).[49,50] This form of the disease has been termed 'generalized PHA1', as salt is wasted from the kidney and colon, as well as from the sweat and salivary glands. Children with arPHA1 have massive renal salt wasting and hyperkalemia that can lead to neonatal death. Affected patients also show evidence of a novel asthma-like syndrome characterized by increased airway surface liquid, indicating a crucial role of pulmonary sodium transport in volume clearance.[51] Patients require lifelong sodium supplementation in addition to potassium-binding resins to maintain electrolyte homeostasis, but even with therapy, they remain at risk of life-threatening hyperkalemia.

Patients with arPHA1 typically have high sweat or salivary sodium chloride,[52] which helps to distinguish them from patients with dominant PHA1. As

Table 3.2 Mendelian disorders of hypotension

Syndrome	Gene	Renin	Aldo	K	Treatment
Recessive PHA1*	α, β, γ ENaC	High	High	High	Salt, potassium-binding resins
Dominant PHA1**	MR	Normal	High	Normal	Salt
Congenital hypoaldosteronism**	Cyp11B2 (AldoS)	High	Low	High	Mineralocorticoid
Gitelman's syndrome*	See Table 3.3	High/normal	High/normal	Low	NSAIDs, amiloride, spironolactone
Bartter's syndrome*	See Table 3.3	High/normal	High/normal	Low	NSAIDs, amiloride, spironolactone

* Autosomal recessive inheritance.
** Autosomal dominant inheritance.
NSAIDS, non-steroidal anti-inflammatory drugs.

will be discussed, patients with Bartter's syndrome type 2 can also present like PHA1, with hyperkalemia and metabolic acidosis; however, after volume repletion, these patients revert to the hypokalemia and alkalosis more typical of Bartter's syndrome.

Autosomal dominant pseudohypoaldosteronism type 1

Unlike the recessive form of the disease, autosomal dominant PHA1 (adPHA1), is generally considered to be mild.[48] At birth, patients might be asymptomatic or quite ill, with failure to thrive and vomiting. They respond well to sodium supplementation, which enables normal growth and development, and are generally able to discontinue salt therapy by the age of five. Studies of extended adPHA1 kindreds have demonstrated that there is no obvious adult phenotype of this disorder; affected adults have normal blood pressure and serum electrolytes when compared to unaffected relatives. The only sign of the disease is asymptomatic hyperaldosteronemia.[53]

AdPHA1 is caused by heterozygous loss-of-function mutations in MR.[54] Only 22 mutations in 24 kindreds have been described, including deletions and frameshift, missense and nonsense mutations. Haploinsufficiency – the loss of one of the two functional genes – is sufficient to cause the adPHA1 phenotype.[53,55] Although it has been proposed that mutations in other genes might cause adPHA1 due to the inability to detect exonic MR mutations in adPHA1 patients,[56,57] to date no conclusive evidence ruling out MR mutations in an adPHA1 kindred has been provided.[53] As such, we believe that mutations in MR represent the principal, if not the only, cause of the adPHA1 phenotype.

It is intriguing to note that up to 30% of adPHA1 patients carry *de novo* mutations in MR.[53] The high frequency of *de novo* mutations suggests impaired reproductive fitness in patients with adPHA1. Although we identified no inability of parents to transmit the disease gene to their children in extended adPHA1 kindreds, we did note a number of neonatal deaths in infants at risk for adPHA1.[53] Consequently, we believe that frequent neonatal mortality might account for the presumed impairment of reproductive fitness. Hence, we recommend prophylactic salt administration to infants at risk of adPHA1.

Congenital hypoaldosteronism

The final step in aldosterone synthesis is performed by the enzyme aldosterone synthase, encoded by the gene *CYP11B2*, which performs the necessary 11-hydroxylase, 18-hydroxylase and 18-oxidation steps. Children who lack this enzyme have isolated hypoaldosteronism. The clinical picture is similar to that seen in adPHA1, in that – as neonates – patients can have hyperkalemia and life-threatening salt wasting that responds well to salt (or 9α-fluorohydroxycortisone) administration. Two forms of the disease have been described – corticosterone methyl oxidase I (CMO I) deficiency and corticosterone methyl oxidase II deficiency (CMO II). Patients with CMO I deficiency have low serum levels of both aldosterone and 18-hydroxycorticosterone, whereas CMO II deficient patients have elevated 18-hydroxycorticosterone levels in the absence of aldosterone secretion. While CMO I and CMO II deficiency were previously thought to be due to distinct disease processes, it is now clear that both entities are caused by mutations in the same *CYP11B2* gene.[58]

Inherited hypokalemic alkalosis (Table 3.3)

In 1962, Bartter described a novel clinical syndrome characterized by hyperplasia of the juxtaglomerular complex, hyperaldosteronism and hypokalemic alkalosis in the absence of hypertension.[59] Subsequent reports of patients with similar syndromes, however, yielded a striking clinical divergence. Whereas hypokalemia and metabolic alkalosis were universally present, other clinical indices, such as age of presentation, divalent ion transport, and nephrocalcinosis, differed markedly among the cases. It has since been realized that there are at least six such disorders featuring inherited hypokalemic alkalosis, which are distinguished by their genetic defects. These will be reviewed below.

Gitelman's syndrome

Gitelman's syndrome is an autosomal recessive disorder characterized by metabolic alkalosis with renal salt wasting, hypocalciuria and hypomagnesemia. Patients with this syndrome typically present at older ages, often in early adulthood, without overt signs of hypovolemia.[60] Gitelman's syndrome is caused by homozygous or compound heterozygous mutations in the *SLC12A3* gene, which encodes NCCT, the thiazide-sensitive NaCl cotransporter of the distal convoluted tubule.[61] To date, scores of disease-causing mutations have been identified in this transporter, and Gitelman's syndrome is considered genetically homogeneous, meaning that this phenotype is caused exclusively by mutations in *SLC12A3*. It should be noted that Jeck et al identified three patients with a clinical picture similar to Gitelman's syndrome who had no mutations in *SLC12A3* but did have mutations in the *CLCNKB* gene, the cause of Bartter's syndrome type 3 (see below). Although their electrolytes were suggestive of Gitelman's syndrome, these patients presented atypically with dehydration, weakness and failure to thrive within the first year of life; only later did they develop the more typical hypomagnesemia and hypocalciuria.[62]

Table 3.3 Inherited hypokalemic alkalosis

Syndrome	Gene	Onset	Urine calcium	Nephrocalcinosis	Associated signs/symptoms
Gitelman's syndrome*	*SLC12A3* (NCCT)	Teens, early adult	Low	No	Weakness, tetany, salt craving
Bartter's type 1*	*SLC12A1* (NKCC2)	Prenatal, neonatal	High	Yes	FTT, polydipsia, polyuria
Bartter's type 2*	*KCNJ1* (ROMK2)	Prenatal, neonatal	High	Yes	Transient hyperkalemia, FTT
Bartter's type 3*	*CLCNKb*	Childhood	Normal	No	
Bartter's type 4*	*BSND* (Barttin)	Prenatal/ neonatal	Normal	No	Sensorineural hearing loss, FTT
Bartter's type 5**	*CASR*	Neonatal	High	Yes	Low serum calcium, high phosphate, low parathyroid hormone

* Autosomal recessive.
** Autosomal dominant.
FTT, failure to thrive.

Identification of the genetic defect causing Gitelman's syndrome has allowed genotype–phenotype correlation studies in expanded pedigrees. Whereas Gitelman's patients appear to be normotensive, their age- and gender-adjusted systolic and diastolic blood pressures are, on average, approximately 8 mmHg lower than heterozygous and wild-type relatives, consistent with the salt wasting phenotype of the disorder.[63] The principal manifestations of the disease – weakness, tetany, salt craving and chondrocalcinosis – are related to the electrolyte abnormalities. The characteristic hypomagnesemia and hypokalemia of Gitelman's syndrome might predispose patients to ventricular tachyarrhythmias and QTc prolongation.[64,65] Treatment is primarily directed at limiting these electrolyte abnormalities, via use of oral potassium and magnesium supplements and spironolactone (or amiloride) to inhibit distal nephron K^+ secretion.

Bartter's syndrome

Bartter's syndrome, like Gitelman's syndrome, is an autosomal recessive disorder characterized by salt wasting in the setting of hypokalemic metabolic alkalosis. In contrast to Gitelman's syndrome, however, Bartter's syndrome typically presents in the first year of life with failure to thrive and signs and symptoms of volume depletion. Levels of prostaglandin E are quite elevated, leading some to term this condition hyperprostaglandin E syndrome. Genetic studies in patients with Bartter's syndrome have revealed five distinct genetic causes, each of which is associated with a slightly different metabolic phenotype. Because the clinical course is principally determined by the genetic defect, we favor a nomenclature in which the Bartter's subtypes are identified by the underlying molecular defect.

Bartter's syndrome, type 1 and type 2 (hyperprostaglandin E syndrome, antenatal Bartter's syndrome) The clinical phenotype of Bartter's syndrome – hypokalemic metabolic alkalosis with renal salt wasting and hypercalciuria – is similar to the picture observed in patients taking the loop diuretic furosemide. Simon et al therefore studied *NKCC2*, the gene encoding the sodium-potassium-2 chloride cotransporter in the thick ascending limb of Henle, and furosemide's site of action. They identified disease-causing mutations in five patients,[66] a finding later confirmed by others.[67] These patients all had a typical presentation: polyhydramnios and prematurity, severe salt wasting and failure to thrive during the neonatal period, severe hypercalciuria and development of nephrocalcinosis.

The identification of mutations in *NKCC2* in affected infants did much to clarify the molecular basis of this disorder. For example, it was now clear that the excess prostaglandin E characteristic of the syndrome did not cause the disease but instead resulted from an underlying defect in tubular sodium transport. However, it soon became clear that most patients with Bartter's syndrome did not have mutations in *NKCC2*, leading to a search for other candidate genes.

As *NKCC2* function in the thick ascending limb is dependent on an apical potassium transporter that recycles potassium to the luminal space, Simon and colleagues investigated *KCNJ1*, a gene encoding the renal apical potassium channel ROMK, in patients with Bartter's syndrome. They identified disease-causing mutations in four Bartter's kindreds,[68] a finding again replicated by others.[69] These findings established ROMK as the apical potassium channel implicated in NKCC2 function and implicated mutations in ROMK as a cause of Bartter's syndrome type 2.

For the most part, patients with NKCC2 and ROMK mutations have similar phenotypes as described above. However, one significant clinical distinction can be made between these two groups of patients. Whereas NKCC2 is expressed solely in the thick ascending loop of Henle, ROMK is also found in the distal nephron, where it functions as an aldosterone-sensitive potassium secretory channel. For this reason, patients with ROMK mutations often present initially with salt wasting and hyperkalemia, a picture much more typical of PHA1. After volume resuscitation, these patients revert to the hypokalemia more typical of Bartter's syndrome but their hypokalemia remains less pronounced than in patients with other forms of Bartter's syndrome.[60]

Bartter's syndrome type 3 ('classic Bartter's syndrome') Simon and colleagues identified *NKCC2* or *ROMK* mutations in only 22 of 66 kindreds with Bartter's syndrome, and used linkage studies to definitively exclude these loci in other kindreds, ensuring further genetic heterogeneity in this disorder. As sodium chloride reabsorption in the thick ascending limb requires transport of these ions across both an apical and basolateral membrane, Simon and colleagues speculated that loss of basolateral chloride channel activity could lead to a Bartter's-like phenotype. They therefore investigated *CLCNKA* and *CLCNKB*, which encode the human homologues of the ClC-K1 and ClC-K2 chloride channels identified in the rat loop of Henle. Mutations were identified in *CLCNKB* in 17 patients, confirming mutations in this channel as the cause of a third distinct subtype of Bartter's syndrome.[70] In comparison to patients with Bartter's syndromes type 1 and 2, where polyhydramnios and premature delivery are the rule, these patients most commonly present with failure to thrive and salt wasting in the first 2 years of life.[60,70] As with types 1 and 2, hypokalemia and alkalosis are characteristic findings, but type 3 can often be clinically distinguished by the absence of hypercalciuria and by preserved urinary concentrating ability. Most notable, however, is the infrequency of nephrocalcinosis, an almost universal finding in types 1 and 2, which is rare in type 3.[60,70] The absence of hypercalciuria likely reflects the expression of CLCNKB in the distal convoluted tubule, an area central to the regulation of renal calcium excretion.

Bartter's syndrome type 4: Bartter's syndrome with sensorineural deafness In 1995, Landau and colleagues described a new form of Bartter's syndrome in which patients have sensorineural deafness in addition to the classic electrolyte features of salt wasting, hypokalemia, hypercalciuria and metabolic alkalosis.[71] Via linkage analysis and positional cloning techniques, Birkenhager et al identified a gene, *BSND*, encoding a novel protein they named barttin, mutations in which were responsible for this phenotype.[72] They found that barttin is expressed exclusively in the kidney and inner ear, consistent with the observed phenotype in these patients. Physiologic analysis confirmed that barttin acts as an essential beta-subunit for CLCNKA and CLCNKB, with which it colocalizes in the basolateral membrane in the renal tubules and in potassium secreting epithelia of the inner ear.[73]

Study of Bartter's syndrome type 4 patients revealed a number of clinical distinctions compared to the other forms of the syndrome. Patients invariably present *in utero* with polyhydramnios as early as 20 weeks, leading to preterm delivery. Like Bartter's type 1 and 2, they have severe salt wasting and a urinary concentrating defect, but they lack hypercalciuria and nephrocalcinosis.

Patients have poor growth and development, which is only partially alleviated via high-calorie diets or parenteral nutrition.[74] Chronic renal failure might be seen[75] but is not a universal finding.[74] Patients have a difficult perinatal course, spending up to a third of their first 2 years in the hospital, most commonly because of fever and vomiting episodes that lead to severe volume depletion and electrolyte imbalances. In addition to the sensorineural deafness, patients have delayed motor development and hypotonia. Finally, it has been proposed that these patients might have a poorer response to indomethacin than is generally observed in other forms of Bartter's syndrome,[75] although this has been disputed.[74]

Bartter's syndrome type 5 The calcium-sensing receptor (CaSR) is a plasma membrane G-protein coupled receptor that is expressed in the parathyroid gland as well as in cells lining the renal tubule. It functions to maintain calcium homeostasis via alterations in parathyroid hormone (PTH) secretion and renal calcium handling. Heterozygous loss-of-function mutations in this gene lead to familial hypocalciuric hypercalcemia. Homozygous mutations cause severe neonatal hyperparathyroidism, characterized by increased PTH secretion due to a loss of normal calcium sensing mechanisms. In contrast, mild activating mutations in the CaSR cause familial hypercalciuric hypocalcemia, with decreased PTH secretion induced by the oversensitive receptor.

Watanabe et al described two patients with striking autosomal dominant hypocalcemia, deficient PTH secretion and other electrolyte abnormalities characteristic of Bartter's syndrome.[76] They screened *CaSR* and identified missense mutations that cosegregated with disease in each patient. *In vitro* studies confirmed that these were strong gain-of-function mutations. Studies in the rat had previously suggested that activation of the CaSR by calcium could inhibit ROMK activity, suggesting that these gain-of-function mutations in CaSR might cause a Bartter's-like phenotype via inhibition of ROMK activity.

As in other forms of Bartter's syndrome, patients with Bartter's syndrome type 5 have an inherited hypokalemic alkalosis. However, unlike the other forms, type 5 is transmitted in an autosomal dominant fashion. The most prominent clinical finding is tetany. Serum calcium levels are low, with a high serum phosphate and an inappropriately low serum PTH level; nephrocalcinosis is common.

Congenital adrenal hyperplasia (Table 3.4)

Although not commonly thought of as Mendelian disorders affecting blood pressure, the congenital adrenal hyperplasias (CAH) are a family of autosomal recessive disorders characterized by impaired biosynthesis of cortisol from cholesterol in the adrenal glands, which produce characteristic effects on blood pressure in affected individuals. Due to the loss of negative feedback, levels of ACTH rise, inducing steroidogenesis in the adrenal gland, with resultant shunting of steroid synthesis into pathways not affected by the enzymatic block. Although patients with CAH are usually characterized by virilization and adrenal insufficiency, each particular phenotype is dependent on the enzymatic step in the pathway that is impaired.

Approximately 90–95% of cases of CAH are due to deficiency of the enzyme 21-hydroxylase (21-OH), which is necessary in both the aldosterone and cortisol biosynthetic pathways. Hence, the immediate precursors in the pathway –

Table 3.4 Congenital adrenal hyperplasia

Enzyme deficiency	Gene	Phenotype	Treatment
11-β hydroxylase	CYP11B1	HTN, salt retention	GC
17-α hydroxylase	CYP17A1	HTN, salt retention	GC
21-α hydroxylase	CYP21	Virilization, salt wasting, hyperkalemia	MC ± GC
3-β OH ketoisomerase	HSD3B	Hypospadias, mild virilization, salt loss	MC ± GC, estrogen
Steroid acute regulatory protein	STAR	All female, severe salt wasting, often lethal	MC + GC
Cholesterol 20-22 desmolase	CYP11A1	All female, severe salt wasting, often lethal	MC + GC

GC, glucocorticoids; MC, mineralocorticoids.

progesterone and 17-hydroxyprogesterone – accumulate and are shunted into the androgen pathway with resultant overproduction of dehydroepiandrosterone, androstenedione and testosterone. Whereas the virilizing effects of these steroids result in the classic signs of ambiguous genitalia in females and precocious puberty in males, the block in aldosterone synthesis results in salt wasting as well. Diagnosis of all forms of 21-OH deficiency is by measurement of 17-hydroxyprogesterone before and after ACTH stimulation. Although much less common, CAH with salt wasting can also be caused by the congenital deficiency of cholesterol 20-22 desmolase, steroid acute regulatory protein, or 3β-hydroxy ketoisomerase,[77–79] enzymes also required for glucocorticoid and mineralocorticoid synthesis.

CAH is relatively common, with an incidence of ~1 : 15 000 live births in the general population, although it is more common in certain homogeneous populations.[80] It is thought to be the most common human autosomal recessive disorder, with a frequency of greater than 1 : 100 in some ethnic groups.[80] The gene for 21-OH, *CYP21*, is located on chromosome 6p within class III HLA. To date, more than 90 allelic variants have been identified, although there are eight specific mutations reported with highest frequency.[81]

In contrast to the salt-wasting subtypes of CAH, deficiencies of either 11α-hydroxylase (*CYP11B1*) or 17α-hydroxylase (*CYP17A1*) lead to hypertension. These account for the remaining 5–8% of cases of CAH. The lack of either enzyme results in increased biochemical shunting to the aldosterone synthesis pathway in the zona glomerulosa. In the case of 11-hydroxylase deficiency, the pathway terminates early at 11-deoxycortisocsterone (DOC), a potent salt retainer, leading to hypertension. Similarly, in the case of 17-hydroxylase deficiency, the excess production of corticosterone and deoxycorticosterone in the zona fasciculata leads to salt retention and hypertension. As with all other forms of CAH, these disorders are treated effectively with physiologic doses of glucocorticoids to suppress the expression of the steroid byproducts.

PERSPECTIVES

The understanding of the monogenic disorders with a primary effect on blood pressure has greatly improved our understanding of the molecular basis of blood pressure regulation, but it is clear that substantial challenges remain. Initially, there was speculation that the well-described, inherited predisposition to essential hypertension might be explained by polymorphisms within the genes described here. A wide variety of studies have evaluated such polymorphisms but most have generally led to disappointment in this regard. However, there are a number of areas in which our understanding of cardiovascular disease has been impacted as a result of the genetic dissection of these disorders.

A variety of mechanisms have been proposed to underlie hypertension – including potassium and calcium balance, and neural, vascular, and endocrine mechanisms – and it is remarkable that all of these disorders affect blood pressure via a single pathway. Disorders that result in increased renal sodium reabsorption increase blood pressure, whereas those that result in decreased renal sodium reabsorption lower blood pressure. These findings coincide with a long line of physiologic research that has implicated renal sodium handling in the maintenance of hypertension, and lend support to the notion that more common forms of hypertension also have an alteration in renal sodium handling at their root.[82,83] Thus, it is not surprising that chlorthalidone, a thiazide diuretic, produces unchanged or even improved clinical outcomes when compared to amlodipine, a calcium channel blocker, and lisinopril, an angiotensin-converting enzyme (ACE) inhibitor, in the Antihypertensive and Lipid-Lowering Treatment to Prevent Heart Attack Trial (ALLHAT).[84] Whereas antihypertensive agents typically function poorly in dialysis patients, it has been shown that long, slow dialysis regimens enabling more effective sodium removal allow for the normalization of blood pressure without medication in this difficult population.[85]

A second finding of clinical relevance gleaned from the study of these disorders is the fact that hypokalemia is not an obligate finding in primary aldosteronism. Screening for aldosteronism had traditionally been restricted to a select group of patients until the demonstration that hypokalemia is not a universal finding in diseases known to be caused by excess aldosterone effect. Through the development and implementation of new screening protocols utilizing the aldosterone–renin ratio, it is now clear that primary aldosteronism is much more common than was previously believed. Some investigators have reported that primary aldosteronism might be present in at least 10% of all essential hypertensives when screened by this newer, more sensitive technique.[84,86,87] Whether this high prevalence is found among all essential hypertensives is not known, but it is clear that primary aldosteronism should be ruled out in any patient with resistant hypertension regardless of the serum potassium level.

A third area of insight derived from our understanding of Mendelian blood pressure regulation disorders is the role of the renin–angiotensin–aldosterone system in mediating cardiovascular disease. In recent years, there has been much interest regarding the role of factors such as renin, angiotensin II and aldosterone in promoting cardiovascular disease and in mediating cardiac and perivascular fibrosis. A review of the disorders described here suggests that the principal pathogenic effect of these hormones might, in fact, be the augmentation of renal sodium reabsorption. The absence of renin, angiotensin II or aldosterone secretion in Liddle syndrome does not seem to prevent stroke, heart failure or kidney failure in affected patients.[88] Conversely, the extraordinarily high circulating levels of renin, angiotensin II and aldosterone in arPHA1 patients do not seem to induce congestive heart failure, stroke or kidney disease, entities that have never been described in these patients. These observations suggest that the pathologic effects of angiotensin II and aldosterone are load dependent, and that the cardiovascular benefits of their blockade might be due, in large part, to inhibition of renal sodium reabsorption. Although there has also been interest in the so-called nongenomic effects of aldosterone, effects mediated via a membrane receptor distinct from MR, the example of adPHA1 patients with normal blood pressure and no known incidence of significant cardiovascular disease despite lifelong elevation of serum aldosterone levels[53] suggests that there are no significant pathologic effects of aldosterone stemming from this pathway.[53]

Although we have made great strides in furthering our understanding of the mechanisms of hypertension through molecular dissection of monogenic forms of blood pressure dysregulation, more work remains to be done, as the etiology of hypertension remains unknown in the vast majority of patients. Improved understanding of the origins of essential hypertension will likely have a profound impact on the prevention and treatment of this common disorder, and the lessons provided from the study of these monogenic disorders provide a major step forward in this pursuit.

References

1. Shimkets RA, Warnock DG, Bositis CM, et al. Liddle's syndrome: heritable human hypertension caused by mutations in the beta subunit of epithelial sodium channel. *Cell* 1994; 79:407–414.
2. Hansson JH, Nelson Williams C, Suzuki H. Hypertension caused by a truncated epithelial sodium chanel gamma subunit: genetic heterogeneity of Liddle syndrome. *Nat Genet* 1995; 11:76–82.
3. Botero-Velez M, Curtis JJ, Warnock DG. Liddle's syndrome revisited – a disorder of sodium reabsorption in the distal tubule. *N Engl J Med* 1994; 330:178–181.
4. Abriel H, Loffing J, Reghun JF, et al. Defective regulation of the epithelial Na$^+$ channel by Nedd 4 in Liddle's syndrome. *J Clin Invest* 1999; 103:667–673.
5. Snyder PM, Price MP, McDonald FJ, et al. Mechanism by which Liddle's syndrome mutations increase activity of a human epithelial Na$^+$ channel. *Cell* 1995; 83:969–978.
6. Freundlich M, Ludwig M. A novel epithelial sodium channel beta-subunit mutation associated with hypertensive Liddle syndrome. *Pediatr Nephrol* 2005; 20:512–515.
7. Geller DS, Farhi A, Pinkerton N, et al. Activating mineralocorticoid receptor mutation in hypertension exacerbated by pregnancy. *Science* 2000; 289:119–123.
8. Rafestin-Oblin M-E, Souque A, Bocchi B, et al. The severe form of hypertension caused by the activating S810L mutation in the mineralocorticoid receptor is cortisone related. *Endocrinology* 2003; 144:528–533.
9. Schmider-Ross A, Wirsing M, Buscher V, et al. Analysis of the S810L point mutation of the mineralocorticoid receptor in patients with pregnancy induced hypertension. *Hypertens Pregnancy* 2004; 23:113–119.
10. Lifton RP, Dluhy RG, Powers M, et al. A chimeric 11 & MAC223;-hydroxylase/aldosterone synthase gene causes glucocorticoid-remediable aldosteronism and human hypertension. *Nature* 1992; 355:262–265.
11. Pascoe L, Jeunemaitre X, Lebrethon MC, et al. Glucocorticoid-suppressible hyperaldosteronism and adrenal tumors occurring in a single French pedigree. *J Clin Invest* 1995; 96:2236–2246.
12. Ulick S, Chan CK, Gill JR. Defective fasciculata zone function as the mechanism of glucocorticoid-remediable aldosteronism. *J Clin Endocrinol Metab* 1990; 71: 1151–1157.
13. Litchfield WR, New MI, Coolidge C, et al. Evaluation of the dexamethasone suppression test for the diagnosis of glucocorticoid-remediable aldosteronism. *J Clin Endocrinol Metab* 1997; 82:3570–3573.
14. Fardella CE, Pinot M, Mosso L, et al. Genetic study of patients with dexamethasone suppressible aldosteronism without the chimeric CYP11B1/CYP11B2 gene. *J Clin Endocrinol Metab* 2001; 86:4805–4807.
15. Stowasser M, Bachmann AW, Huggard PR, et al. Treatment of familial hyperaldosteronism Type 1: only partial suppression of adrenocorticotropin required to correct hypertension. *J Clin Endocrinol Metab* 2000; 85:3313–3318.

16. Pitt B, Zannad F, Remme WJ, et al. The effect of spironolactone on morbididty and mortality in patients with severe heart failure. *N Engl J Med* 1999; 341:709–717.
17. Brilla CG, Weber KT. Mineralocorticoid excess dietary sodium and myocardial fibrosis. *J Lab Clin Med* 1992; 120 893–901.
18. Ulick S, Levine LS, Gunczler P, et al. A syndrome of apparent mineralocorticoid excess associated with defects in the peripheral metabolism of cortisol. *J Clin Endocrinol Metab* 1979; 49:757–764.
19. Shackleton CH, Honour JW, Dillon MJ, et al. Hypertension in a four year old child: gas chromatographic and mass spectrometric evidence for deficient hepatic metabolism of steroids. *J Clin Endocrinol Metab* 1980; 50:786–772.
20. Oberfield SE, Levine LS, Carey RM, et al. Metabolic and blood pressure responses to hydrocortisone in the syndrome of apparent mineralocorticoid excess. *J Clin Endocrinol Metab* 1983; 56:332–339.
21. J'Arriza JL, Weinberger C, Cerelli G, et al. Cloning of human mineralocorticoid receptor complementary DNA: structural and functional kinship with the glucocorticoid receptor. *Science* 1987; 237:268–275.
22. Mune T, Rogerson FM, Nikkila H, et al. Human hypertension caused by mutations in the kidney isosyme of 11-beta-hydroxysteroid dehydrogenase. *Nat Genet* 1995; 10:394–399.
23. Stewart PM, Wallace AM, Valentino R, et al. Mineralocorticoid activity of liquorice: 11-beta-hydroxysteroid dehydrogenase deficiency comes of age. *Lancet* 1987; 2:821–824.
24. New MI, Wilson RC. Steroid disorders in children: congenital adrenal hyperplasia and apparent mineralocorticoid excess. *Proc Natl Acad Sci U S A* 1999; 96:12790–12797.
25. Li A, Tedde R, Krozowski ZS, et al. Molecular basis for hypertension in the 'type II' variant of apparent mineralocorticoid excess. *Am J Hum Genet* 1998; 63:370–379.
26. Wilson RC, Dave-Sharma S, Wei J, et al. A genetic defect resulting in mild low-renin hypertension. *Proc Natl Acad Sci U S A* 1998; 95:10200–10205.
27. Palermo M, Cossu M, Shackleton CHL. Cure of apparent mineralocorticoid excess by kidney transplantation. *N Engl J Med* 1998; 339:1787–1788.
28. Paver WK, Pauline GJ. Hypertension and hyperpotassaemia without renal disease in a young male. *Med J Aust* 1964; 35:305–306.
29. Gordon RD. The syndrome of hypertension and hyperkalaemia with normal glomerular filtration rate: Gordon's syndrome. *Aust N Z J Med* 1986; 16:183–184.
30. Mansfield TA, Simon DB, Farfel Z, et al. Multilocus linkage of familial hyperkalaemia and hypertension, pseudohypoaldosteronism type II, to chromosomes 1q31-42 and 17p11-q21. *Nat Genet* 1997; 16:202–205.
31. Disse-Nicodeme S, Archard J.-M, Desitter I, et al. A new locus on chromosome 12p13.3 for pseudohypoaldosteronism type II, an autosomal dominant form of hypertension. *Am J Hum Genet* 2000; 67:302–310.
32. Xu B, English JM, Wilsbacher JL, et al. WNK1 a novel mammalian serine/threonine protein kinase lacking the catalytic lysine in subdomain II. *J Biol Chem* 2000; 275:16795–16801.
33. Wilson FH, Disse-Nicodeme S, Choate KA, et al. Human hypertension caused by mutations in WNK kinases. *Science* 2001; 293:1107–1112.
34. Yang CL, Angell J, Mitchell R, Ellison DH. WNK kinases regulate thiazide-sensitive Na–Cl cotransport. *J Clin Invest* 2003; 111:1039–1045.
35. Wilson FH, Kahle KT, Sabath E, et al. Molecular pathogenesis of inherited hypertension with hyperkalaemia: the Na–Cl cotransporter is inhibited by wild-type but not mutant WNK 4. *Proc Natl Acad Sci U S A* 2003; 100:680–684.
36. Kahle KT, Wilson FH, Lalioti M, et al. Regulation of diverse ion transport pathways by WNK 4 kinase: a novel molecular switch. *Trends Endocrinol Metab* 2005; 16:98–103.
37. Mayan H. Pseudohypoaldosteronism type II: marked sensitivity to thiazides, hypercalciuria, normomagnesemia, and low bone mineral density. *J Clin Endocrinol Metab* 2002; 87:3248–3254.
38. Levy D, De Stefano AL, Larson MG, et al. Evidence for a gene influencing blood pressure on chromosome 17: genome scan linkage results for longitudinal blood pressure phenotypes in subjects from the Framingham Heart Study. *Hypertension* 2000; 36:477–483.
39. Bilginturan N, Zileli S, Karacadag S, Pirnar T. Hereditary brachydactyly associated with hypertension. *J Med Genet* 1973; 10:253–259.
40. Chitayat D, Grix A, Balfe JW, et al. Brachydactyly – short stature-hypertension (Bilginturan) syndrome: report on two families. *Am J Med Genet* 1997; 73:279–285.
41. Hattenbach L-O, Toka HR, Toka O, et al. Absence of hypertensive retinopathy in a Turkish kindred with autosomal dominant hypertension and brachydactyly. *Br J Ophthalmol* 1998; 82:1363–1365.
42. Schuster H, Wienker TF, Bähring S, et al. Severe autosomal dominant hypertension and brachydactyly in a unique Turkish kindred maps to human chromosome 12. *Nat Genet* 1996; 13:98–100.

43. Schuster H, Wienker TF, Toka HR, et al. Autosomal dominant hypertension and brachy-dactyly in a Turkish kindred resembles essential hypertension. *Hypertension* 1996; 28:1085–1092.
44. Gong M, Zhang H, Schulz H, et al. Genome-wide linkage reveals a locus for human essential (primary) hypertension on chromosome 12p. *Hum Mol Genet* 2003; 12:1273–1277.
45. Stowasser M, Gordon RD, Tunny TJ, et al. Familial hyperaldosteronism type II: five families with a new variety of primary aldosteronism. *Clin Exp Pharmacol Physiol* 1992; 19:319–322.
46. Lafferty AR, Torpy DJ, Stowasser M, et al. A novel genetic locus for low renin hypertension:familial hyperaldosteronism type II maps to chromosome 7 (7p22). *J Med Genet* 2000; 37:831–835.
47. Cheek DB, Perry JW. A salt-wasting syndrome in infancy. *Arch Dis Child* 1958; 33:252–256.
48. Hanukoglu A. Type I pseudohypoaldostreronism includes two clinically and genetically distinct entities with either renal or multiple target organ defects. *J Clin Endocrinol Metab* 1991; 73:936–944.
49. Chang SS, Grunder S, Hanukoglu A. Mutations in subunits of the epithelial sodium channel cause salt wasting with hyperkalemic acidosis. *Nat Genet* 1996; 12:248.
50. Strautnieks SS, Thompson RJ, Gardiner RM, Chung E. A novel splice-site mutation in the gamma subunit of the epithelial sodium channel gene in the pseudohypoaldosteronism type I families. *Nat Genet* 1996; 13:248–250.
51. Kerem E, Bistritzer T, Hanukoglu A. Pulmonary epithelial sodium-channel dysfunction and excess airway liquid in pseudohypaldosteronism. *N Engl J Med* 1999; 341:156–162.
52. Hanukoglu A, Bistritzer T, Rakover Y, Mandelberg A. Pseudohypoaldosteronism with increased sweat and saliva electrolyte values and frequent low respiratory tract infections mimicking cystic fibrosis. *J Pediatr* 1994; 125:752–757.
53. Geller DS, Rodriguez-Soriano J, Boado AV, et al. Autosomal dominant pseudohypoaldosteronism type I: mechanisms, evidence for neonatal lethality and phenotypic expression in adults. *J Am Soc Nephrol* 2006; 17:1429–1436.
54. Geller DS, Rodriguez-Soriano J, Boado AV, et al. Mutations in the mineralocorticoid receptor gene cause autosomal dominant pseudohypoaldosteronism type I. *Nat Genet* 1998; 19:279–281.
55. Sartorato P, Lapeyraque A-L, Armanini D, et al. Different inactivating mutations of the mineralocorticoid receptor in fourteen families affected by type I pseudohypoaldosteronism. *J Clin Endocrinol Metab* 2003; 88:2508–2517.
56. Viemann M, Peter M, Lopez-Siguero JP, et al. Evidence for genetic heterogeneity of pseudohypoaldosteronism type I: identification of a novel mutation in the human mineralocorticoid receptor in one sporadic case and no mutations in two autosomal dominant kindreds. *J Clin Endocrinol Metab* 2001; 86; 2056–2059.
57. Huey CL, Riepe FG, Sippell WG, Yu ASL. Genetic heterogeneity in autosomal dominant pseudohypoaldosteronism Type I: exclusion of Claudin-8 as a candidate gene. *Am J Nephrol* 2004; 24:483–487.
58. Mitsuuchi Y, Kawamoto T, Naiki Y, et al. Congenitally defective aldosterone biosynthesis in humans: the involvement of point mutations of the P-450C18 gene (CYP11B2) in CMOII deficient patients. *Biochem Biophys Res Commun* 1992; 182:974–979.
59. Bartter FC, Pronove P, Gill JR Jr, Maccardle RC. Hyperplasia of the juxtaglomerular complex with aldosteronims and hypokalemic aldosteronism and hypokalemic alkalosis: a new syndrome. *Am J Med* 1962; 33:811–828.
60. Peters M, Jeck N, Reinalter S, et al. Clinical presentation of genetically defined patients with hypokalemic salt-losing tubulopathies. *Am J Med* 2002; 112:183–190.
61. Simon DB, Nelson-Williams C, Bia MJ, et al. Gitelman's variant of Bartter's syndrome, inherited hypokalemic alkalosis is caused by mutations in the thiazide-sensitive Na–Cl cotransporter. *Nat Genet* 1996; 12:24–30.
62. Jeck N, Konrad M, Peters M, et al. Mutations in the chloride channel gene CLCNKB, leading to a mixed Bartter–Gitelman phenotype. *Pediatr Res* 2000; 48:754–758.
63. Cruz DN, Simon DB, Nelson-Williams C, et al. Mutations in the Na–Cl cotransporter reduce blood pressure in humans. *Hypertension* 2001; 37:1458–1464.
64. Pachulski RT, Lopez F, Sharaf R. Gitelman's not-so-benign syndrome. *N Engl J Med* 2005; 353:850–851.
65. Nakane E, Kono T, Sasaki I, et al. Gitelman's syndrome with exercise-induced ventricular tachycardia. *Circ J* 2004; 68:509–511.
66. Simon DB, Karet FE, Hamdan JM, et al. Bartter's syndrome, hypokalemic alkalosis with hypercalciuria, is caused by mutations in the Na–K–2Cl cotransporter NKCC2. *Nat Genet* 1996; 13:183–188.
67. Vargas-Poussou R, Feldmann D, Vollmer M. Novel molecular variants of the Na-K-2Cl cotransporter gene are responsible for antenatal Bartter syndrome. *Am J Hum Genet* 1998; 62:1332-1340.

3

MONOGENIC DISORDERS OF BLOOD PRESSURE REGULATION

68. Simon DB, Karet FE, Rodriguez-Soriano J, et al. Genetic heterogeneity of Bartter's syndrome revealed by mutations in the K+ channel, ROMK. *Nat Genet* 1996; 14:152–156.
69. International Collaborative Study Group for Bartter-like syndromes. Mutations in the gene encoding the inwardly-rectifying renal potassiuim channel, ROMK, cause the antenatal variant of Bartter syndrome: evidence for genetic heterogeneity. *Hum Mol Genet* 1997; 6:17–26.
70. Simon DB, Bindra RS, Mansfiled TA. Mutations in the chloride channel gene, CLCNKB, cause Bartter's syndrome type III. *Nat Genet* 1997; 17:171–178.
71. Landau D, Shalev H, Ohaly M, Carmi R. Infantile variant of Bartter syndrome and sensorineural deafness:a new autosomal recessive disorder. *Am J Med Genet* 1995; 59:454–459.
72. Birkenhager R, Otto E, Schurmann MJ, et al. Mutation of BSND causes Bartter syndrome with sensorineural deafness and kidney failure. *Nat Genet* 2001; 29:310–314.
73. Estevez R, Boettger T, Stein V, et al. Barttin is a Cl⁻ channel beta-subunit crucial for renal Cl⁻ reabsorption and inner ear K+ secretion. *Nature* 2001; 414:558–561.
74. Shalev H, Ohali M, Kachko L, Landau D. The neonatal variant of Bartter syndrome and deafness; preservation of renal function. *Pediatrics* 2003; 112:628–633.
75. Jeck N, Reinalter SC, Henne T, et al. Hypokalaemic salt-losing tubulopathy with chronic renal failure and sensorineural deafness. *Pediatrics* 2001; E5:108.
76. Watanabe S, Fukumoto S, Chang H, et al. Association between activating mutations of calcium–sensing receptor and Bartter's syndrome. *Lancet* 2002; 360:692–694.
77. Bose HS, Sugawara T, Strauss JF 3rd, Miller WL. The pathophysiology and genetics of congenital lipoid adrenal hyperplasia. International Congenital Lipoid Adrenal Hyperplasia Consortium. *N Engl J Med* 1996; 335:1870–1878.
78. Bongiovanni AM. The adrenogenital syndrome with deficiency of 3β-hydroxysteroid dehydrogenase. *J Clin Invest* 1962; 41:2086–2089.
79. Rheaume E, Simard J, Morel Y, et al. Congenital hyperplasia due to point mutations in the type II 3 beta-hydroxysteroid dehydrogenase. *Nat Genet* 1992; 1:239–245.
80. Speiser PW, Dupont B, Rubinstein P, et al. High frequency of nonclassical steroid 21-hydroxylase deficiency. *Am J Hum Genet* 1985; 37:650–667.
81. Friaes A, Rego AT, Aragues JM, et al. CYP21A2 mutations in Portuguese patients with congenital adrenal hyperplasia: identification of two novel mutations and characterisation of four different partial gene conversions. *Mol Genet Metab* 2006; 16 E-publishing.
82. Guyton AC. Blood pressure control: special role of the kidneys and body fluids. *Science* 1991; 252:1813–1816.
83. Lifton RP, Gharavi A, Geller DS. Molecular mechanisms of human hypertension. *Cell* 2001; 104:545–556.
84. The ALLHAT Officers and Coordinators for the ALLHAT Collaborative Research Group. Major outcomes in high-risk hypertensive patients randomized to angiotensin–converting enzyme inhibitor or calcium channel blocker vs diuretic. *JAMA* 2002; 288:2981–2997.
85. McCormick BB, Pierrato A, Fenton S, et al. Review of clinical outcomes in nocturnal haemodialysis patients after renal transplantation. *Nephrol Dial Transplant* 2004; 19:714–719.
86. Stowasser M, Gordon RD, Gunase Kera TG, et al. High rate of detection of primary aldosteronism including surgically treatable forms, after 'non-selective' screening of hypertensive patients. *J Hypertens* 2003; 21:2149–2157.
87. Young WF Jr. Primary aldosteronism: a common and curable from of hypertension. *Cardiol Rev* 1999; 7:207–214.
88. Warnock DG, Bubien JK. Liddle syndrome: clinical and cellular abnormalities. *Hosp Pract (Office edn)* 1994; 29:95–98.

4 | Genome scans in hypertension

Chris Wallace, MZ. Xue, Mark Caulfield and Patricia B. Munroe

INTRODUCTION

High blood pressure (BP), or hypertension, is an important risk factor for heart attacks, stroke and kidney failure. It is a major concern for public health, estimated to cause 4.5% of the current global disease burden. It is prevalent not only in developed countries but also in many developing countries.[1] The cause of hypertension remains unclear, although many drugs that act to decrease blood pressure have been developed.[2]

Hypertension is a complex disorder and, as with other multifactorial diseases, many risk factors that influence its pathogenesis – including environmental and genetic factors – have been identified. The former include controllable risk factors such as stress, salt consumption, diet, alcohol consumption, weight and exercise. Other (uncontrollable) risk factors include age, a family history of hypertension and ethnic background. It has been shown there is a family predisposition to high levels of systolic and diastolic blood pressure (SBP and DBP, respectively), which strongly suggests that genes are involved in human susceptibility to hypertension.[3]

Blood pressure depends on the interplay between multiple genes in the human genome and multiple environmental factors. These genes have not yet been identified, but the evidence suggests that they are distributed over many chromosomes. Identification will improve understanding of the pathogenesis of hypertension and help determine treatment pathways.

In this chapter, we review studies which have searched the whole human genome for the genes influencing essential hypertension (EH). We begin by discussing the BP phenotypes (traits) used in these studies and contrast the gene-by-gene and whole genome search approaches before addressing the studies themselves. Our emphasis is on explaining the methods used as well as the results found, so we begin with an introduction to the methodological issues and organize the review according to the methods employed and populations studied. We then compare the results across studies and explore some of the design issues that might explain the lack of consistent findings. Finally, we summarize our thoughts on the future directions opening to researchers in this field, with the continued improvement in both molecular genetic technology and our knowledge of the human genome.

HETEROGENEITY OF HYPERTENSION AND STUDY DESIGN

It is estimated that the genes involved in essential hypertension are heterogeneous (differ) between affected individuals and that multiple genes contribute to hypertension in a single patient. Heterogeneity is increased between studies because of sample differences in ethnicity and body weight; this can make genetic analyses of human hypertension and their replication difficult.[4,5] Steps are usually taken in the recruitment stage to reduce these problems by excluding those individuals with known causes of hypertension, diabetics and those with high levels of the risk factors listed above, such as older or obese individuals. The aim is to ensure the individuals being studied are likely to have raised BP because they carry genetic variants rather than non-genetic causes.

BLOOD PRESSURE PHENOTYPES

In any genetic study, we require some measurement of the phenotype (trait) thought to be under genetic influence and we aim to determine whether there exists a relationship between genetic data and that phenotype. Several different BP phenotypes have been used in genome-wide studies, broadly split into quantitative (numerical) and qualitative (categorical) phenotypes; in the sections below, their definitions and a brief summary of the evidence for their heritability is given.

Heritability is a useful measure of 'how genetic' a trait is. A 100% heritable trait would be caused solely by genes, whereas 0% heritability would imply that a trait is solely due to environmental causes. However, members of the same family tend to share their environment, which can lead to inflated estimates of heritability if this is not properly accounted for. For this reason, twin studies (comparing mono- and dizygous twins) are often preferred to family and population studies. These allow quantification of the shared genetic and environmental risk factors – we assume all twins share all their environment and that monozygous twins share all their genes whereas dizygous twins share only 50%.

Quantitative phenotypes

In the genetic analysis of BP, commonly used phenotypes include SBP, DBP, pulse pressure (PP) and mean arterial pressure (MAP). Recently, ambulatory blood pressure (ABP) has also been analyzed as a quantitative trait. Genetic analysis has shown these phenotypes differ in their heritability.

Systolic and diastolic blood pressure

Both SBP and DBP have been estimated to be about 50% heritable. A study of Caucasian twins estimated the heritability of SBP to be between 52% and 66% and that of DBP between 44% and 66%.[6] Similar heritabilities have been found in twin and family studies of European and African Americans.[7–9]

Pulse pressure

Pulse pressure is the difference between systolic and the diastolic readings. It is correlated with SBP (which is possibly suggestive of common causes) and seems to be an indicator of aortic stiffness and inflammation in the blood vessel walls. However, little is known about its genetic basis. Estimates of PP heritability show more between population variability than those of SBP and DBP – from 51% and 53% in White[10] and European[11] Americans respectively, to 25% in Mexican Americans[12] and 13% in Nigerians.[13]

BP phenotypes tend to show large intraindividual variation over time, and even the more reliable ABP measures are subject to short-term influences by factors such as dietary salt or alcohol, antihypertensive medication and levels of exercise.[14] This can introduce considerable noise into trait measures, which in turn can obscure genotype-phenotype relationships.

Blood pressure as a qualitative phenotype: hypertension

Although BP measures are continuous quantitative traits, they can be divided into categorical qualitative traits, with the common division being based on the two diagnostic categories of hypertension and normotension. The British Hypertension Society defines hypertension as SBP ≥ 140 and/or DBP ≥ 90 mmHg.[15] Nonhypertensives are termed 'normotensive'. Note that there is no real dividing line between normal and high BP; hypertension is arbitrarily defined at a value at which target organs (such as the heart, kidney and brain) are possibly damaged; this definition is needed for practical reasons in the assessment and treatment of patients.[16] When hypertension is used as a phenotype, many individuals will be on antihypertensive medications by the time they are recruited[17] and it is important to ascertain as best as possible that the premedicated BP met whatever definition of hypertension was used by the study.

Essential hypertension is characterized as high blood pressure with no known identifiable cause. Estimates of the heritability of EH have varied between 20% (in family studies) to 60% in twin studies,[18] similar to the quantitative BP phenotypes.

THE SEARCH FOR HYPERTENSIVE GENES

The candidate gene approach

The candidate gene strategy has been the traditional approach in genetic studies of human EH. Genes that are possible candidates are selected on the basis of the role the proteins they encode play in pathways involved in the regulation of BP or BP-related phenotypes (such as salt sensitivity or Na^+–Li^+ countertransport). An effective approach is to search for an association between different variants of candidate genes and hypertension. This approach can demonstrate that an allele has a different frequency distribution in hypertensive and normotensive groups.

An alternative list of possible candidates can be generated by considering those genes involved in Mendelian forms of hypertension. These tend to be traits for which hypertension is just part of the phenotype and it is in the study of such traits that the first successful genome screens have been conducted. Generally, just a few large multicase families are studied and often different loci are implicated in different families (emphasizing the problems likely to be found in analysis of EH families). More than 15 genes are involved in Mendelian BP-related diseases,[19–23] which include glucocorticoid-remediable aldosteronism, Liddle's syndrome, apparent mineralocorticoid excess, an activating mutation of the mineralocorticoid receptor and pseudohypoaldosteronism type 2. Although the genetic mutations identified as causing these diseases have strong effects, resulting in phenotypes of which high BP is only one factor, other less severe mutations in the same genes might also have lesser effects on BP and so should be considered as good candidates for analyses of EH.

Candidate genes are selected by virtue of their physiological function, and this means such studies are limited by what is currently known about the function of genes involved in the pathogenesis of EH. Numerous candidates have been evaluated in many populations and positive association results have been obtained. However, the results are not consistent between studies and common variants in Mendelian BP genes have not been found to explain EH.[24] This might be explained by differences in genetic background for various populations but it is also likely that at least some results are false positives.

The genome scanning approach

In recent years there has been a tendency to look for an alternative strategy in the hunt for human BP genes. The method of genome-wide scanning or whole-genome linkage analysis is such an alternative and is the focus of this chapter. This method corresponds to a systematic genotyping of hundreds of polymorphic markers spaced evenly throughout the genome in related individuals who have either been measured for a quantitative trait or share a qualitative trait.

Such linkage analysis has been used, with considerable success, in the search for disease-causing genes relating to simple Mendelian traits. If two loci lie close together on the same chromosome, they will tend to segregate together (that is, be passed down from parent to offspring together) and are said to be 'linked'. The probability of this happening is greater, and so linkage is 'tighter', the closer they are. With the development of maps of genetic markers spanning the whole genome, researchers have taken advantage of this property to search the entire genome for regions linked to many diseases, including hypertension.

Underlying all methods to test for linkage is the principle that relatives who have similar traits should have inherited genes influencing the trait, and the genetic material around it, from a common ancestor. In regions containing such genes they would then share more genetic material than expected.

GENOME-WIDE LINKAGE ANALYSES

Methods of linkage analysis exist for both qualitative and quantitative traits. To test for linkage between a binary trait (e.g. hypertensive or normotensive) and a genetic region, two or more affected relatives are recruited and genetic markers are tested with the hope of finding regions that tend to be shared among them and that therefore might contain a disease-related gene. Additional (unaffected) family members are useful to help resolve the inheritance of these genetic markers and should also be recruited, where possible, to increase the potential information in the sample. A common design is to recruit a number of pairs of affected siblings (sibpairs); in this case their parents provide all the additional information necessary, but if they are unavailable (as commonly happens for late-onset disorders), unaffected siblings will also be useful. For a quantitative trait (e.g. SBP), the trait is measured among all family members, and the aim is to find regions where genetic sharing is related to the phenotypic relationship between individuals. Thus, a relatively small chromosomal region could be identified as containing a putative trait-related gene. Such a region might be in the order of 5–10 cM for monogenic diseases but tends to be substantially larger (up to 30 cM) for a complex trait. This region can then be searched systematically for that gene.

Methods can be classified broadly into two groups: mode of inheritance-based methods (often called model-based) and model-free methods (sometimes called nonparametric). The evidence for linkage is often presented as a LOD ('log-odds') score for model-based or qualitative-trait analysis, or as a P value in model-free analysis of quantitative traits. With all locations on the genome being tested simultaneously, the thresholds at which to declare significant linkage are not clear. Certainly, a threshold such as $P < 0.05$ would result in many false positives. Theoretical arguments (assuming 'perfect information') led to the conclusion that a threshold of LOD > 4 (equivalent to $P < 10^{-4}$) corresponded to genome-wide significance,[25] but other authors have argued that such a threshold is overly conservative and a threshold of 3.2[26] is more commonly used, with a LOD > 1.9 taken to be 'suggestive' linkage (not significant, but worth follow-up investigation, e.g. typing more genetic markers in the region or in additional families). The problem with defining a single threshold that can be applied to all studies arises because studies differ in terms of the family structures studied and the amount of genetic information extracted. Other authors have suggested using simulation methods either to estimate thresholds[27] or to count the number of regions expected to exceed some threshold[28] in each individual study. These methods provide more accurate determination of statistical significance but they are time consuming and not generally available in packaged software, which probably explains their lack of common use.

Model-based linkage analysis

Under model-based analysis, we posit a model for the genetic determination of the trait of interest, e.g. dominant. This is then used to infer the (unobserved) disease genotype and test whether this locus (with unknown position) is linked to any region in our map of genetic markers (with known position). This is a powerful method when the mode of inheritance for a trait is known, because it makes use of this information. However, common complex traits such as EH do not follow simple Mendelian patterns of inheritance, meaning the disease genotype cannot be inferred from the phenotype. This can be due to a number of factors, including the trait being under the control of multiple genes; uncertain diagnosis; genetic heterogeneity; variable age of onset; or the existence of nongenetic risk factors. Model-based methods that assume an incorrect mode of inheritance can be biased and – more often – model-free methods are used for complex traits. Despite this, several model-based analyses of BP and EH have been conducted.

Ten extended families from the San Antonio Family Heart Study (SAFHS) were studied to test for linkage to SBP, DBP and PP under the assumption that each trait in turn could be explained by a two-allele, single-locus Mendelian model.[12,29] These models were estimated by segregation analysis, which finds the genetic model that best explains the observed pattern of disease transmission. Such modeling allows the effects of age, body mass index (BMI) and sex to be included in the analysis, but the valididty of analyzing three related complex traits as independent Mendelian traits is not clear. The results for the correlated traits of SBP and PP were similar, finding suggestive linkage to 18q23 and 21q22 for both and to 7q22 and 8q24 for PP. The results differed for DBP, finding significant linkage to 2p11 (LOD = 3.92) and suggestive linkage to 2q12.

Significant linkage of hypertension to 2p12 was also found by a Chinese study, which considered a single large family (94 individuals) together with 32 nuclear families;[30] however, there were flaws in the statistical methods used. It was assumed that all alleles of any one marker had equal frequencies in the population, which can lead to false positive results,[31] and no justification was given for the genetic model assumed. Results of model-based analysis depend on the model used and, when the true model is not (or cannot be) known, it is common either to estimate the model using segregation analysis (as in the analysis of the SAFHS data) or to consider a range of models and report the results under each.[32,33] As neither of these approaches were explored, their results should be treated with caution.

However, a nearby (but not overlapping) region on chromosome 2p was also flagged in the analysis of a single large pedigree from the isolated Sardinian population containing 35 EH-affected members.[34] Both model-based and model-free analyses were used and the strongest evidence for linkage was found to a region on chromosome 2p24-2p25 (LOD between 1.5 and 2.1 under a range of models). This is not significant in itself, but stronger evidence came from the nonparametric analysis which obtained P values between 10^{-3} and 10^{-4} across a range of statistics.

Some supporting evidence for the existence of a PP-related gene on chromosome 8 was found in a study of 26 extended Utah pedigrees.[11] The method used is more robust to model misspecification, and four genetic models were considered. Simulation was used to determine the thresholds for genome-wide significance and two regions of suggestive linkage on chromosomes 8p and 12q (LOD > 2.5) were reported. Although these regions did not overlap with those flagged in the SAFHS families, there was modest evidence for linkage (LOD > 1.5) to chromosome 8q24.

The results of these studies are summarized in Table 4.1; we suggest one should be cautious about drawing conclusions in the absence of a formal meta-analysis but regions on chromosomes 2p and 8q do seem to be implicated.

Model-free analysis of qualitative phenotypes

Because of the problems applying model-based methods to complex traits, many researchers prefer to use model-free methods. Note that 'model-free' does not mean nonparametric in the statistical sense, rather that no genetic model for disease is assumed; instead, genetic markers are used to trace which regions affected individuals have inherited from common ancestors. This observed

Table 4.1 Summary of model-based and model-free genome scans of hypertension and BP listing regions of suggestive and (in bold) genome-wide significant linkage found in each study

Study	Population	Number/type families	Trait and linked regions (if any)
Model-based analyses			
Atwood et al[12,29]	Mexican American	637 individuals from 10 families	PP: 7q22, 8q24, 18q23, 21q22 DBP: **2p11**, 2q12, 8q24 SBP: 18q23, 21q22
Angius et al[34]	Sardinian	Single large pedigree	EH: 1p36, 2p21-2p25, 13q22, **15q25**, 17p12
Gong et al[30]	Chinese	1 large kindred, 32 nuclear families	EH: **12p12**
Camp et al[11]	Utah	1454 individuals from 26 families	PP: 8q21-p12, 12q23
Model-free analyses: Family Blood Pressure Program			
Krushkal et al[38] (ED pairs from Rochester arm of GENOA)	Non-Hispanic WA	69 ED sibpairs	SBP: 2p21-22, 5q33-34, **6q23-24**, 15q25-26
Ranade et al[41] (SAPPHIRe)	Chinese and Japanese	Extreme-value subset of 1425 sibpairs	EH: 9q34, 10p14
Kardia et al[42] (GENOA)	AA and WA	450 AA and 539 WA sibpairs	EH: none
Rao et al[43] (HyperGEN)	AA and WA	650 AA and 915 WA sibpairs	EH: 2p22
Morrison et al- (nonobese AA from HyperGen, GENOA, GenNet)	AA	275 sibships	EH: **2q36**
Province et al[45] (GENOA, SAPPHIRe, HyperGEN GenNet meta-analysis)	AA, WA, Chinese and Japanese	6245 relatives	None
Model-free analyses: European			
Perola et al[46]	Finnish	47 sibpairs	EH: 1q31, 2q24-32, **3q24 (AT1)**, 22q12, Xp11
Von Wowern et al[47]	Scandinavian	91 nuclear families	EH: 2p11-2q14, **14q13-q23**
Kristjansson et al[48]	Icelandic	490 hypertensives from 120 families	EH: 18q21
Sharma et al[49]	British Caucasian	263 nuclear families	EH: 11q24
Caulfield et al[50] (BriGHT)	British Caucasian	2010 ASPs, 1599 nuclear families	EH: 2q24, 5q13, **6q27**, 9q34
Model-free analyses: Chinese			
Xu et al[39,40]	Chinese	377 families	SBP: 3p26, 11q12, 16q12, 17p12 DBP: **15q26**
Zhu et al[51]	Chinese	In three stages: 283, 637 and 777 sibpairs	EH: 2q21-2q24

AA, African American; DBP, diastolic blood pressure; EH, essential hypertension; PP, pulse pressure; SBP, systolic blood pressure; WA, white American.

inheritance by descent (IBD) sharing is compared to that expected given only the relationships of the affected relatives. If the affected relatives inherited the same genetic disease variant, we would expect the observed IBD to exceed that expected in the neighborhood of the disease-related gene. Methods to detect the departure of observed IBD from that expected include scoring[35] and maximum likelihood.[36] For convenience, and to allow for comparison with model-based tests, evidence for linkage is often converted to a nonparametric linkage (NPL) LOD score, or presented as an MLS score, which can be interpreted in the same way. They are also sometimes presented as NPL Z scores, for which the same thresholds do not apply; the associated P value must be referred to the thresholds described earlier to determine genome-wide significance. This is an important point because Z-scores are generally higher then LOD scores; a Z score of 3.7 corresponds to a P value of 10^{-4}.

Extreme phenotype sibpair studies

Hypertensives are simply those individuals in the upper tail of the BP distribution, and two early studies sought to compare those in the upper and lower tails (hypertensives and low normotensives) to search for genetic differences between the two. Such selection (not studying those in the centre of the distribution) has been shown to have increased power because it is those individuals in the tails of the distribution who provide most information.[37]

The first such scan[38] studied 69 extreme discordant (ED) sibpairs identified from the Rochester arm of the GENOA study, part of the Family Blood Pressure Program (FBPP). This is a resource of non-Hispanic white Americans ascertained without regard to health status. They found significant evidence for linkage ($P < 10^{-4}$) in the region of chromosome 6q23, but also some suggestive evidence ($P < 10^{-3}$) on chromosomes 15q26, 5q34 and 2p22. An extension of this design was used in a Chinese population with not only ED pairs, but also high and low concordant (HC and LC) pairs identified for both SBP and DBP.[39] No significant evidence for linkage was found, but follow-up of a suggestive region, with a redefinition of 'extreme' (now including BMI and sex as well as age) and additional markers found genome-wide significant linkage (MLS = 3.77) on chromosome 15q26 among 53 LC DBP pairs.[40] Interestingly, this region had the second highest MLS in the initial study. Stronger evidence was initially found on chromosome 16q12 among LC SDP pairs, but the redefinition of 'extreme' caused the number of these pairs to fall from 39 to 18; which was too few to study. Note that both of these potential loci were associated with the lower extreme of the BP distribution; despite ascertainment of more HC pairs, only suggestive evidence for linkage was found on chromosome 17p12 and 10p12 for DBP and SBP respectively (MLS = 2.07 and 2.33).

Another member of the FBPP is SAPPHIRe, which recruited 1425 sibpairs of Chinese and Japanese origin living in Taiwan, San Francisco or Hawaii. This is an unusual study design (mixing Chinese and Japanese populations); most studies aim to recruit individuals from a genetically homogenous background to reduce the genetic heterogeneity in the sample and thus the risk of missing a real result because different genetic variants are carried in different populations. There is a real risk that allele frequencies might differ between the populations, which can lead to incorrect inference of IBD sharing. This can be overcome if the marker allele frequencies are estimated separately in each population and used to estimate IBD sharing, before the likelihood is maximized over the entire sample. A study of ED, HC and LC sibpairs from this resource found a region of suggestive linkage on chromosome 10p14 (LOD = 2.5 in a combined analysis).[41] However, the possibility of differences in marker allele frequencies by ethnicity was not allowed for, which must throw doubt on this result.

Comparison of these three studies is complicated not just by the different populations studied, but also by the different criteria for 'extreme' – the GENOA study used the upper and lower twentieth, the Chinese the upper and lower tenth and SAPPHIRe the upper twentieth and lower thirtieth age-sex specific percentiles. However, it is interesting that 15q26 was flagged by the first two (better designed) studies, despite the population differences.

Although the most extreme percentiles offer the most powerful comparison, they contain fewer individuals and so there is a trade-off with sample size. ED pairs are rare and difficult to collect, and it is not always clear that the increase in power will justify their recruitment (e.g. the GENOA resource contained 3974 members of 583 multigenerational pedigrees but only 69 ED pairs were identified). As the cost of genotyping has come down, so it has become relatively more costly to phenotype so many pairs whose genes will not be studied. Instead, researchers have focused on just the upper tail of the BP distribution, selecting either those individuals diagnosed with clinical hypertension or those whose BP exceeds some study-defined threshold. Still, the principle, that more extreme cases are likely to provide more information for genetic studies is well established and many researchers aim to recruit those with higher BP measures, or lower age of onset (or both).

Other members of the Family Blood Pressure Program (North American populations)

The Rochester arm of the GENOA resource was later studied jointly with its Jackson arm (which recruited African–American siblings).[42] A less extreme phenotype was studied – clinical diagnosis of hypertension before 60 years of age – and this resulted in a larger resource (450 and 539 sibpairs in the Jackson and Rochester collections). However, analysis found not even one region of suggestive hypertension, illustrating the additional power that might be found by using more extreme phenotypes.

Another FBPP member is the HyperGEN network, which recruited 650 African and 915 white American hypertensive sibpairs, of whom over 80% have severe hypertension (SBP ≥ 160 or DBP ≥ 100). Again, a genome scan found no strong evidence for linkage in either group, with only one LOD score > 1.5 found; this among African–Americans on chromosome 2p22 (MLS = 2.08).[43]

One reason for the lack of linkage in these two studies might be the inclusion of obese individuals. BMI was not reported by the HyperGEN authors but the mean BMI was > 30 in the GENOA collections. As we mentioned above, weight is an important risk factor for hypertension, therefore obese individuals are commonly excluded from genetic studies. The African–American siblings from these two studies, together with those from a third arm (GenNet) have subsequently been reanalyzed. An additional restriction was placed that the sibpairs must also have BMI ≤ 30, resulting in a total of 275 sibships.[44] With this reduced sample, significant evidence *was* found for linkage on chromosome 2q (LOD = 3.59), with nearly all the evidence coming from the GENOA subset (LOD = 4.07). That this result was found only in nonobese sibpairs emphasizes the need to exclude those individuals with other causes of hypertension, such as obesity, in order not to dilute any genetic signal to a point where it becomes undetectable.

The FBPP also undertook a meta-analysis of the data from all four networks.[45] This is an unusual step because of the different populations from which the networks drew their families. The hypothesis underlying such an analysis must be that these populations carry variants in the same genes that act to influence BP. If this was really the underlying hypothesis then perhaps unifying the study design in each arm would have been useful, as it would have allowed a (more powerful) joint analysis of the entire resource. Poor design of both the network arms (e.g. not excluding obese individuals) and the strategy of combining the analysis of such different populations probably explains why no regions of even suggestive linkage were found in the combined analysis.

European populations

European studies tend to have employed stricter case definitions and exclusion criteria, which might explain the more convincing evidence for linkage which has been found. A study of 47 Finnish nondiabetic sibpairs who were diagnosed with hypertension before the age of 50 found strong evidence for linkage with an intragenic marker in the angiotensin II receptor type 1 (AT1) gene on chromosome 3q21 (MLS = 3.38); evidence was higher still among the 19 sibpairs from the south-west of the country (MLS = 4.04).[46] Highly suggestive linkage was also found in this group on chromosome 2q31 (MLS = 2.96). Both these results are unusually high for such a small sample in a complex trait; the authors explain this with reference to the relative isolation of the Finnish population, suggesting that there may be fewer disease-predisposing variants so each is more likely to be detected. Their strict, early onset, case definition might also have helped because it led them to recruit those more powerful 'extreme' cases. However, they also acknowledge that: 'It is quite possible, and even probable, that some of the loci showing some evidence for linkage to hypertension in our genome-wide scan represent false-positive findings'.

A larger study of 91 Scandinavian hypertensive sibships (mean 2.7 affecteds per family) found some evidence for linkage to chromosome 14q21 (LOD = 2.7).[47] Again, a fairly strict phenotype definition was used, including only those with onset of hypertension (SBP ≥ 160 or DBP ≥ 90) before age 50, but included 21 type II diabetics. Larger still was an Icelandic study of 120 extended families containing 490 hypertensives (SBP ≥ 160 or DBP ≥ 95).[48] Although the researchers did not exclude those with late-onset hypertension, the use of extended families gave this study a large increase in power and the only region showing evidence for linkage was highly significant on chromosome 18q21 (MLS = 4.6).

The first study of EH among British hypertensives recruited only 169 pairs of siblings and defined hypertensive individuals as those on antihypertensive medication with no exclusion criteria. Only one region of weakly suggestive linkage was found on chromosome 11q24.[49] A much larger study has since been undertaken in this population, studying 2010 affected sibling pairs with a strictly defined phenotype designed to capture the individuals in the top fifth percentile of the United Kingdom BP distribution, and excluding those with secondary hypertension, diabetes or high levels of controllable risk factors.[50] Initial results identified two regions of suggestive linkage on chromosomes 6q27 and 9q34 (MLS = 3.21 and 2.24 respectively); these and two other regions with MLS > 1.57 are being followed up using an increased density of genetic markers (Caulfield & Munroe, personal communication).

Chinese populations

The largest Chinese genome scan to date employed a three-stage design, using 283 affected sibpairs to screen the genome, and then followed up a region on chromosome 2 in further independent sets of 637 and 777 sibpairs.[51] This is an unusual design because the three sets of siblings were not analyzed jointly, even for the chromosome 2 region. Initial evidence for linkage found in the stage I pairs ($P = 0.002$) was not replicated in stage II ($P > 0.02$) but was in stage III ($P = 0.0009$). It would have been interesting to conduct a joint analysis of all sets because this would provide more power to confirm positive linkage.

Analysis of quantitative phenotypes

Fully quantitative traits should provide more information than a dichotomized phenotype, but there are additional problems introduced by the variability of BP measurements as described earlier. Two methods are commonly used: Haseman-Elston (HE) regression[52] and variance components (VC).[53,54]

In HE analysis, the aim is to search for regions where the genetic similarity between relative pairs is related to their phenotypic similarity. This is done by regressing the squared trait difference for the relative pairs on the proportion of alleles' shared IBD. If a marker is linked to the trait, high levels of IBD sharing should be associated with a small difference in trait values, and the regression slope should be negative. Thus, linkage can be tested with a regression t-test. Few assumptions are made so this method is applicable to all quantitative traits, but it is restricted to the analysis of sibling pair data.

An alternative is to decompose the variance of the trait into genetic and nongenetic factors and estimate these by maximum likelihood. This VC method has some advantages over HE – it is considerably more powerful for Gaussian (normal) data and can be applied to pedigrees as well as siblings. However, it has two major disadvantages also. A heavy reliance on normality assumptions means it can fail dramatically when these assumptions are violated and there are difficulties applying it to selected traits[55] (e.g. if we wanted to use BP measurements from families recruited because they were suffering from hypertension).

VC methods have been the primary choice for genetic analysis of BP measures but the checking of normality in these analyses, if even considered, is generally given only the briefest mention ('the phenotype was approximately normal') without any formal test of normality. This is an important point, so it is worth repeating. If VC is used for non-normal data, the false-positive rate will increase[56] and so the results of analyses of traits for which normality has not been tested must be viewed with a level of skepticism.

Further, the different VC analyses in this field have used a variety of phenotypes (including SBP and DBP,[9,57–63] longitudinal SBP and DBP,[8] PP,[10] postural changes in SBP and DBP,[64,65] exercise changes in resting SBP and DBP[59] and exercise BP.[66] We have decided not to review such studies here and instead have focused our attention on the more well-defined phenotype of hypertension. This is due partly to the difficulty in comparing the results of studies of such varied traits and the problems with the VC methods commonly used. Also, in our opinion, hypertension is a better defined phenotype, which suffers less from problems of variation in BP measurement. We wished to use the space available to explore studies of hypertension in greater depth. Readers who wish for more detail on genetic analysis of quantitative BP traits should refer to recent reviews.[67,68]

RECONCILING RESULTS FROM DIFFERENT STUDIES

If hypertension is genetic, why haven't more loci been found?

Given the number of studies reviewed here, it is perhaps surprising that so few genetic loci have been identified at a genome-wide significant level. One explanation is that hypertension is not genetic at all, and all results that have been found are false. This is countered, however, by the clear evidence from heritability studies, which show that up to half of BP variation is inherited. If we accept that hypertensive loci do exist, one explanation for them remaining as yet undiscovered is found in the design of many studies. If only half of BP variation is inherited, the rest must be environmental, and many of these causes are known. In the UK, approximately 53% of 54- to 65-year-olds, and 71% of those aged over 75, have hypertension.[69] This is similar to most Western countries but contrasts with populations living in rural, non-Western settings. For example, a study of the Xhosa people of Southern Africa found that their BP did not rise with age (although it did among those members who live in an urban setting).[70] Such studies suggest that lifelong exposure to risk factors present in Western and urban environments leads to hypertension.

So if we want to discover the genetic causes, we must study the 'genetic' (rather than 'environmental') cases. To do so, we must focus on those extreme cases who have early-onset disease and an absence of obvious nongenetic risk factors, such as obesity. Indeed, it is the studies of such extreme phenotypes that have published the most significant findings.

The GENOA arm of the FBPP study is a useful example of how genetic signals can be missed behind environmental noise if these simple guidelines in study design are not followed. Although not a huge sample, around 1000 sibpairs were collected, about half African and half white American. The only criterion for recruitment was a clinical diagnosis of hypertension before the age of 60. The authors acknowledge that only 27% of American hypertensives have their BP adequately controlled, but the mean BP in their sample was a fairly respectable 139/80 mmHg, suggesting that there might have been some overdiagnosis and certainly that less extreme cases were being studied. Further, the mean BMI was > 30, so that a large proportion of the cases had an important nongenetic risk factor. Analysis of each group found no regions of even suggestive linkage. Refined analyses of the extreme white American[38] and the nonobese African–American[44] siblings each found a region of genome-wide significant linkage despite the reduced sample size; both regions were completely missed in the analysis of the complete data.[42] We have singled out the GENOA study because missed linkage has been demonstrated, but most studies suffer from some design problems, implying that truly linked regions could have been missed.

Why do different studies find different loci?

Fig. 4.1 shows the location of all the significant and suggestive linkages reported in the papers discussed here. Linkage analysis is not good at localizing

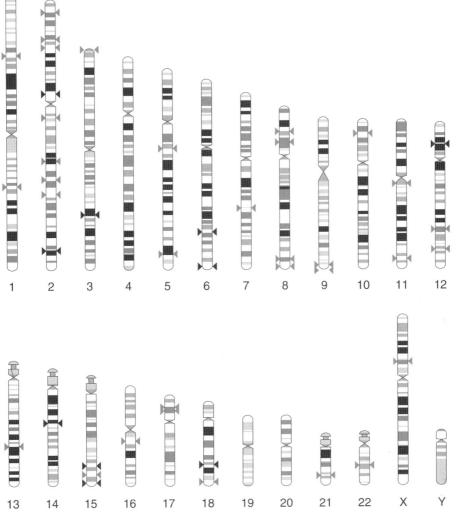

Fig. 4.1 An idiogram of the human chromosomes. Regions of suggestive and significant linkage to hypertension listed in Table 4.1 are indicated by gray and black triangles, respectively.

genes – LOD score peaks are generally long (20–30 cM is not unusual) and often the gene causing the linkage will lie at the edge or even outside of such a peak,[71] so we must be generous when considering whether two studies do indeed overlap. Chromosome 2, for example, has nine 'hits' and there are three studies reporting linkage peaks relatively close together on chromosome 15, two of which met genome-wide significance. Even so, many apparently linked regions appear isolated. As all studies are attempting to study the same or related phenotypes, why do their results not coincide? One reason is that many of the studies will have missed real evidence of linkage because of poor study design or small sample size. Another is that many of the reported linkage regions will be false positives. Additionally, this is a complex trait that is under the control of several genes and those subsets of genes that contain important phenotype-affecting variants might vary between populations.

Given these considerations it is not so surprising that results differ between studies. Still, we would expect that if genes that have the potential to affect human BP do exist, regions close to these genes would be flagged in more than one study, perhaps even across different populations, and Fig. 4.1 allows us to identify a few regions that fit this pattern. Chromosome 15q is probably the most promising and there are two or three less well-defined regions on chromosome 2 – one on each arm and possibly one centromeric as well as a region on 18q. Finally, we might include 8p, 8q, 9q and 12q, although none of these really have strong support. More formally, a recent meta-analysis of nine genetic studies of hypertension and BP among Caucasians found evidence for new regions of linkage of EH and DBP to chromosomes 3p14-q12 ($P = 0.0001$) and 2p12-q22 ($P = 0.0005$).[72]

Once a linkage peak is identified, it is generally subjected to further follow-up work, trying to extract more information either by recruiting additional families or by typing further genetic markers in a region (to better characterize the inheritance patterns within families already studied). Linkage is not a precise tool for detecting the genes at work in complex disease. As well as the problems with localization, it is suitable only for variants with a reasonably strong signal. Another method is association analysis–testing either known candidate genes in the region of interest or searching the whole region for polymorphisms that differ in frequency between cases and controls. The same phenomenon gives rise to linkage disequilibrium (LD) at the population level – essentially because all living humans are members of the same large family. However, in the population, there have been many more meioses and so LD extends over much shorter genetic distances. This allows association analyses to better localize any disease-related gene, but requires many more genetic markers to be typed. Association analysis is also capable of detecting genes with smaller effects than linkage. Such follow-up work will reveal which of the linked regions do contain BP genes.

SUMMARY

Despite the relatively recent availability of the tools necessary for genome-wide scans for hypertension, many studies have been conducted, each differing in its phenotype definition and methods of analysis used. Some studies have suffered from poor design, including vague phenotype definition, lack of exclusion criteria or low sample size. We place our greatest belief in the results from those with good design. Despite these differences, chromosome 15q appears to be implicated repeatedly, as does 2p, with other results also worthy of follow up. More work is needed before the genes that control hypertension are identified but a critical review of published studies demonstrates the utility of genome-wide searches to identify good candidate regions, which will be searched at a finer resolution using association analysis tools.

The case-control samples needed for association analysis should be easier to collect than multiply affected family samples but, because of the much higher numbers of polymorphisms needed to scan any region, to date they been used only in candidate gene and small region-wide studies. However, it is likely that the next generation of genome scans will be based on association rather than linkage methods. There are now many identified single nucleotide polymorphisms (SNPs) across the genome, and, as the cost of high throughput SNP-typing technology continues to decrease, projects are underway to identify further SNPs and discover the range of LD between them.[73]

Association studies offer increased power over linkage analysis for detecting genes with smaller effect, but there remain issues that require resolution. Not least are the effects of population substructure. Most human populations are actually collections of smaller subpopulations. If disease prevalence differs between these subpopulations then some subpopulations will be oversampled when cases are recruited and others oversampled in the control group. If genetic polymorphisms not related to disease also differ between these subpopulations, then these will appear to differ in frequency between cases and controls and so appear to be spuriously associated with disease. It was worries such as these that led to the development of family-based association testing (e.g. the transmission disequilibrium test, which is valid regardless of substructure).[74] Such concerns have been thought to be overstated for studies that use carefully defined populations to avoid gross levels of structure[75,76] but there is an increasing expectation that even modest levels of population structure cannot be safely ignored for the larger sample sizes needed for genome-wide studies.[77] Several statistical methods have been proposed to account for substructure,[78–80] but their effectiveness will not be properly assessed until genetic data from the first large-scale studies are available.

Competing models are proposed for the genetic architecture of complex traits: that common diseases are caused by ancient common variants [the common disease, common variant (CDCV) hypothesis][81,82] or that they are caused by multiple rare variants (MRV).[83,84] Examples of both already exist, with the common e4 allele at APOE, which is associated with Alzheimer's disease,[85,86] providing support for the former and the multiple Crohn's disease-associated alleles at NOD2[87,88] providing support for the latter. As more complex disease genes are found, it is likely they will cover a spectrum from common to rare variants, but whereas methods are well developed for assessing association under the CDCV, further work is needed to develop robust statistical methods for the identification of rare variants.

All these challenges are surmountable, and whole-genome SNP association analysis offers great promise to those who continue to search for the elusive BP genes.

References

1. World Health Organization, International Society of Hypertension Writing Group. 2003 World Health Organization (WHO)/International Society of Hypertension (ISH) statement on management of hypertension. *J Hyperten* 2003; 21:1983–1992.
2. Staessen JA, Wang J, Bianchi G, et al. Essential hypertension. *Lancet* 2003; 361:1629.
3. Cusi D, Bianchi G. A primer on the genetics of hypertension. *Kidney Int* 1998; 54:328–342.
4. Corvol P, Persu A, Gimenez-Roqueplo A-P, et al. Seven lessons from two candidate genes in human essential hypertension: angiotensinogen and epithelial sodium channel. *Hypertension* 1999; 33:1324–1331.
5. Nabika T. From animal models to humans. *Clin Exper Pharmacol Physiol* 1999; 26:541–543.
6. Evans A, van Baal GCM, McCarron P, et al. The genetics of coronary heart disease: the contribution of twin studies. *Twin Res* 2003; 6:432–441.
7. Snieder H, Harshfield GA, Treiver FA. Heritability of blood pressure and hemodynamics in African– and European–American youth. *Hypertension* 2003; 41:1196–1201.
8. Levy D, DeStefano AL, Larson MG, et al. Evidence for a gene influencing blood pressure on chromosome 17: genome scan linkage results for longitudinal blood pressure phenotypes in subjects from the Framingham Heart Study. *Hypertension* 2000; 36:477–483.
9. Turner ST, Kardia SLR, Boerwinkle E, et al. Multivariate linkage analysis of blood pressure and body mass index. *Genet Epidemiol* 2004; 27:64–73.

10. DeStefano AL, Larson MG, Mitchell GF, et al. Genome-wide scan for pulse pressure in the National Heart, Lung and Blood Institute's Framingham Heart Study. *Hypertension* 2004; 44:152–155.

11. Camp NJ, Hopkins PN, Hasstedt SJ, et al. Genome-wide multipoint parametric linkage analysis of pulse pressure in large, extended Utah pedigrees. *Hypertension* 2003; 42:322–328.

12. Atwood LD, Samollow PB, Hixson JE, et al. Genome-wide linkage analysis of pulse pressure in Mexican Americans. *Hypertension* 2001; 38:425–428.

13. Adeyemo AA, Omotade OO, Rotimi CN, et al. Heritability of blood pressure in Nigerian families. *J Hypertens* 2002; 20:859–863.

14. Geleijnse JM, Kok FJ, Grobbee DE. Impact of dietary and lifestyle factors on the prevalence of hypertension in Western populations. *Eur J Public Health* 2004; 13(3):235–239.

15. Williams B, Poulter NR, Brown MJ, et al. British Hypertension Society guidelines. Guidelines for management of hypertension: report of the fourth working party of the British Hypertension Society, 2004 – BHS IV. *J Hum Hypertens* 2004; 18:139–185.

16. Carrtero OA, Oparil S. Essential hypertension. Part 1: definition and etiology. *Circulation* 2000; 101:329–335.

17. Burt VL, Cutler JA, Higgins M, et al. Trends in the prevalence, awareness, treatment, and control of hypertension in the adult US population: data from the health examination surveys, 1960 to 1991. *Hypertension* 1995; 26:60–69.

18. Staessen JA, Wang J, Bianchi G, et al. Essential hypertension. *Lancet* 2003; 361:1629–1641.

19. Lifton RP, Gharavi AG, Geller DS. Molecular mechanisms of human hypertension. *Cell* 2001; 104:545–556.

20. Wilson FH, Disse-Nicodeme S, Choate KA, et al. Human hypertension caused by mutations in WNK kinases. *Science* 2001; 293:1107–1112.

21. Hopkins PN, Hunt SC. Genetics of hypertension. *Genet Med* 2003; 5:413–429.

22. Johnson D, Kan S, Oldridge M, et al. Missense mutations in the homeodomain of HOXD13 are associated with brachydactyly types D and E. *Am J Hum Genet* 2003; 72:984–997.

23. Carvajal CA, Gonzalez AA, Romero DG, et al. Two homozygous mutations in the 11 beta-hydroxysteroid dehydrogenase type 2 gene in a case of apparent mineralocorticoid excess. *J Clin Endocr Metab* 2003; 85:2501–2507.

24. Genetic Association Database.Online. Available: http://geneticassociationdb.nih.gov/

25. Lander ES, Kruglyak L. Genetic dissection of complex traits: guidelines for interpreting and reporting linkage results. *Nat Genet* 1995; 11:241–247.

26. Suarez BK, Hampe CL. Linkage and association. *Am J Hum Genet* 1994; 54:554–559.

27. Sawcer S, Jones HB, Judge D, et al. Empirical genome-wide significance levels established by whole genome simulations. *Genet Epidemiol* 1997; 14:223–229.

28. Wiltshire S, Hattersley AT, Hitman GA, et al. A genome-wide scan for loci predisposing to type 2 diabetes in a UK population (the diabetes UK Warren 2 repository): analysis of 573 pedigrees provides independent replication of a susceptibility locus on chromosome 1q. *Am J Hum Genet* 2001; 69:553–569.

29. Atwood LD, Samollow PB, Hixson JE, et al. Genome-wide linkage analysis of blood pressure in Mexican Americans. *Genet Epidemiol* 2001; 20:373–382.

30. Gong M, Zhang H, Schulz H, et al. Genome-wide linkage reveals a locus for human essential (primary) hypertension on chromosome 12p. *Hum Mol Genet* 2003; 12:1273–1277.

31. Freimer NB, Sandkuijl LA, Blower SM. Incorrect specification of marker allele frequencies: effects on linkage analysis. *Am J Hum Genet* 1993; 52:1102–1110.

32. Greenberg DA, Abreu PC, Hodge SE. The power to detect linkage in complex disease by means of simple LOD-score analyses. *Am J Hum Genet* 1998; 63:870–879.

33. Durner M, Vieland VJ, Greenberg DA. Further evidence for the increased power of LOD scores compared with nonparametric methods. *Am J Hum Genet* 1999; 64:281–289.

34. Angius A, Petretto E, Maestrale GB, et al. A new essential hypertension susceptibility locus on chromosome 2p24-p25, detected by genome-wide search. *Am J Hum Genet* 2002; 71:893–905.

35. Whittmore AS, Halpern J. A class of tests for linkage using affected pedigree members. *Biometrics* 1994; 50:118–127.

36. Risch N. Linkage strategies for genetically complex traits. I. Multilocous models. *Am J Hum Genet* 1990; 42:222–228.

37. Williamson CG. Linkage analysis of quantitative traits: increased power by using selected samples. *Am J Hum Genet* 1991; 49:786–796.

38. Krushkal J, Ferrell R, Mockrin SC, et al. Genome-wide linkage analyses of systolic blood pressure using highly discordant siblings. *Circulation* 1999; 99:1407–1410.

39. Xu X, Rogus JJ, Terwedow HA, et al. An extreme-sibpair genome scan for genes regulating blood pressure. *Am J Hum Genet* 1999; 64:1694–1701.

40. Xu X, Yang J, Rogus J et al. Mapping of a blood pressure quantitative trait locus to chromosome 15q in a Chinese population. *Hum Mol Genet* 1999; 8:2551–2555.

41. Ranade K, Hinds D, Hsiung CA, et al. A genome scan for hypertension susceptibility loci in populations of Chinese and Japanese origins. *Am J Hypertens* 2003; 16:158–162.

42. Kardia SL, Rozek LS, Krushkal J, et al. Genome-wide linkage analyses for hypertension genes in two ethnically and geographically diverse populations. *Am J Hypertens* 2003; 16:154–157.
43. Rao DC, Province MA, Leppert MF, et al. A genome-wide affected sibpair linkage analysis of hypertension:the HyperGEN network. *Am J Hypertens* 2003; 16:148–150.
44. Morrison AC, Coper R, Hunt S, et al. Genome scan for hypertension in nonobese African Americans: the National Heart, Lung, and Blood Institute Family Blood Pressure Program. *Am J Hypertens* 2004; 17:834–838.
45. Province MA, Kardia SL, Ranade K, et al. A meta-analysis of genome-wide linkage scans for hypertension: The National Heart, Lung and Blood Institute Family Blood Pressure Program. *Am J Hypertens* 2003; 16:144–147.
46. Perola M, Kainulainem K, Pajukanta P, et al. Genome-wide scan of predisposing loci for increased diastolic blood pressure in Finnish siblings. *J Hypertens* 2000; 18:1579–1585.
47. Van Wowern F, Bengtsson K, Lindgren CM, et al. A genome-wide scan for early onset primary hypertension in Scandinavians. *Hum Mol Genet* 2003; 12:2077–2081.
48. Kristjansson K, Manolescu A, Kristinsson A, et al. Linkage of essential hypertension to chromosome 18q. *Hypertens* 2002; 39:1044–1049.
49. Sharma P, Fatibene J, Ferraro F, et al. A genome-wide search for susceptibility loci to human essential hypertension. *Hypertens* 2002; 35:1291–1296.
50. Caulfield M, Munroe P, Pembroke J, et al. Genome-wide mapping of human loci for essential hypertension. *Lancet* 2003; 361:2118–2123.
51. Zhu DL, Wang HY, Xiong MW, et al. Linkage of hypertension to chromosome 2q14-q23 in Chinese families. *J Hypertens* 2001; 19:55–61.
52. Haseman JK, Elston RC. The investigation of linkage between a quantitative trait and a marker locus. *Behav Genet* 1972; 2:3–19.
53. Amos C I. Robust variance-components approach for assessing genetic linkage in pedigrees. *Am J Hum Genet* 1994; 54:535–543.
54. Almasy L, Blangero J. Multipoint quantitative-trait linkage analysis in general pedigrees. *Am J Hum Genet* 1998; 62:1198–1211.
55. Feingold E. Methods for linkage analysis of quantitative trait loci in humans. *Theor Popul Biol* 2001; 60:167–180.
56. Allison DB, Neale MC, Zannolli R, et al. Testing the robustness of the likelihood-ratio test in a variance –component quantitative-trait loci-mapping procedure. *Am J Hum Genet* 1999; 65:531–544.
57. Cheng LS, Davis RC, Raffel LJ, et al. Coincident linkage of fasting plasma insulin and blood pressure to chromosome 7q in hypertensive Hispanic families. *Circulation* 2001; 104:1255–1260.
58. Hunt SC, Ellison RC, Atwood LD, et al. Genome scans for blood pressure and hypertension – The National Heart, Lung, and Blood Institute Family Heart Study. *Hypertension* 2002; 40:1–6.
59. Rice T, Rankinen T, Chagnon YC, et al. Genomewide linkage scan of resting blood pressure – HERITAGE family study. *Hypertension* 2002; 39:1037–1043.
60. Thiel BA, Chakravarti A, Cooper RS, et al. A genome-wide linkage analysis investigating the determinants of blood pressure in whites and African Americans. *Am J Hypertens* 2003; 16:151–153.
61. Cooper RS, Luke A, Zhu X, et al. Genome scan among Nigerians linking blood pressure to chromosomes 2, 3, and 19. *Hypertension* 2003; 40:629–633.
62. Harrap SB, Wong ZY, Stebbing M, et al. Blood pressure QTLs identified by genome-wide linkage analysis and dependence on associated phenotypes. *Physiol Genomics* 2002; 8:99–105.
63. Hsueh WC, Mitchell BD, Schneider JL, et al. QTL influencing blood pressure maps to the region of PPH1 on chromosome 2q31-34 in Old Order Amish. *Ciculation* 2000; 101:2810–2816.
64. Pankow JS, Rose KM, Oberman A, et al. Possible locus on chromosome 18q influencing postural systolic blood pressure changes. *Hypertension* 2000; 36:471–476.
65. Harrap SB, Cui JS, Wong ZY, et al. Familial and genomic analyses of postural changes in systolic and diastolic blood pressure. *Hypertension* 2004; 43:586–591.
66. Rankinen T, An P, Rice T, et al. Genomic scan for exercise blood pressure in the Health, risk Facotrs, Exercise Training and Genetics (HERITAGE) family study. *Hypertension* 2001; 38:30–37.
67. Samani NJ. Genome scans for hypertension and blood pressure regulation. *Am J Hypertens* 2003; 16:167–171.
68. Mein CA, Caulfield MJ, Dobson RJ, et al. Genetics of essential hypertension. *Hum Mol Genet* 2004; 13:R169–R175.
69. Health Survey for England – trends. 2002. Online. Available: http://www.dh.gov.uk/assetRoot/04/06/60/94/04066094.xls
70. Sever PS, Gordon D, Peart WS, et al. Blood pressure and its correlates in urban and tribal Africa. *Lancet* 1980; 12(2):60–64.

71. Hovatta I, Lechtermann D, Juvonen H, et al. Linkage analysis of putative schizophrenia gene candidate regions on chromosomes 3p, 5q, 6p, 8p, 20p, 22q in a population-based sampled Finnish family set. *Mol Psychol* 1998; 3:452–457.

72. Koivukoski L, Fisher SA, Kanninen T, et al. Meta-analysis of genome-wide scans for hypertension and blood pressure in Caucasians shows evidence of susceptibility regions on chromosomes 2 and 3. *Hum Mol Benet* 2004; 13(19):2325–2332.

73. The International HapMap Project. Online. Available: http://www.hapmap.org

74. Ewens WJ, Spielman RS. The transmission/disequilibrium test: history, subdivision, and admixture. *Am J Hum Genet* 1995; 57(2):455–464.

75. Ardlie KG, Lunetta KL, Seielstad M. Testing for population subdivision and association in four case-control studies. *Am J Hum Genet* 2002; 71:304–311.

76. Wacholder S, Rothman N, Caporaso N. Counterpoint:bias from population stratification is not a major threat to the validity of conclusions from epidemiological studies of common polymorphisms and cancer. *Cancer Epidemiol Biomarkers Prev* 2002; 11:513–520.

77. Marchini J, Cardon LR, Phillips MS, Donnelly P. The effects of human population structure on large genetic association studies. *Nat Genet* 2004; 36(11):1129–1130.

78. Devlin B, Roeder K. Genomic control for association studies. *Biometrics* 1999; 55:997–1004.

79. Pritchard JK, Stephens M, Rosenberg NA, et al. Association mapping in structured populations. *Am J Hum Genet* 2000; 67:170–181.

80. Hoggart CJ, Parra EJ, Shriver MD, et al. Control of confounding of genetic associations in stratified populations. *Am J Hum Genet* 2003; 72:1492–1504.

81. Chakravarti A. Population genetics:making sense out of sequence. *Nat Genet* 1999; 21:56–60.

82. Reich D, Lander E. On the allelic spectrum of human disease. *Trends Genet* 2001; 17:502–510.

83. Pritchard J, Cox N. The allelic architecture of human disease genes: common disease – common variant. . . or not? *Hum Mol Genet* 2002; 11:2417–2423.

84. Terwilliger J, Haghighi F, Hiekkalinna T et al. A biased assessment of the use or SNPs in human complex traits. *Curr Opin Genet Dev* 2002; 12:726–734.

85. Coredr E, Saunders A, Strittmatter W et al. Gene dose of apolipoprotein-e type-4 allele and the risk of Alzheimer's disease in late-onset families. *Science* 1993; 261:921–923.

86. Fullerton S, Clark A, Weiss K et al. Apolipoprotein e variation at the sequence haplotype level: implications for the origin and maintenance of a major human polymorphism. *Am J Hum Genet* 2000; 67:881–900.

87. Hugot JP, Chamaillard M, Zouali H et al. Association of NOD2 leucine-rich repeat variants with susceptibility to Crohn's disease. *Nature* 2001; 411:599–603.

88. Ogura Y, Bonen DK, Inohara N et al. A frameshift mutation in nod2 associated with susceptibility to Crohn's disease. *Nature* 2001; 411:603–606.

5 | Genetics of stroke

Pankaj Sharma

INTRODUCTION

Stroke is the most common cause of disability, the second greatest cause of dementia and the third largest cause of death in the Western world. It consumes around 7% of the entire NHS budget in the UK and the economic burden to the USA is in excess of $50 billion per year, comprising 700,000 stroke cases per year and 4.4 million stroke survivors.

The etiological causes underlying stroke can broadly be divided into those that are predetermined (e.g. age and gender) and those that are modifiable, such as hypertension and diabetes. The complexity in characterizing the underlying genetic defects is compounded by the fact that stroke is a heterogeneous syndrome, being approximately 85% ischemic in nature with most of the remainder hemorrhagic. Notwithstanding the fact that the stroke syndrome is arguably one of the more complex of the polygenic disorders, the genetics of stroke has received considerable attention in recent years. There is now little doubt that a genetic contribution to human sporadic stroke exists, although there is debate as to the extent of that involvement and the attributable risk of any stroke susceptibility gene.

This chapter reviews the background evidence for a genetic involvement in stroke, discusses the strategies available to identify those genes and reviews the susceptibility genes themselves.

EVIDENCE FOR THE GENETIC BASIS OF ISCHEMIC STROKE

Animal studies

Work on rat models has demonstrated the extent of stroke heritability and, as such, the animal literature is well ahead of parallel human work. Genome-wide multipoint linkage analysis has identified three rat chromosomal regions potentially containing stroke influencing genes in the spontaneous hypertensive rat-stroke prone (SHRSP) using a high salt, low potassium diet rat model.[1] The three genes asserted their risk independent of BP and together accounted for ~ 28% of the genetic variance of stroke susceptibility.

Another study using a different stroke-inducing mechanism in the SHRSP was designed to find genetic components involved in large infarct volumes. It found a highly significant quantitate trait locus on rat chromosome 5 that is estimated to account for ~ 67% of the total variance of the disease.[2] A trend of increasing infarct size with SHRSP gene dosage has supported the notion that genes may not only contribute to stroke onset but may also affect the eventual infarct size.[3]

In addition to the qualitative and quantitative effects of cerebral infarction, some recent data suggest that genes might influence functional recovery in the SHRSP compared to reference strain rat models;[4] such data in humans have yet to be conclusively demonstrated.

Human epidemiological studies

The long-established Framingham study has examined patterns of familial aggregation of stroke.[5] Among three generations, investigators showed that a history of paternal [relative risk (RR) 2.4] or maternal (RR 1.4) stroke, or a transient ischemic attack (TIA), was associated with an increased prevalence of these diseases in their offspring. Similarly, when examining the family histories of 90 patients with cerebral infarction, a significant positive family history for stroke was found in 47% of patients compared with 24% of controls.[6]

Several other studies have also supported a familial clustering of cerebral infarction. A Finnish study observed that a positive parental history of stroke was itself a stroke-risk predictor,[7] whereas a study based on patient questionnaire responses found that 25% of men and 35% of women reported a positive family history of stroke.[8] Such a family history was an independent predictor of stroke in females and of ischemic heart disease (IHD) in males. Interestingly, a maternal history of stroke is known to be a strong independent risk factor for strokes in middle-aged men.[9] A study that asked patients who had suffered a TIA about family history of coronary heart disease (CHD) and stroke showed an inherited predisposition for stroke, especially in the older age group.[10] From a large study of 30 000 subjects, the adjusted odds ratio (OR) of stroke in those with a positive paternal (OR = 2.0) and maternal (OR = 1.41) history was not altered by conventional risk factors including cholesterol, cigarette smoking status, CHD history, hypertension and diabetes.[11]

Finally, a family history of stroke is usually more frequently elucidated in large- and small-vessel stroke than in cardioembolic stroke.[12] This effect is amplified when vascular events occur before the age of 65 years, with OR = 2.93 [95% confidence interval (CI) 1.68–5.13] for large-vessel disease and OR = 3.15 (95% CI 1.81–5.50) for small-vessel disease.[13]

Twin studies

Classic genetic studies also support a genetic basis for sporadic ischemic stroke. The most compelling data perhaps come from the National Academy of Sciences National Research Council, which estimates concordance rates for stroke of 17.7% in monozygotic (MZ) twins and 3.6% for dizygotic (DZ) twins, with an RR of 4.3.[14] A more recent study using a Danish twin register reported similar concordance rates for stroke death at 10% in monozygotic (MZ) and 5% in dizygotic (DZ) pairs. The age- and sex-adjusted relative risk of stroke death in MZ compared with DZ twins was 2.1 (95% CI 1.3–3.3). Further analyses showed heritability indices of 0.32 for stroke death and 0.17 for stroke hospitalization.[15]

Although concordance rates for the MZ twins are relatively low (implicating a reasonable environmental component), their rates are high compared to the DZ twins, supporting a hypothesis for a genetic contribution to the prevalence of stroke.

MONOGENIC CAUSES OF STROKE

The single-gene disorders provide tantalizing insights into the possible mechanisms contributing to and underlying the more common phenotype. Two familial causes of ischemic stroke in adults have been identified; these are discussed below.

MELAS

Mitochondria produce ATP via oxidative phosphorylation and, as such, play a critical role in cell metabolism. Abnormalities in mitochondrial DNA (mtDNA) result in a variety of diseases involving many organs.[16] Human mtDNA has a failure replication failure rate of 1020 times that of genomic DNA, presumably due to the lack of proof reading polymerase enzymes.[16] MELAS (mitochondrial myopathy, encephalopathy, lactic acidosis, and stroke-like episodes) is one of the syndromes that occur as a result of mitochondrial mutations, the most common mutation (in around 80% of cases) being A3243G, although only 50% of patients with this mutation have strokes[17] (Fig. 5.1) and other molecular variants or mitochondrial haplotypes might influence the actual clinical phenotype.[18] The stroke deficits often improve but can lead to a progressive encephalopathy. Interestingly, some patients suffer from hemicranial headaches, which are indistinguishable from migraine. The finding of abnormal mitochondrial genome in the vascular endothelium of cerebral vessels might be the pathological basis for the stroke and the migrainous headaches.

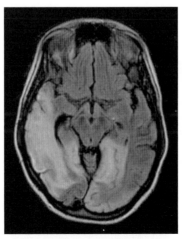

Fig. 5.1 MRI brain of patient presenting with multiple strokes with A3243G proven mutation causing MELAS.

CADASIL

Cerebral autosomal dominant arteriopathy with subcortical infarcts and leukoencephalopathy (CADASIL) is an inherited arterial disease whose acronym was first coined by Tournier-Lasserve et al.[19] The defect has been identified to the transmembrane protein *Notch3* gene (chromosome 19q12), which is believed to be involved in the specification of cell fate during development. Mutations mostly cluster around exons 3 and 4, either creating or destroying a cysteine residue. The clinical features observed include subcortical ischemic events in 84%, progressive or stepwise subcortical dementia with pseudobulbar palsy in 31%, migraine with aura in 22% and mood disorders with severe depressive episodes in 20%[20] and, more recently, seizures[21] in 10%.[22] The mean age of onset of symptoms is 45 years and most patients die by 65 years, as there is no available treatment. Importantly, CADASIL mutations have not been found to occur in common sporadic stroke.[23,24]

Few patients have come to autopsy but the pathological features include reduplication of the elastic media and granular material in the media of affected arteries. The cerebral arteriopathy is slowly progressive, resulting in thickening and fibrosis of small and medium-sized penetrating arteries with consequent narrowing of their lumen. MRI findings in CADASIL include symmetrical and extensive hyperintense signal within the cerebral white matter on T2-weighted images (Fig. 5.2) and well-defined hypointense lesions on T1-weighted images, suggestive of infarcts within the deep white matter and basal ganglia and hyperintensities in the white matter of the anterior temporal lobe using diffusion-weighted imaging.[25]

Other monogenic diseases associated with stroke

Like MELAS and CADASIL, which cause stroke-like symptoms, several other monogenic syndromes can mimic stroke. Familial hemiplegic migraine can result in transient focal neurological hemiparesis during migraine aura. It is an autosomal dominant disease with the genetic defect identified at the calcium channel *CACNA1A* gene on chromosome 19p13, although two other loci are likely to exist elsewhere.[26]

Ischemic events are not alone in possessing a likely underlying genetic etiology. Three other genes causing cerebral bleeding have been identified. Cystatin C gene[27] and Alzheimer amyloid gene[28] have both been identified in hereditary cerebral hemorrhage, whereas the *CCM1* gene as been found to be pathological

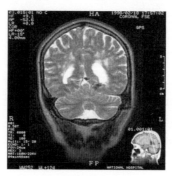

Fig. 5.2 T2-weighted MRI image of patient with CADASIL (with permission).

in hereditary cavernous angiomas.[29] Familial intracranial aneurysms have been linked to chromosomes 5q22-31, 7q11,[30,31] 14q22,[30] 19q12-13 and Xp22,[32,33] although finding the actual genes themselves is proving more difficult.

HUMAN GENETIC STUDIES

Over the last few years, numerous genetic studies in human stroke have been conducted, invariably using the candidate-gene-allele-based case-control model. Investigators have tried to determine the frequency of a variant allele within a candidate gene between an affected cohort compared to an unrelated, unaffected cohort, on the premise that the disease allele will be present in the affected group more often than would be predicted by Mendelian inheritance. This candidate gene approach allows us to identify possible genes based on our knowledge of the pathogenesis and pathophysiology of the condition. However, the number of subjects required by such an approach is quite large; for example, to detect a positive association of an allele that has a background rate of, say, 0.1 (i.e. a clinically relevant frequency) would require ~350 patients and an equal number of well-matched controls.[34] The power of this study would not only depend on the frequency of the risk allele but also on the relative risk conferred by this allele and on the chosen type-1 and type-2 errors. Even then, a negative association study does not exclude a suspect allele. Conversely, a positive study does not confirm the allele in question is necessarily disease causing; it might be in linkage disequilibrium with a nearby gene that has a functional variant on the candidate gene being explored, or on the nearby gene itself.[35] Notwithstanding these limitations, the relative ease with which patients can be recruited for this model, and the widespread availability of PCR molecular biology techniques, have led to a proliferation of publications on the genetics of stroke (Fig. 5.3).

Many of these studies have done much to further confuse, rather than enhance, our understanding by being underpowered and having conflicting results. One method of improving the statistical power of these small studies, allowing plausible candidate genes to be excluded, causative genes to be identified with reliability and genetic risks to be quantified with a greater degree of precision is to perform a meta-analysis. We have recently performed such an analysis for all genes that have been studied in ischemic stroke.[36] In total, 120

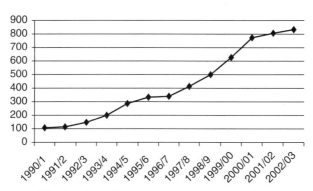

Fig. 5.3 Number of publications in stroke genetics per year.

case-control studies in Caucasians where the diagnosis of stroke was confirmed on neuroimaging and analyzed as a dichotomous trait were enrolled. This totaled 75 702 adult subjects (18 123 cases and 57 579 controls) in 32 genes (51 polymorphisms). Eight (53%) of the 15 meta-analyses had more than 1000 cases and seven (47%) had at least one study with a sample size greater than 1000 subjects. The results indicate that seven of the 15 (46.6%) candidate polymorphisms analyzed significantly increased the risk of stroke among individuals of European ancestry (Table 5.1). In four of these meta-analyses (*ACE-I/D, Factor-V Leiden, MTHFR/C677T* and *Prothrombin/G20210A*) the mean number of cases included per gene was more than 3000 subjects, allowing reasonably precise estimates of the effect of these genes to be made. The individual risk provided by any one of these candidate-genes was moderate (Fig. 5.4).

Other genetic markers that were associated with an increase in the risk for stroke but for which the data set was much smaller, were *glycoprotein Iβ-α*[Thr→Met] or *HPA-2* (OR 1.55), plasminogen activator inhibitor-1 (PAI-1) promoter 4G/5G insertion/deletion (OR 1.47), and *GpIβ-αKozak* sequence (OR 1.88). No significant associations were observed for three genes with a large data set: apolipoprotein E/ε4ε3ε2, *factor-XIII/Val→Leu* and *glycoprotein IIIa/Leu33*Pro or *HPA-1* polymorphisms.

The population attributable risks for the four positive and most investigated candidates *ACE-I/D, MTHFR/C677T, Factor-V Leiden* and *prothrombin/G20210A* following the models of inheritance shown in Table 5.1 were 4.54%, 3.31%, 2.16% and 1.30% respectively. This low level of risk is not surprising as the genetic contribution of any single gene towards a complex disease is unlikely to act in a simple Mendelian fashion but rather with epistatic (gene–gene or gene–environmental interactions) effects. Nevertheless, given the high incidence of stroke, if these estimates are correct they suggest that variants in four common genes might contribute to between 9000 and 32 000 strokes in the United States[36] and to between 2000 and 8000 in the UK each year. The results, however, can be extrapolated only to Caucasian populations; ethnic minorities have different inherited risk profiles[37] and similar analyses in different ethnic groups are awaited.

Association or causal?

Association studies do not prove causality. The role of *MTHFR/C677T*, with its OR for ischemic stroke of 1.24, deserves further discussion and serves as a paradigm for this question. Although it is known that the *MTHFR* gene partly determines homocysteine levels,[38] establishing causality has proved difficult and has been in part hampered by the fact that these factors tend to be associated with the presence of established risk factors, e.g. smoking, hypertension, cholesterol, with which they might be confounded.[39] Unlike many of the other genes with similar OR, folic acid is a readily available pharmacological intervention that will reduce homocysteine. The TT polymorphism increases homocysteine levels by ~2 μmol/L.[38,40] Consequently, the C677T polymorphism produces a natural (Mendelian) randomization.[41] As carriage of *MTHFR/C677T* is randomly assigned at meiosis, any association between this variant and homocysteine should be largely free from confounding by other determinants of homocysteine levels or risk factors for stroke. Any association between genotype and disease would therefore be predictable from the association between genotype and

Table 5.1 Odds ratio of candidate genes in ischemic stroke. (With permission of *Archives of Neurology* 61 : 1652.)

Gene (no. of studies)	Polymorphism	Genetic model	Frequency of variant at risk, %[*]	Cases, total no.	Controls, total no.	OR (95% CI)	P_{Het} Value
Factor V Leiden (26)[16–47]	Arg506Gln	Dominant	6.5	4588	13798	1.33 (1.12–1.58)	.03
MTHFR (22)[20,25–30,34,38,40,42–56]	C677T	Recessive	13.7	3387	4597	1.24 (1.08–1.42)	.22
Prothrombin (19)[†]	G20210A	Dominant	2.9	3028	7131	1.44 (1.11–1.86)	.91
ACE (11)[38,64–73]	I/D	Recessive	26.4	2990	11305	1.21 (1.08–1.35)	.47
Factor XIII (6)[74–79]	Val→Leu	Recessive	6.6	2166	1950	0.97 (0.75–1.25)	.08
Apolipoprotein E (10)[50,56,80–87]	ε4, ε3, ε2	Allele ε4 vs others	29.3	1805	10921	0.96 (0.84–1.11)	.02
Glycoprotein IIIa (9)[23,88–95]	Leu33Pro	Dominant	27.3	1467	2537	1.11 (0.95–1.28)	.76
eNOS (3)[94–98]	Glu298Asp	Recessive	12.5	1086	1089	0.98 (0.76–1.26)	.40
PAI1 (4)[74,90–101]	4G/5G	Recessive	18.9	842	1189	1.47 (1.13–1.92)	.75
GPIBA (3)[102–104]	VNTR	D/D vs others	2.08	816	719	0.81 (0.39–1.70)	.78
Glycoprotein IIb (3)[88,89,91]	Ile→Ser	Recessive	13.9	770	1090	0.99 (0.74–1.32)	.42
GPIBA(4)[88,91,102,104]	Thr→Met[‡]	Dominant	13.4	564	962	1.55 (1.14–2.11)	.68
Factor VII (3)[33,105,106]	A1/A2	Dominant	24.8	545	504	1.11 (0.83–1.48)	.20
GPIBA (3)[102,107,108]	Kozak sequence	T/T vs C/C + C/T	71.7	350	549	1.88 (1.28–2.76)	<.001
LPL (3)[108–111]	Asn291Ser	Dominant	4.78	452	8879	1.27 (0.80–2.01)	.73

Abbreviations: *ACE*, gene encoding angiotensin-converting enzyme; CI, confidence interval; *D/D*, deletion/deletion; *eNOS*, endothelial nitric oxide synthase; *GPIBA*, gene encoding glycoprotein Ib-α; I/D, insertion/deletion; *LPL*, gene encoding lipoprotein lipase; *MTHFR*, gene encoding methylenetetrahydrofolate reductase; OR, odds ratio; *PAI1*, gene encoding plasminogen activator inhibitor 1; *P P* for heterogeneity; VNTR, variable number tandem repeat.

[*]Derived from control subjects.

[†]References 17, 20, 22, 23, 26, 28–30, 32, 34, 38, 40, 57–63.

[‡]Also known as the *HPA2* polymorphism.

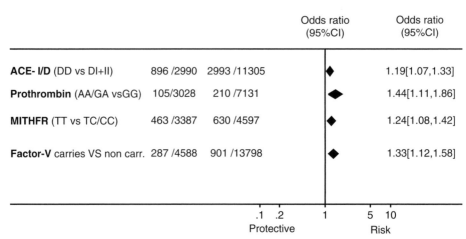

			Odds ratio (95%CI)	Odds ratio (95%CI)
ACE- I/D (DD vs DI+II)	896 /2990	2993 /11305		1.19[1.07,1.33]
Prothrombin (AA/GA vsGG)	105/3028	210 /7131		1.44[1.11,1.86]
MITHFR (TT vs TC/CC)	463 /3387	630 /4597		1.24[1.08,1.42]
Factor-V carries VS non carr.	287 /4588	901 /13798		1.33[1.12,1.58]

```
            .1   .2        1        5   10
            Protective              Risk
```

Fig. 5.4 Odds ratio of four extensively investigated genes in ischemic stroke.

homocysteine level, and homocysteine level and disease. This 'triangulation' (or comparison of risk estimates) between (1) genotype, (2) biochemical marker and (3) disease,[42] is the principle of 'Mendelian randomization'.[43] However, because any effect of homocysteine and genotype is likely to be small, very large numbers of patients are required to demonstrate this relationship. A meta-analysis of studies examining the association between *MTHFR* and stroke has demonstrated that subjects homozygous for *MTHFR/TT* have a significantly greater mean homocysteine level (1.93 μmol/L) and risk of stroke (OR 1.26; 95% CI 1.14–1.40) than those who are homozygous for *MTHFR/CC*.[44] As the two types of study conducted by these investigators have different sources of error, the consistency in results supports a causal role for homocysteine.[41] Commentators have further noted that this finding is likely to be robust compared with the underestimates obtained from observational studies, which correlate a single measurement of homocysteine with stroke risk.[41] The findings therefore suggest that lowering homocysteine by ~3 μmol/L with vitamin B therapy should reduce the population stroke risk by ~20%, although this remains to be proved in large-scale, prospective, adequately dosed, double-blind studies.[45] Notwithstanding this therapeutic caveat, the genetic–epidemiological strategy to discriminate between causal and noncausal associations has been argued to be potentially one of the most significant genetic contributions to complex disorders to date.[39]

OTHER GENETIC STRATEGIES FOR STROKE

Several criticisms of case control models should be borne in mind. The assignment of the control is always potentially contestable but, more importantly, a small sample of the overall population is necessarily studied. Clearly, it is logistically impractical to study whole large populations and studying isolated populations is an alternative. These populations are often closed communities and suffer from low migration rates and hence little admixture and thus may represent a more realistic picture.

Genome-wide studies

By utilizing the genealogical database of an isolated population for stroke a whole genome scan could be possible. Investigators have used such a strategy by using genetic data from an isolated Icelandic population.[46] Going against conventional wisdom, the investigators combined all stroke subtypes (hemorrhagic, ischemic stroke and TIAs), reasoning that as pedigrees could contain both broad types of stroke, the underlying genetic mechanisms might be similar. After all, cerebral arteries leak and cause cerebral hemorrhage because of previous ischemic damage.[47] Under this strategy, a maximum LOD score of 4.4 on 5q12 was achieved[46] and the gene encoding phosphodiesterase 4D (*PDE4D*) has recently been identified as the likely causative gene.[48] Three common haplotypes of *PDE4D* were identified as conferring high risk (RR 1.46, present in 16% of population) or low/protective risk (RR 0.7), relative to the wild-type haplotype present in 55% of the population. *PDE4D* is widely expressed and known to be an important regulator of intracellular levels of cAMP,[49] which is known to be altered in acute stroke[50] for several possible reasons.[51,52]

PDE4D was strongly associated with cardiogenic and carotid forms of stroke, which should intuitively be two distinct pathological processes. It has been argued that perhaps genetic predisposition to a cardiovascular/cerebrovascular disease ought to be seen in terms of overall vascular risk profile rather than highly specific pathophysiological processes.[52] The finding of the *ALOX5AP* gene as a susceptibility gene for both myocardial and cerebral infarction[53] with a near doubling in risk for either disease seems to support this view.

CONCLUSIONS

There is a genetic basis for stroke, albeit a moderate one. The strategies for dissecting-out the underlying genetic etiology for stroke are finally beginning to bear fruit. Genes have been identified in familial ischemic stroke, linkage to familial cerebral hemorrhagic diseases has been established and the genetics of common sporadic stroke has come of age now that comprehensive and systematic meta-analysis have provided robust and reliable attributable risk estimates. As national DNA repositories, such as the UK Biobank, begin to emerge, we can expect further genetic advances to take place ultimately leading to novel therapeutic targets.

References

1. Rubattu S, Volpe M, Kreutz R, et al. Chromosomal mapping of quantitative trait loci contributing to stroke in a rat model of complex human disease. *Nature Genet* 1996; 13:42929–42934.
2. Jeffs B, Clark JS, Anderson NH, et al. Sensitivity to cerebral ischaemic insult in a rat model of stroke is determined by a single genetic locus. *Nat Genet* 1997; 16:464–467.
3. Coyle P, Odenheimer DJ, Sing CF. Cerebral infarction after middle cerebral artery occlusion in progenies of spontaneously stroke-prone and normal rats. *Stroke* 1984;15:711–716.
4. McGill JK, Gallagher L, Carswell HVO, et al. Impaired functional recovery after stroke in the stroke-prone spontaneously hypertensive rat. *Stroke* 2005; 36:135–141.
5. Kiely DK, Wolf PA, Cupples LA, et al. Familial aggregation of stroke. The Framingham Study. *Stroke* 1993; 24:1366–1371.
6. Graffagnino C, Gasecki AP, Doig GS, Hachinski VC. The importance of family history in cerebrovascular disease. *Stroke* 1994; 25:1599–1604.

7. Jousilahti P, Rastenyte D, Tuomilehto J, et al. Parental history of cardiovascular disease and risk of stroke. A prospective follow-up of 14371 middle-aged men and women in Finland. *Stroke* 1997; 28:7361–7366.

8. Khaw KT, Barrett-Connor E. Family history of stroke as an independent predictor of ischemic heart disease in men and stroke in women. *Am J Epidemiol* 1986; 123:59–66.

9. Welin L, Svardsudd K, Wilhelmsen L, et al. Analysis of risk factors for stroke in a cohort of men born in 1913. *N Engl J Med* 1987;317:521–526.

10. Brass LM, Shaker LA. Family history in patients with transient ischemic attacks. *Stroke* 1991; 22:837–841.

11. Liao D, Myers R, Hunt S, et al. Familial history of stroke and stroke risk. The Family Heart Study. *Stroke* 1997; 28:10908–10912.

12. Schulz UGR, Flossmann E, Rothwell PM. Heritability of ischemic stroke in relation to age, vascular risk factors, and subtypes of incident stroke in population-based studies. *Stroke* 2004; 35:419–424.

13. Jerrard-Dunne P, Cloud G, Hassan A, Markus HS. Evaluating the genetic component of ischemic stroke subtypes: a family history study. *Stroke* 2003; 34:6364–6369.

14. Brass LM, Isaacsohn JL, Merikangas KR, Robinette CD. A study of twins and stroke. *Stroke* 1992; 23:221–223.

15. Bak S, Gaist D, Sindrup SH, et al. Genetic liability in stroke: a long-term follow-up study of Danish twins. *Stroke* 2002; 33:369–374.

16. Leonard JV, Schapira AH. Mitochondrial respiratory chain disorders I: mitochondrial DNA defects. *Lancet* 2000; 355:920099–920304.

17. Pulkes T, Sweeney MG, Hanna MG. Increased risk of stroke in patients with the A12308G polymorphism in mitochondria. *Lancet* 2000; 356:9247068–9247069.

18. Majamaa K, Finnila S, Turkka J, Hassinen IE. Mitochondrial DNA haplogroup U as a risk factor for occipital stroke in migraine. *Lancet* 1998; 352:912655–912656.

19. Joutel A, Bousser MG, Biousse V, et al. A gene for familial hemiplegic migraine maps to chromosome 19. *Nature Genet* 1993; 5:40–45.

20. Chabriat H, Vahedi K, Iba-Zizen MT, et al. Clinical spectrum of CADASIL: a study of 7 families. *Lancet* 1995; 346:934–939.

21. Sharma P, Wang T, Brown MJ, Schapira AH. Fits and strokes. *Lancet* 2001; 358:927620.

22. Dichgans M, Mayer M, Uttner I, et al. The phenotypic spectrum of CADASIL: clinical findings in 102 cases. *Ann Neurol* 1998; 44:531–539.

23. Wang T, Sharma SD, Fox N, et al. Description of a simple test for CADASIL disease and determination of mutation frequencies in sporadic ischaemic stroke and dementia patients. *J Neurol Neurosurg Psychiatry* 2000; 69:552–554.

24. Dong Y, Hassan A, Zhang Z, et al. Yield of screening for CADASIL mutations in lacunar stroke and leukoaraiosis. *Stroke* 2003; 34:103–105.

25. O'Sullivan M, Jarosz JM, Martin RJ, et al. MRI hyperintensities of the temporal lobe and external capsule in patients with CADASIL. *Neurology* 2001; 56:528–534.

26. Ducros A, Denier C, Joutel A, et al. The clinical spectrum of familial hemiplegic migraine associated with mutations in a neuronal calcium channel. *N Engl J Med* 2001; 345:17–24.

27. Palsdottir A, Abrahamson M, Thorsteinsson L, et al. Mutation in cystatin C gene causes hereditary brain haemorrhage. *Lancet* 1988; 2:861103–861104.

28. Levy E, Carman MD, Fernandez-Madrid IJ, et al. Mutation of the Alzheimer's disease amyloid gene in hereditary cerebral hemorrhage, Dutch type. *Science* 1990; 248:4959124–4959126.

29. Laberge-le-Couteulx S, Jung HH, Labauge P, et al. Truncating mutations in CCM1, encoding KRIT1, cause hereditary cavernous angiomas. *Nature Genet* 1999; 23:289–293.

30. Onda H, Kasuya H, Yoneyama T, et al. Genomewide-linkage and haplotype-association studies map intracranial aneurysm to chromosome 7q11. *Am J Hum Genet* 2001; 69:404–419.

31. Farnham JM, Camp NJ, Neuhausen SL, et al. Confirmation of chromosome 7q11 locus for predisposition to intracranial aneurysm. *Hum Genet* 2004; 114:350–355.

32. van der Voet M, Olson JM, Kuivaniemi H, et al. Intracranial aneurysms in Finnish families: confirmation of linkage and refinement of the interval to chromosome 19q13.3. *Am J Hum Genet* 2004; 74:564–571.

33. Yamada S, Utsunomiya M, Inoue K, et al. Genome-wide scan for Japanese familial intracranial aneurysms: linkage to several chromosomal regions. *Circulation* 2004; 110:24727–24733.

34. Sharma P. Genes for ischaemic stroke: strategies for their detection. *J Hypertens* 1996; 14:377–385.

35. Holopainen P, Arvas M, Sistonen P, et al. CD28/CTLA4 gene region on chromosome 2q33 confers genetic susceptibility to celiac disease. A linkage and family-based association study. *Tissue Antigens* 1999; 53:570–575.

36. Casas JP, Hingorani AD, Bautista LE, Sharma P. Meta-analysis of genetic studies in ischaemic stroke: 32 genes involving 18,000 cases and 58,000 controls. *Arch Neurol* 2004; 61:1652–1662.

37. Lisabeth LD, Ireland JK, Risser JMH, et al. Stroke risk after transient ischemic attack in a population-based setting. *Stroke* 2004; 35:8842–8846.

38. Wald DS, Law M, Morris JK. Homocysteine and cardiovascular disease: evidence on causality from a meta-analysis. *Br Med J* 2002; 325:7374202.

39. Keavney B. Genetic epidemiological studies of coronary heart disease. *Int J Epidemiol* 2000; 31:430–436.

40. Klerk M, Verhoef P, Clarke R, et al. MTHFR 677C → T polymorphism and risk of coronary heart disease: a meta-analysis [see comment]. *JAMA* 2002; 288:16023–16031.

41. Hankey GJ, Eikelboom JW. Homocysteine and stroke. *Lancet* 2005; 365:194–195.

42. Smith GD, Ebrahim S. 'Mendelian randomization': can genetic epidemiology contribute to understanding environmental determinants of disease? *Int J Epidemiol* 2003; 32:1–22.

43. Little J, Khoury MJ. Mendelian randomisation: a new spin or real progress? *Lancet* 2003; 362:930–931.

44. Casas JP, Bautista LE, Smeeth L, et al. Homocysteine and stroke: evidence on a causal link from mendelian randomisation. *Lancet* 2005; 365:945524–945532.

45. Toole JF, Malinow MR, Chambless LE, et al. Lowering homocysteine in patients with ischemic stroke to prevent recurrent stroke, myocardial infarction, and death: the Vitamin Intervention for Stroke Prevention (VISP) randomized controlled trial [see comment]. *JAMA* 2004; 291:565–575.

46. Gretarsdottir S, Sveinbjornsdottir S, Jonsson HH, et al. Localization of a susceptibility gene for common forms of stroke to 5q12. *Am J Hum Genet* 2002; 70:593–603.

47. Dickinson CJ. Genetics of stroke. *Lancet* 2004; 364:943481.

48. Gretarsdottir S, Thorgeirsson G, Reynisdottir S, et al. The gene encoding phosphodiesterase 4D confers risk of ischemic stroke. *Nat Genet* 2003; 35:131–138.

49. Xu RX, Hassell AM, Vanderwall D, et al. Atomic structure of PDE4: insights into phosphodiesterase mechanism and specificity. *Science* 2000; 288:5472822–5472825.

50. Buttner T, Hornig CR, Busse O, Dorndorf W. CSF cyclic AMP and CSF adenylate kinase in cerebral ischaemic infarction. *J Neurol* 1986; 233:597–603.

51. Iadecola C, Zhang F, Xu S, et al. Inducible nitric oxide synthase gene expression in brain following cerebral ischemia. *J Cerebral Blood Flow Metab* 1995; 15:378–384.

52. Sharma P. Cracking the genetics of cerebrovascular disease. *Lancet* 2004; 363:1839–1840.

53. Helgadottir A, Manolescu A, Thorleifsson G, et al. The gene encoding 5-lipoxygenase activating protein confers risk of myocardial infarction and stroke. *Nate Genet* 2004;36: 333–339.

6 | Genetics of pre-eclampsia

Fiona Broughton Pipkin and Linda Morgan

INTRODUCTION

Some hypertension occurs in ~10% of pregnancies. However, in 1–3%, hypertension is associated with proteinuria (pre-eclampsia; PE) and is a manifestation of extensive endothelial dysfunction. In these women, the global nature of endothelial damage results in a multisystem disorder that can include renal impairment, hepatocellular damage, platelet activation, hemolysis and, rarely, convulsions. It arises, apparently *de novo*, in women thought previously to be in normal health, can reach life-threatening intensity within a few days and usually begins to resolve shortly after delivery of the placenta.

For research purposes, the broad consensus diagnosis of PE requires the occurrence of a blood pressure of 140/90 mmHg on at least two occasions separated by at least 6 hours after the twentieth week of pregnancy in a woman known to have been normotensive before this time and in whom the blood pressure returns to normal by 6–12 weeks after delivery. This hypertension must be accompanied by significant proteinuria (300 mg/L or 500 mg/24 h) in the absence of urinary tract infection;[1,2] edema is now not used as a diagnostic criterion. Elements of the syndrome can occur in the absence of clinical hypertension, and hypertension and/or proteinuria in pregnancy are not always associated with PE; it can also be superimposed on essential hypertension or renal disease. There is currently no biochemical marker to reliably identify women with the syndrome. In some, PE might be the result of pregnancy unmasking latent hypertension, as it can unmask latent diabetes, but other women can pass the rest of their lives with normal blood pressures.

An associated condition is the HELLP syndrome (hemolysis, elevated serum liver enzyme concentrations and a low platelet count). The outcome differs across populations. A study of a predominantly African–American population in the Southern US reported 'a high incidence' of maternal complications,[3] whereas in the UK, a large prospective study reported disease-specific morbidities of 1 : 250 for severe PE and 1 : 2000 for HELLP.[4]

Placentation is abnormal in women who suffer PE. Normal placentation involves the remodeling of the spiral arteries into thin-walled, large-bore vessels.[5] This is achieved by the highly invasive cytotrophoblast, which changes phenotype to a vascular form.[6] These changes are much reduced in PE placentae, and in those associated with intrauterine growth restriction (IUGR).[5,7] Any study of the causes of PE needs to take these abnormalities into account. However, there is no suitable way of investigating early placentation in pregnancies that are subsequently affected by PE. Furthermore, although much is known of the pathology and biochemistry of established PE, it is difficult to distinguish between cause and effect. The window of opportunity for functional studies is small, as the phenotype is transient, usually resolving fully following delivery. However, maternal and fetal genotypes remain unaltered by the condition and can be studied at any time before, during or after the affected pregnancy. Functional correlates of genetic variation can be studied *in vitro*, providing insights into disease mechanisms and identifying potential targets for therapeutic interventions.

This chapter considers the evidence that PE has an inherited component, the strategies that can be adopted in the search for susceptibility genes and gives an overview of published association studies of candidate genes, grouped by their physiological effects in relation to the known pathophysiology of PE. Two exhaustive reviews of published studies to late 2001 were published in 2002;[8,9] this chapter largely concentrates on the more recent data.

EVIDENCE THAT PE HAS AN INHERITED COMPONENT

Until very recently, the diagnosis of PE recorded in older datasets was variable and unreliable. Even so, epidemiological studies have consistently shown a 3- to 5-fold increase in the risk of PE or eclampsia in first-degree relatives of affected women.[10–17]

Initial attempts to identify a model of inheritance by segregation analysis of extended families assumed that PE was due to a single gene. A number of models were suggested by various datasets, including a maternal recessive gene or a maternal dominant gene with partial penetrance.[15,16] The fetal genotype is one factor that might affect the penetrance of maternal genes. When three sets of data were tested against six possible models of single gene inheritance, the model that fitted the data best was that of fetal and maternal homozygosity for a shared recessive gene.[18] The diversity of models suggested by pedigree analysis implies that PE is not inherited as a Mendelian disorder, although it might be due to a single gene in some families. Thus a more complex model would include interplay between maternal and/or fetal genes and genetic interactions with environmental factors.

The ratio of the risk to sibs of affected women to the risk in the general population is known as the sibling relative risk (λ_s). A λ_s for PE of 3–5 is comparable to that for type 2 diabetes ($\lambda_s \sim 3.5$)[19] and considerably lower than that for type 1 diabetes ($\lambda_s \sim 15$). λ_s reflects both genetic and shared environmental factors such as diet, socioeconomic circumstances and exposure to infective agents. Comparison of concordance for disease in dizygotic (DZ) twins with that in monozygotic (MZ) twins, sharing respectively 50% and 100% of their genes, allows the dissection of genetic and environmental influences on the risk of disease.

Evidently, only parous female twin pairs are informative, so even studies based on large twin registries have lacked statistical power. A study from the

Swedish Twin Register, which includes data from all twin births in Sweden (avoiding possible ascertainment bias inherent in voluntary twin registries[20]) and the Medical Birth Register, which covers 99% of all births, provided 917 pairs of parous MZ sisters, including eight who were concordant for PE and 47 who were discordant.[21] Amongst 1199 pairs of DZ twins, two pairs were concordant and 59 were discordant for PE. Their estimate of the heritability of PE was 0.54 [confidence interval (CI) 0–0.71] and for gestational hypertension (GH) was 0.24 (CI 0–0.53). When GH was considered as a mild form of PE, the heritability was 0.47 (CI 0.13–0.61).

In a novel statistical approach to the problem of estimating heritability in PE, data from 239 193 sib pairs and their partners who had had between one and three pregnancies (total 774 858) recorded in the Swedish Birth Registry between 1987 and 1997 were analysed;[22] 20 358 were complicated by PE. The calculated heritability due to maternal genetic effects was 0.35, with narrow confidence intervals of 0.33–0.36. They also estimated heritability due to fetal genes, whether maternally or paternally inherited, as 0.20 (CI 0.11–0.24).

A study of data from the Medical Birth Registry of Norway reported that women who conceived by a man who previously fathered a PE pregnancy in a different woman had an odds ratio of 1.8 (CI 1.2–2.6) for developing PE.[23] Another study of 1777 pregnancies used the Utah Population Database, which recorded whether either parent had been born from a PE pregnancy.[24] This reported that a man who had been born of a PE pregnancy had a 2.1-fold (CI 1.0–4.3) increase in risk of fathering a PE pregnancy. These studies support a rôle for paternally inherited fetal genes.

Interplay between maternal and fetal genes is consistent with the two-stage model hypothesis of the etiology of PE. The first stage involves placentation (see above) with interactions between fetally derived trophoblast and maternal uterine tissue. Complex mechanisms ensure that the foreign paternally encoded antigens do not cause maternal rejection of the trophoblast in healthy pregnancies. It is proposed that impaired placentation results in poor placental perfusion, and the generation of free radicals. Fragments of trophoblast and oxidized lipids, which are released into the maternal circulation in healthy pregnancies, are present in higher concentrations in PE pregnancies.[25] The second stage would involve the maternal response to the pregnancy. If a woman is unable to mount an effective response to circulating factors derived from the placenta, endothelial damage results and the syndrome of PE ensues.[26] Maternal genes could play a critical role in this response.

IDENTIFICATION OF SUSCEPTIBILITY GENES FOR PE

Genome screening

Genome screening involves a search for genetic data to inform pathophysiological hypotheses (see Chapter 4). Currently, this approach requires a number of families with more than one member affected by the condition. The identification of extended pedigrees affected by PE presents problems, because neither males nor nulliparous females are informative. Furthermore, classical linkage analysis requires specification of the model of inheritance, which is uncertain in PE; misspecification of the model results in loss of power to detect susceptibility loci. Model-free approaches to linkage analysis have been used for the study of PE, including affected sibpair analysis. As family sizes in the Western world decrease, identification of pairs of sisters affected by PE becomes increasingly time-consuming and expensive.

Nevertheless, a number of genome-wide linkage screens for maternal susceptibility genes have been published. The first report included 15 Australian families and implicated a locus on chromosome 4q;[27] this was later given some support by a study of 15 Finnish families.[28] Analysis of Scandinavian and Dutch populations variously identified segregation at chromosomes 2p12, 2p25, 9p1 and 10q22 but no other evidence of linkage to chromosome 4q.[28–31] One study[29] included two large multicase families, which showed strong linkage to chromosome 2p. When the data were reanalyzed without these two families there was no evidence of linkage. This might simply reflect the greater statistical power of linkage analysis in large pedigrees; however, it might suggest that in these two families PE is a Mendelian disorder due to a gene on chromosome 2. Available data are thus inconclusive.

Lack of consistent reproducibility of linkage studies has bedeviled research into such complex disorders as nonpregnant hypertension. The relatively low power of linkage studies to detect genes with small effects has contributed to this. Susceptibility genes for most complex disorders will probably be associated with a locus specific risk for disease of around 1.5, well below the limits of detection of many linkage studies. A further limitation of linkage studies is their low resolution; susceptibility loci might extend over 50 cM (~50 million bases) of the genome, and include many putative susceptibility genes. Refining susceptibility loci requires a finer net of DNA markers, which can be applied to populations rather than pedigrees. The development of extensive databases of single nucleotide polymorphisms (SNPs) (see: http://www.snp.cshl.org) and haplotype mapping of the human genome (see: http://www.hapmap.org), together with recent advances in genotyping technology, have raised hopes that it will be possible in the near future to conduct genome-wide screens using SNP genotyping applied to DNA collections from unrelated individuals.

Candidate genes

Candidate gene analysis uses pathophysiological knowledge to suggest likely genes for analysis. The choice is influenced by the current understanding of the pathophysiology of the disorder, and is supported if the gene lies within a region identified by linkage studies. Most published studies have used a case-control design, comparing the frequencies of allelic variants in women with PE and normotensive pregnancies. Although there have been many published reports of association between genetic variants and PE (e.g. see ref. 8), none has been consistently replicated in independent studies. Aspects of study design might contribute to this; a careful definition of inclusion criteria for cases and controls is vital, and subtle ethnic stratification of groups must be avoided. Furthermore, very few researchers report the performance characteristics of their genotyping assays – specifically, the rate of misgenotyping – or the quality assurance procedures that they adopted. The most important cause of poor reproducibility of results of candidate gene studies, in PE as in all complex disorders, is almost certainly the reporting of false-positive results, based on insufficiently stringent criteria for statistical significance. With over 20 000 genes and 2 million SNPs available, multiple testing will inevitably result in a plethora of results that achieve P values of < 0.05. Identifying the optimum method of statistical correction that will minimize both false-positive and false-negative results is the subject of current debate.[32,33] What is clear, however, is that sample sizes in the hundreds, possibly thousands, are required to provide robust studies of genetic variants that are likely to have small individual effects. This calls for collaborative approaches between multiple research groups with an interest in PE.

One further aspect of study design needs to be considered in disorders of pregnancy. How are the effects of fetal and maternal genes to be distinguished? A genetic variant associated with PE, which is active in the fetus, will be present at increased frequency not only in affected babies but also in the parents from whom it was inherited. Similarly, a variant that is active in the mother will also be overrepresented in her offspring. A strategy known as transmission disequilibrium testing addresses this problem.[34] This approach is based on the expectation that heterozygous parents have a probability of 0.5 of transmitting either allele to their offspring. Significant deviations from this expected frequency in child–parent trios affected by PE indicate that the allele that is overtransmitted is associated with disease, and is active in the offspring.

CANDIDATE GENES IN RELATION TO PATHOPHYSIOLOGY

PE should be considered as a syndrome, probably initiated in the first weeks of pregnancy, rather than a disease. The control of the systemic arterial blood pressure is multifactorial, and both the endocrinological and the complex autonomic control mechanisms change significantly during normotensive and hypertensive pregnancy.[35,36] There are probably multiple susceptibility genes for PE, which vary by ethnicity and by environmental exposure. Research using tightly phenotyped subgroups might allow the identification of a more limited set of genes predisposing to that phenotype.[37] Such an approach is being used for the ongoing multicentre UK Genetics of PE Study (GOPEC).

This section focuses on the potential involvement of polymorphisms in candidate genes, where those polymorphisms are known to be associated with a change in protein structure or gene regulation, which is associated with a functional effect relevant to the PE phenotype. As noted above, until very recently there was ambiguity in the definition of 'PE' used in a number of studies, with some evidently including, or indeed mainly comprising, women with GH, rather than PE. Given the different long-term outcomes of such women, such data should be regarded with caution.

The renin–angiotensin–aldosterone system

Although initially described as a classic circulating hormone, angiotensin II (ANG II) is now also known to have autocrine and paracrine effects. All components of the renin–angiotensin–aldosterone system (RAAS) are present in human endometrium and decidua.[38] mRNAs for renin, angiotensinogen (AGT), angiotensin-converting enzyme (ACE) and the ANG II type 1 receptor (AT1R) are present in decidua from at least as early as 5 weeks gestation.[39,40] Renin and AGT are localized around the spiral arteries, which are not yet fully remode[...] whereas AT1Rs are found mainly in decidual perivascular stromal cells.[...]

suggests that locally generated ANG II might be involved in the spiral artery remodeling that is central to successful placentation and impaired in PE. Furthermore, autoantibodies agonistic to the AT1R have been demonstrated in almost all women with PE,[41] and these decrease trophoblast invasiveness *in vitro*.[42]

Angiotensinogen

Polymorphisms in the *AGT* gene in relation to hypertension and cardiovascular disease are discussed elsewhere in this volume (see Chapter 7). The widely-studied *AGT* 235Met>Thr polymorphism is significantly more prevalent in female than in male subjects with essential hypertension[43] with both plasma [AGT] and the probability of hypertension running with allele number.[43] A significantly higher frequency of the 235Thr allele was initially reported in 41 PE women (in Utah, USA) than in either women with GH or controls.[44] A number of other studies have since addressed this polymorphism, with rather more than half failing to identify an association (see ref. 8), although haplotype analysis in some populations has suggested associations with PE.[45] There is a wide ethnic variation in allele frequency, which might account for the difference, and it is interesting that one of the strongest associations has been revealed in a group of Japanese women of higher body mass index (BMI) and a preference for salty dishes.[46] The Thr allele is present at a frequency of 0.84 in the Japanese population. IUGR is very prevalent in PE. The 235Thr allele has also been reported in significant excess in association with nonhypertensive IUGR.[47]

A subset of nonpregnant patients with essential hypertension (EHT) show a reduced response of the renal blood flow to ANG II infusion during a period of high salt intake and a reduced aldosterone response to ANG II during a low salt intake ['nonmodulating (NM) hypertension'].[48] NM hypertension is associated with the 235Thr allele.[49] A significant association has been reported between the Thr allele and a low plasma volume (PV) in nulligravid women.[50] The PV rises significantly over the first 6 weeks of human pregnancy, in parallel with increases in plasma renin activity and aldosterone (ALD) concentration[51] and cardiac output.[51–53] There is thus a proactive response to the stimulus of conception, which is 'perceived' as a state of underfilling. However, in established pregnancy hypertension, PV is reduced,[54,55] and in a proportion of such women remains low months into the puerperium.[56] Women with pregnancy-associated hypertension have a decreased plasma renin : ALD ratio compared with normotensive women.[57]

Angiotensin receptors

At least four types of receptor for ANG II have been described. AT1R is the most prevalent in adult tissues, where it mediates the vasoconstrictor and growth-promoting effects of ANG II. Very little is known about the functional effects of receptor polymorphisms at the molecular level (see Chapter 3). A number of groups have studied polymorphisms in the *AGTR1* gene (chromosome 3q21-q25) in relation to PE, but none has identified a significant effect of any polymorphism in isolation.[45,58–61] Haplotype analysis of *AGTR1* polymorphisms has also failed to reveal any association.[61] Interestingly, however, a small study has reported that women with PE and the *AGT* 235Thr/Thr genotype were significantly more likely to carry the 1166C allele of the 1166A>C polymorphism of the *AGTR1* gene than normotensive pregnant women.[60] This allele has been reported to be associated with decreased endothelium-dependent and endothelium-independent vasodilatation in healthy nonpregnant subjects.[62]

A number of polymorphisms outside the coding region of the *AGTR2* gene (chromosome Xq24-q25) have been described. The AT2R is expressed at a high density during fetal development, but this expression declines rapidly after birth (reviewed in ref. 63). The AT2R in many respects counters the effects of ANG II mediated through the AT1Rs, inhibiting vascular and perivascular cell growth and proliferation, promoting apoptosis, inhibiting extracellular matrix proteins and being associated with vasodilatation.[63] The only published study of the *AGTR2* genotype in relation to PE[61] reported a significant difference in maternal haplotype distribution between normotensive and PE pregnancies. The mechanism of this effect is not known, but it may be through alteration in the balance of expression of the two main receptor subtypes.

Angiotensin-converting enzyme

Plasma concentrations of ACE fall in the first half of normal pregnancy, before rising to term;[64] data in hypertensive pregnancy are less clear-cut, with both no change and a small increase being reported.[65,66] However, as human placental tissue contains both ACE mRNA[67] and protein,[68] and is highly vascularized, it is possible that ACE might influence placentation. The *ACE* gene (chromosome 17q23) has a well-documented insertion : deletion (I/D) polymorphism in intron 16,[69] which accounts for half of the variance in plasma [ACE]. This has been the subject of considerable study in relation to nonpregnant hypertension (see Chapter 4). Studies of the I/D genotype in PE have almost all described no significant association.[45,59,60,70,71] Differences were reported in a group of parous Italian women with a history of PE, between those who did and did not develop PE in a subsequent pregnancy,[72] but their long-term likelihood of nonpregnant hypertension also differed, making interpretation difficult.[73]

Aldosterone

Women with established PE have a nearly four-fold lower excretion of tetrahydro-aldosterone, suggesting a reduction in CYP11B2 (aldosterone synthase) activity.[74] There is also evidence for a reduction in methyl oxidase activity. The enzyme CYP11B2 catalyses the final steps of aldosterone biosynthesis and has 11β-hydroxylase, 18β-hydroxylase and 18-methyl oxidase activities. The *CYP11B2* gene (chromosome 8q22) has several polymorphisms which have been related to various forms of nonpregnant human hypertension. In a recent study of two Swiss populations, a significantly increased proportion of women with PE carried one or more polymorphisms in *CYP11B2* than matched controls.[74] Interestingly, a previously described polymorphism in exon 7, the 386Val>Ala polymorphism, was detected in 17% of the PE women but none of the controls. This polymorphism has been associated with reduced CYP11B2 activity. Study of other functional polymorphisms in the aldosterone synthase cascade is merited given the reduced plasma volume of PE.

Endothelial cell function

Nitric oxide

Nitric oxide (NO) is a highly potent, locally synthesized vasodilator. Its local synthesis makes it very difficult to study in human pregnancy and there are conflicting data, suggesting either that synthesis is decreased (potentially causal) or increased (counterbalancing a vasoconstricted state) in PE. The interaction of NO and superoxide produces the anion peroxynitrite (ONOO), which is pro-oxidant and can cause vascular damage. Peroxynitrite can be detected histochemically by localization of nitrotyrosine residues. In PE, increased staining for nitrotyrosine is localized in villous vascular endothelium and the surrounding vascular smooth muscle.[75,76] However, NO synthase staining was simultaneously identified in the endothelium of stem villous vessels, which might be an adaptive response to the increased resistance. Thus an increase in nitric oxide synthesis might in fact be worsening oxidative damage (see below).

Although a number of polymorphisms in the endothelial NO synthase (*NOS3*) gene (chromosome 7q36) have been described as having clinical significance, there is very marked ethnic differentiation in allele frequency,[77] which might imply a different rôle when interacting with the rest of the genotype. Furthermore, smoking can differentially interact with *NOS3* polymorphisms,[78] and it is rare for reported studies to stratify by smoking habit.

Affected pedigree member analysis in 50 families from Scotland and Iceland suggested linkage between the *NOS3* locus, and a familial GH[79] variant within exon 7 (nucleotide 894G>T) has been identified, which results in the missense polymorphism 298Glu>Asp. This is associated with increased proteolytic cleavage and decreased bioavailability. Reduced flow-mediated vasodilatation has been reported in first trimester pregnancy[80] in normal women carrying the Asp allele. The frequency of the 298Asp variant was reported as being significantly higher in a group of predominantly primigravid Japanese women with severe pre-eclampsia than in controls,[81] and homozygosity for Asp was associated with a 6-fold increase in the risk of PE in a Colombian population.[82] However, no such association has been reported in Western European, Hispanic/White US or Bangladeshi populations,[83-85] in all of which the Asp variant is present in markedly higher frequency.

A further polymorphism, 786T>C, is present in the promoter region of *NOS3*, and studies *in vitro* suggest that it is associated with reduced activity. This has not been associated with PE.[82,83]

Another polymorphism in this gene is a variable number of tandem repeats (VNTR) in intron 4, the *NOS3*A* polymorphism. This polymorphism has been associated with an increased risk of PE in a small study of predominantly Mexican Hispanic women[86] but not in Colombian women of various ancestry, including Hispanic White.[82] Functional effects for this intronic polymorphism have not been described, and it may be acting as a marker for a functional polymorphism elsewhere in the gene.

Curiously, known polymorphisms, with functional correlations, in the prostacylin- and kallikrein-generating systems, appear not to have been studied in relation to PE, even though prostacyclin excretion, like that of kallikrein, is significantly reduced in the first trimester in women who go on to develop PE.[87] Here, perhaps, is another area for investigation.

RECEPTOR-COUPLED G-PROTEINS

The main role of the trimeric G-proteins is to convert signals from the cell surface into a cellular response. The G-protein family is big and very variable, and the type of α, β and γ subunits in any G-protein determine its specificity. There is a common polymorphism (825C>T) in exon 10 of the gene for the β3 subunit (chromosome 12p13), which is associated with increased G-protein activation and has been linked to hypertension, dyslipidemia, insulin resistance and obesity.[88] However, a single case-control study in PE did not identify any association.[89]

Endogenous oxidant/antioxidant systems

It is likely that the initiation of maternal perfusion of the placenta does not occur until the end of the first trimester.[90] This would result in a fairly rapid increase in local oxygen tension, which should be accompanied by increased expression and activity of such antioxidants as glutathione peroxidase, catalase and the various forms of superoxide dismutase.[91] If this antioxidant response were reduced, then the cascade of events leading to impaired placentation could be initiated. Lipid peroxidation has been a candidate causative agent for the endothelial damage of PE for more than 20 years.[92] Evidence for reduced antioxidant activity in PE has recently been reviewed;[93] however, genetic studies are surprisingly limited. For example, catalase has not been studied at all in this context, and there is only one very small study of any of the superoxide dismutases.

The cytosolic glutathione-S-transferases (GSTs) form a large family. The P class is the form expressed in highest levels outside the liver, and is expressed at a high level in human placental tissues.[94] To date, there appears to be only one study of a possible role for polymorphisms in this family in relation to PE, reporting on 170 women with a history of PE, 90 of whom had had HELLP syndrome and 109 of whom were healthy control women. Of the polymorphisms examined, only the glutathione-S-transferase P1b/1b genotype (chromosome 11q.13) was present in higher frequency in previously PE women.[95] This has been associated with lower glutathione-S-transferase activity.

Several polymorphisms have been described in the gene for the p22phox subunit of NADPH/NADH oxidase (CYBA; chromosome 16q.24), which is part of the cascade of superoxide generation. One (242C>T) in exon 4, results in an amino acid substitution (72His>Tyr), which has been associated with worsening atherosclerosis in populations at risk.[96] This polymorphism was, however, recently reported to show no evidence of an association with either PE or HELLP/PE.[97]

Prothrombotic polymorphisms

Abnormalities of the clotting cascade are well known in women with PE.[98] A subset of women develop frank thrombocytopenia, often in association with HELLP. The endothelial damage of PE is associated with an altered phenotype from anticoagulant to procoagulant and decreased endothelially mediated vasorelaxation. It is not known whether this phenotype is present before PE pregnancy or secondary to damage initiated during placentation. However, there is reduced expression of such endothelial anticoagulant factors as protein S and antithrombin III in the face of increases in the procoagulatory plasminogen-activator inhibitor-1 (PAI-1), von Willebrand factor, endothelin and fibronectin.[99,100] It is therefore not surprising that a number of functional polymorphisms, with clinical correlates in nonpregnant subjects, should have been studied in relation to PE.

5,10-Methylene tetrahydrofolate reductase

Homocysteine (HCy) is a demethylated metabolite of the essential amino acid methionine. Hyperhomocysteinemia is associated with procoagulatory changes and decreased endothelially mediated vasorelaxation, as well as increased lipid peroxidation, serum uric acid and triglycerides. Even moderately raised plasma [HCy] is associated with endothelial damage, thought to be via increased hydrogen peroxide formation. Normal pregnancy is associated with decreased plasma [HCy] from the first trimester,[101] but a proportion of women with PE have concentrations similar to those of nonpregnant women.[102]

5,10-Methylene tetrahydrofolate reductase (MTHFR) catalyzes the reduction of 5,10-methylenetetrahydrofolate to 5-methyltetrahydrofolate, which is the main circulatory form of folate and the carbon donor for the remethylation of homocysteine to methionine. There are two common functional polymorphisms of *MTHFR* (chromosome 1p36.3), 677C>T[103] and 1298A>C,[104] which specify thermolabile enzymes with mildly reduced activity and hence increased [HCy] when folate status is low.[105] The allele frequency of 677T varies very widely with ethnicity, from 9% in Indonesians[106] to 58% in Peruvians.[107]

The 677T polymorphism has been the subject of more than 50 published studies in relation to PE since the first reports in 1997 suggested an association.[108,109] However, these have been contradictory, even when corrected for folate status, smoking habit and parity. Recent meta-analyses[110,111] using data from 'hypertensive' and control women, reported a small overall increase in risk [odds ratio (OR) 1.21; 95% confidence interval (CI) 1.01–1.44] in association with the T allele, with little change when the analysis was confined to women with PE (OR 1.40; 95% CI 1.08–1.83) or severe PE (OR 1.4; 95% CI 0.9–2.0). These analyses include women from a wide variety of ethnic backgrounds and parities, with significant between-study heterogeneity. They support the impression that, overall, any contribution of polymorphisms in the MTHFR gene to the risk of developing PE must be very small. However, three studies have reported nonsignificant increases in 677T-allele frequency in multiparous women with PE by comparison with primiparous women.[108,109,112] PE/eclampsia presenting only in the first pregnancy has a different long-term prognosis from repeated PE.[113,114] There is no convincing evidence linking the 677T polymorphism with HELLP in populations in the Southern USA[115] or Western Europe.[116]

No evidence was found suggesting an increased prevalence of paternally inherited 677T alleles in the fetuses of PE women compared to controls.[106] The 1298A>C polymorphism appears only to have been reported in two studies,[116,117] and neither alone nor in combination with 677C>T was there an association with PE and/or eclampsia.

Factor V

The functional point mutation at nucleotide 1691G>A (exon 10) of the *FV* gene (chromosome 1q23) causes the substitution of Gln for Arg at position 506 and resistance to activated protein C (the 'factor V Leiden' mutation).[118] The mutation seems to be relatively recent and of Western European origin; the allele is absent or present only at very low frequency in the south and east of Europe.[119] Activated protein C resistance has been associated with one-fifth of deep vein thromboses in those under 70, and homozygotes are said to be at 80-fold higher risk of nonpregnant venous thrombosis.[119] The allele frequency in control pregnant women

(1.5–9.2%) is sufficiently low[83,115,120] that small studies would be of inadequate power. A number of studies initially reported an association between factor V Leiden and PE and/or HELLP (see ref. 8) but more recent studies, from different populations, have mostly not confirmed this.[112,121,122] Recent meta-analyses[110,111] report pooled OR of 1.8 (95% CI 1.1–2.89) for the association of factor V Leiden and all cases of PE and 2.2 (95% CI 1.3–3.9) for severe PE. Again, the authors comment on significant between-study heterogeneity, possibly resulting from publication bias.

Prothrombin (factor 2)

Prothrombin is the proenzyme for thrombin and, once activated, converts fibrinogen to fibrin. It has been implicated in maintaining vascular integrity during development and postnatal life. There is a single nucleotide polymorphism (20210G>A) in the 3′ UTR of *F2* (chromosome 11p11-q12), which is associated with an increase in plasma thrombin activity[123] via a higher transcription rate. Unlike factor V Leiden, the prevalence is higher in southern than northern Europe (3% cf 1.7%) but, again, is very low indeed in Asia and Africa.[124] As has been so often the case, early, small-scale studies suggested an association but subsequent larger ones have not supported this.[115,125,126] A very recent meta-analysis[111] also failed to identify a significant association of this polymorphism and either all PE (OR 1.4; 95% CI 0.7–2.6) or severe PE (OR 2.0; 95% CI 0.9–4.2).

Glycoprotein IIIa

Integrins are integral cell-surface proteins made up of an α and a β chain. Platelet glycoprotein IIIa (GPIIIa) is the integrin β chain β3, which links with the αIIb chain in platelets. The αvβ3 integrin is expressed by trophoblasts as they invade the spiral arteries,[127] and there is a failure of this expression in PE.[128] A functional polymorphism in exon 2 of the platelet *ITGB3* (chromosome 17q21.32; 98C>T) results in two distinct forms of the GPIIb/IIIa antigen on platelets and has been associated with increased risk of stroke in young women. A study in an East Anglian population reported an increased T-allele frequency in PE,[125] but a study of Zulu women with severe PE did not identify any such association.[129] The T-allele frequencies were identical in both control groups (14%).

Plasminogen activator-inhibitor-1

Increased plasminogen activator-inhibitor-1 (PAI-1) is a cause of decreased fibrinolysis and the ratio of PAI-1 to PAI-2 is raised before PE can be diagnosed in a proportion of women with a prior history of the disease.[130] Increased plasma PAI-1 has also been associated with increased resistance to blood flow in the placental circulation in PE.[131] There is an insertion polymorphism in the promoter region of the *PAI-1* gene (chromosome 7q21.3-q22; 4G/5G) such that homozygosity for 4G is associated with significantly increased plasma PAI-1 by comparison with homozygosity for 5G,[132] probably through a direct effect on transcription.[133] The 4G form is present in a significant proportion (25–50%) of Western populations. This polymorphism has been studied by a number of groups in relation to PE, but although the first published study – from Japan – reported an association between the 4G/4G genotype and PE,[134] this has not been confirmed in other studies.[83,115,122,135]

Thrombin-activatable fibrinolysis inhibitor

Two polymorphisms (−438 G>A and 1040C>T) have been reported in the gene encoding thrombin-activatable fibrinolysis inhibitor (TAFI) (*CPB2*, chromosome 13q14.11). These might predispose to both deep vein thrombosis and pulmonary embolus in nonpregnant subjects.[136] However, a study from the Netherlands failed to identify any association of either with PE.[122]

Combinations of polymorphisms in the coagulation cascade

Nonpregnant patients who carry a combination of prothrombotic polymorphisms are at greater risk of venous thromboembolism than those who carry only one such polymorphism.[137] However, no interaction has been identified between the factor V Leiden and MTHFR 677C>T polymorphisms in PE[112,121,122] or when the two TAFI polymorphisms were included.[122]

In conclusion, there is some evidence from meta-analyses, with their attendant problems of cross-study heterogeneity, of trends towards increasing risk of PE with the carriage of one or more of the known polymorphisms that, in nonpregnant subjects, contribute to a hypercoagulable state. It might be that when two or more such polymorphisms are carried, the risk is additive, or even multiplicative. However, the wide variability in allele frequency in different populations, and the effects of dietary intake, suggest that any screening program focused on these polymorphisms is unlikely to be cost-effective except in high-risk populations.

HELLP is relatively uncommon and its study is therefore even more difficult, but where sample sizes are above 50 the evidence suggests that it is also probably not associated with carriage of a thrombophilic polymorphism.[115,116]

INFLAMMATORY MEDIATORS

There is evidence for an exacerbated systemic inflammatory response in PE.[138] Tumor necrosis factor α (TNFα) is mainly secreted by macrophages and is involved in the regulation of a variety of biological processes, including cell proliferation and differentiation, apoptosis, immunoregulation, lipid metabolism and coagulation. Increased plasma concentrations, and placental mRNA and protein expression, have been consistently reported in PE; receptors are also said to be increased.[139] The *TNF* gene (chromosome 6p21.3) lies within the major histocompatibility complex, close to the gene encoding lymphotoxin α, (*LTA*; also known as TNFβ). A number of polymorphisms in the 5′ flanking region of *TNF* are associated with altered rates of mRNA transcription. The polymorphism −308G>A results in the alleles *TNFA-1* (G) and *TNFA-2* (A). There is a gradient in TNFα secretion by genotype, such that homozygotes for *TNFA-2* have the highest secretion rates, at least from peripheral blood mononuclear cells.[140] Curiously, however, it was the major allele that was associated with PE in a small, case-control study,[141] although larger studies, including the investigation of multi-alleleic haplotypes, did not confirm this observation.[142,143] A recent study, while again not identifying any association with PE, did report a weak association of the *TNFA-2* allele and eclampsia.[144] The very low incidence of eclampsia makes any study of its genetics extremely difficult.

Both TNFα and ANG II can influence the production and/or release of the proteolytic matrix metalloproteinases (MMPs), which have been implicated in trophoblast invasion, and hence placentation. MMP-1 has been implicated in normal placentation, and decidual concentrations are lower in PE;[145] MMP-2 can also influence vascular reactivity both through the synthesis of vasoconstrictors such as medium endothelin and through the metabolism of vasodilators such as calcitonin gene-related peptide. MMP-2 release is increased from umbilical venous endothelial cells when harvested from PE pregnancies.[146]

To date, only one small study[147] has addressed the possible contribution of a polymorphism, the insertion/deletion polymorphism at −1607 in the *MMP-1* gene (chromosome 11q22.3) in any of the *MMP* genes to PE. This is associated with increased transcription, but no association with hypertension in pregnancy was identified. The study group included women with GH and eclampsia, as well as PE.

The role of the inflammatory cytokine and immunological modulator interleukin-1β (IL-1β) in PE is uncertain. Two functional polymorphisms in *IL1B* (chromosome 2q.14) in the promoter region (−511C>T) and in exon 5, and one in the IL-1β receptor antagonist gene (*IL1RN*), which directly antagonizes the proinflammatory effects of IL-1β, have been studied in relation to PE. However, studies in three populations did not identify any direct association between individual polymorphisms and PE or HELLP.[148–150]

THE IMMUNE SYSTEM

It is thought that PE might arise partly as a result of an abnormal maternal immune response to paternally derived antigens on the trophoblast. PE is primarily a disease of first pregnancy, but a new partner for a subsequent pregnancy[151] and gamete donation[152] increase the risk, observations supporting the general hypothesis. However, despite nearly 40 years of investigation into a possible immune contribution to pathology, no clear-cut evidence has emerged.[139]

Human leukocyte antigen-G (HLA-G) is a nonclassical MHC class Ib antigen expressed on the fetally derived extravillous trophoblast. HLA-G might inhibit activation of maternal decidual T and natural killer (NK) cells. Lack of expression of this antigen has been associated with inadequate placentation and PE.[153] Trophoblastic HLA-G expression has been shown to induce IL-3 and IL-1β release from mononuclear cells, while decreasing release of TNFα.[154] There is a single base-pair deletion in exon 3 (1597 delC), which is a null mutation for the full-length HLA-G1 protein, and that might, therefore, be associated with inadequate placentation. However, one small study failed to show any association.[155,156]

A recent study from Denmark, building on earlier, smaller studies, evaluated the 14 basepair (bp) sequence insertion polymorphism in the 3′ UTR of exon 8 of *HLA-G* and the synonymous codon 93 (CAC/CAT) polymorphism in exon 3, in 110 primiparous mother : father : baby triads (40 severe PE and 70 control).[157] A significantly increased allele frequency of the 14 bp insertion was reported in the babies of PE mothers, with 30% of the babies being homozygous for the polymorphism, compared with 7% in the control babies. This insertion was associated with lower HLA-G expression and its placental distribution reported to differ between samples from PE and normotensive women.[158] A similar trend was identified for the codon 93 CAT variant, which is in linkage disequilibrium with the 14 bp insertion. Transmission disequilibrium testing (TDT) revealed a significantly greater paternal : fetal transmission of the insertion polymorphism in PE.

As well as HLA-G, fetal trophoblast cells express polymorphic HLA-C antigens, ligands for killer cell immunoglobulin-like receptors (KIR) expressed by maternal decidual NK cells, which have the morphological appearance of large granular lymphocytes.[159] The KIR locus is very polymorphic, at both gene and allele level. There are two main KIR haplotype groups, type A and type B.[160] A recent study has suggested that if a mother lacked most or all activating KIR (AA genotype) and the fetus carried HLA-C belonging to the HLA-C2 group, the likelihood of pre-eclampsia was much increased.[161]

An intriguing observation linking an immunomodulator with a decreased risk of PE has recently been published. IL-10 downregulates the expression of T-helper 1 (Th1) cytokines and stimulates Th2 and humoral immune responses, and thus has actions directly opposed to those of TNFα. Not unexpectedly, it inhibits endometrial invasion by cytotrophoblasts.[162] There is a functional polymorphism in the promoter region of *IL-10* (chromosome 1q31-q32; − 2849G>A), such that AA homozygotes have significantly lower blood leukocyte IL-10 responsiveness to endotoxin than AG or GG genotypes; women with this genotype are also more likely to have impaired fertility.[163] However, a recent case-control study of 157 women with PE and their controls identified a three-fold lower incidence of PE (OR 0.29; 95%CI 0.10–0.83) in women homozygous for the A allele.[164] This discrepancy deserves further study, as sub-fecundity has been associated with an increased, not decreased, risk of PE over the years.[165]

OBESITY AND LIPIDS

Insulin resistance and dyslipidemia are features of PE (reviewed in ref. 166) and a high BMI – before or in early pregnancy – is a well-documented risk factor for the disease.[167] Leptin rises in normal pregnancy and is raised further in PE.[168] An interesting study reported that PE women who had begun pregnancy with a BMI of ≤ 25 kg/m^2 had higher mean second-trimester leptin concentrations than controls,[169] whereas those who had BMI greater than this had lower mean leptin concentrations than controls.

There is a tetranucleotide repeat (TTTC)n in the 3′-flanking region of *LEP* (chromosome 7q31.3), which has been associated with hypertension independently of obesity.[170] Two alleles of the polymorphism have been described, based on repeat length: class I (repeats < 160 bp) and class II (repeats = 160 bp). Some distortion of allele frequency has been reported in a preliminary study of this polymorphism in women with PE, class I allele frequency being significantly greater than in controls ($n = 80$ and $n = 78$, respectively).[171] This group again reported significantly raised plasma leptin in women with PE, but did not stratify the hormonal results by genotype.

Lipoprotein lipase (LPL; chromosome 8p22) hydrolyses circulating lipoprotein triglycerides, and a number of functional polymorphisms have been described which reduce its activity. The 9A>G polymorphism in exon 2 and the 291A>G polymorphism in exon 6 are relatively common, result in amino acid substitution and are associated with nonpregnant dyslipidemia, including decreased high-density lipoprotein (HDL) cholesterol, increased small, dense low density lipoproteins (LDLs) and increased triglycerides.[172] A significantly increased G-allele carrier frequency in the 291A>G polymorphism has been linked to a four-fold increase in the incidence of PE,[173] whereas heterozygosity at 9A>G is associated with a five-fold increase. Cholesteryl ester transfer protein (CETP; chromosome 16q.21) facilitates reverse cholesterol transport. Non-pregnant subjects carrying the *CETP* TaqIB polymorphism are more likely to have increased CETP activity and lower HDL cholesterol concentrations, and a dose-related fall in apoB/apoA$_1$ ratio per B2 allele.[174] This association has not been found in women with PE.[175] A polymorphism (2488C>T) in the apolipoprotein B gene (*APOB*; chromosome 2p24-p23) is associated with increased serum triglyceride and cholesterol concentrations,[176] such as are found in PE. It is not, however, directly associated with the disease.[45] Two polymorphisms in the apolipoprotein E gene (*APOE*; chromosome 19q13.2) result in three common alleles, the ε2, ε3 and ε4 alleles, and the efficiency of intestinal cholesterol absorption increases in this allelic order.[177] Published data disagree in their estimates of the impact of this polymorphism on PE. A relatively small study from Hungary reported an association between 'severe PE' (clinical data not provided) and the ε2 allele.[178] However, a similarly-sized study from Portugal, with less severe disease, did not identify such an association;[175] nor did a larger study of Finnish women.[179]

The β3 adrenergic receptor is found mainly in adipose tissue and contributes to regulation of the rate of lipolysis. The polymorphism 190T>C in *ADRB3* (chromosome 8p12-p11.2) results in an amino acid substitution (64Trp>Arg) in the first intracellular loop, with possible functional significance, which has been linked with early-onset diabetes and obesity outside pregnancy.[180] However, a study of 173 PE women and 179 controls, predominantly Caucasian, failed to identify any association between the mutant allele and either PE or the response to a glucose tolerance test.[181]

CONCLUSION

Significant insights into the mechanisms of PE have been gained through the application of molecular techniques to the study of gene transcription in pregnancy. The availability of microchip array technology will lead to further understanding in the years to come. By contrast, although attempts have been made over the last decade to unravel the contribution of inherited genetic variation to the pathology of PE, it is clear that any effect of the candidate genes studied so far is small. The marked differences in some allele frequencies with ethnicity, the effects of environment : polymorphism interaction and variation in phenotyping the clinical condition, all compound the difficulties of such studies. Family-based linkage studies are currently the only practical approach to genome-wide screening as a mechanism for the identification of susceptibility loci. Within a few years it is likely that genome-wide association studies will become technically and economically viable. If this opportunity is to be fully exploited it will be vital to conduct large, carefully designed studies of an appropriate power for the multiple hypotheses (i.e. genes) being tested. The study of carefully selected candidate genes, informed by increasing understanding of the pathology of the condition, remains an important approach that invites collaboration between interested research groups at national and international level.

References

1. National High Blood Pressure Education Program Working Group. Report of the National High Blood Pressure Education Program Working Group on high blood pressure in pregnancy. *Am J Obstet Gynecol* 2000; 183:S1–S22.
2. Higgins JR, de Swiet M. Blood-pressure measurement and classification in pregnancy. *Lancet* 2001; 357(9250):131–135.
3. Sibai BM, Ramadan MK, Usta I, et al. Maternal morbidity and mortality in 442 pregnancies with hemolysis, elevated liver enzymes, and low platelets (HELLP syndrome). *Am J Obstet Gynecol* 1993; 169(4):1000–1006.
4. Waterstone M, Bewley S, Wolfe C. Incidence and predictors of severe obstetric morbidity: case-control study. *Br Med J* 2001; 322(7294):1089–1093.
5. Brosens JJ, Pijnenborg R, Brosens IA. The myometrial junctional zone spiral arteries in normal and abnormal pregnancies: a review of the literature. *Am J Obstet Gynecol* 2002; 187(5):1416–1423.
6. Zhou Y, Fisher SJ, Janatpour M, et al. Human cytotrophoblasts adopt a vascular phenotype as they differentiate. A strategy for successful endovascular invasion? *J Clin Invest* 1997; 99(9):2139–2151.
7. Lim KH, Zhou Y, Janatpour M, et al. Human cytotrophoblast differentiation/invasion is abnormal in pre-eclampsia. *Am J Pathol* 1997; 151(6):1809–1818.
8. Lachmeijer AM, Dekker GA, Pals G, et al. Searching for preeclampsia genes: the current position. *Eur J Obstet Gynecol Reprod Biol* 2002; 105(2):94–113.
9. Wilson ML, Goodwin TM, Pan VL, Ingles SA. Molecular epidemiology of preeclampsia. *Obstetr Gynecol Survey* 2003; 58(1):39–66.
10. Adams E, Finlayson A. Familial aspects of pre-eclampsia and hypertension in pregnancy. *Lancet* 1961; ii:1375–1378.
11. Chesley L, Cosgrove R, Annitto J. Pregnancies in the sisters and daughters of eclamptic women. *Obstet Gynecol* 1962; 20:39–46.
12. Chesley LC, Annitto JE, Cosgrove RA. The familial factor in toxemia of pregnancy. *Obstet Gynecol* 1968; 32(3):303–311.
13. Cooper DW, Liston WA. Genetic control of severe pre-eclampsia. *J Med Genet* 1979; 16(6):409–416.
14. Sutherland A, Cooper DW, Howie PW, et al. The indicence of severe pre-eclampsia amongst mothers and mothers-in-law of pre-eclamptics and controls. *Br J Obstet Gynaecol* 1981; 88(8):785–791.
15. Chesley LC, Cooper DW. Genetics of hypertension in pregnancy: possible single gene control of pre-eclampsia and eclampsia in the descendants of eclamptic women. *Br J Obstet Gynaecol* 1986; 93(9):898–908.
16. Arngrimsson R, Bjornsson S, Geirsson R, et al. Genetic and familial predisposition to eclampsia and pre-eclampsia in a defined population. *Br J Obstet Gynaecol* 1990; 97(9):762–769.
17. Cincotta RB, Brennecke SP. Family history of pre-eclampsia as a predictor for pre-eclampsia in primigravidas. *Int J Gynecol Obstet* 1998; 60(1):23–27.
18. Liston WA, Kilpatrick DC. Is genetic susceptibility to pre-eclampsia conferred by homozygosity for the same single recessive gene in mother and fetus? *Br J Obstet Gynaecol* 1991; 98(11):1079–1086.
19. McCarthy M, Menzel S. The genetics of type 2 diabetes. *Br J Clin Pharmacol* 2001; 51(3):195–199.
20. Thornton JG, Macdonald A. Twin mothers, pregnancy hypertension and pre-eclampsia. *Br J Obstet Gynaecol* 1999; 106(6):570–575.
21. Salonen Ros H, Lichtenstein P, Lipworth L, Cnattingius S. Genetic effects on the liability of developing pre-eclampsia and gestational hypertension. *Am J Med Genet* 2000; 91(4):256–260.
22. Pawitan Y, Reilly M, Nilsson E, et al. Estimation of genetic and environmental factors for binary traits using family data. *Stat Med* 2004; 23(3):449–465.
23. Lie RT, Rasmussen S, Brunborg H, et al. Fetal and maternal contributions to risk of pre-eclampsia: population based study. *Br Med J* 1998; 316(7141):1343–1347.
24. Esplin MS, Fausett MB, Fraser A, et al. Paternal and maternal components of the predisposition to preeclampsia. *N Engl J Med* 2001; 344(12):867–872.
25. Redman C, Sargent I. Placental debris, oxidative stress and pre-eclampsia. *Placenta* 2000; 21:597–602.
26. Roberts J, Hubel C. Is oxidative stress the link in the two-stage model of pre-eclampsia? *Lancet* 1999; 354:788–789.
27. Harrison GA, Humphrey KE, Jones N, et al. A genomewide linkage study of pre-eclampsia/eclampsia reveals evidence for a candidate region on 4q. *Am J Hum Genet* 1997; 60(5):1158–1167.
28. Laivuori H, Lahermo P, Ollikainen V, et al. Susceptibility loci for preeclampsia on chromosomes 2p25 and 9p13 in Finnish families. *Am J Hum Genet* 2003; 72(1):168–177.

29. Arngrimsson R, Sigurardottir S, Frigge ML, et al. A genome-wide scan reveals a maternal susceptibility locus for pre-eclampsia on chromosome 2p13. *Hum Mol Genet* 1999; 8(9):1799–1805.

30. Lachmeijer AM, Arngrimsson R, Bastiaans EJ, et al. A genome-wide scan for preeclampsia in the Netherlands. *Eur J Hum Gen* 2001; 9(10):758–764.

31. Oudejans CB, Mulders J, Lachmeijer AM, et al. The parent-of-origin effect of 10q22 in pre-eclamptic females coincides with two regions clustered for genes with down-regulated expression in androgenetic placentas. *Mol Hum Reprod* 2004; 10(8):589–598.

32. Colhoun H, McKeigue P, Davey Smith G. Problems of reporting genetic associations with comlex outcomes. *Lancet* 2003; 361:865–872.

33. Wacholder S, Chanock S, Garcia-Closas M, et al. Assessing the probability that a positive report is false: an approach for molecular epidemiology studies. *J Natl Cancer Inst* 2004; 96:434–442.

34. Spielman RS, McGinnis RE, Ewens WJ. Transmission test for linkage disequilibrium: the insulin gene region and insulin-dependent diabetes mellitus (IDDM). *Am J Hum Genet* 1993; 52(3):506–516.

35. Broughton Pipkin F. Maternal physiology in pregnancy. In: Chamberlain G, Steer P, eds. *Turnbull's obstetrics. 3rd edn.* London: Churchill Livingstone; 2001:71–91.

36. Rang S, Wolf H, Montfrans GA, Karemaker JM. Non-invasive assessment of autonomic cardiovascular control in normal human pregnancy and pregnancy-associated hypertensive disorders: a review. *J Hypertens* 2002; 20(11):2111–2119.

37. Williams GH, Fisher NDL. Genetic approach to diagnostic and therapeutic decisions in human hypertension. *Curr Opin Nephrol Hypertens* 1997; 6:199–204.

38. Hagemann A, Nielsen AH, Poulsen K. The uteroplacental renin–angiotensin system: a review. *Exp Clin Endocrinol* 1994; 102(3):252–261.

39. Morgan T, Craven C, Ward K. Human spiral artery renin–angiotensin system. *Hypertension* 1998; 32(4):683–687.

40. Morgan T, Craven C, Nelson L, et al. Angiotensinogen T235 expression is elevated in decidual spiral arteries. *J Clin Invest* 1997; 100(6):1406–1415.

41. Wallukat G, Homuth V, Fischer T, et al. Patients with preeclampsia develop agonistic autoantibodies against the angiotensin AT1 receptor. *J Clin Invest* 1999; 103(7):945–952.

42. Xia Y, Wen H, Bobst S, et al. Maternal autoantibodies from preeclamptic patients activate angiotensin receptors on human trophoblast cells. *J Soc Gynecol Invest* 2003; 10(2):82–93.

43. Jeunemaitre X, Soubrier F, Kotelevtsev YV, et al. Molecular basis of human hypertension: role of angiotensinogen. *Cell* 1992; 71(1):169–180.

44. Ward K, Hata A, Jeunemaitre X, et al. A molecular variant of angiotensinogen associated with preeclampsia. *Nat Genet* 1993; 4(1):59–61.

45. Levesque S, Moutquin JM, Lindsay C, et al. Implication of an AGT haplotype in a multigene association study with pregnancy hypertension. *Hypertension* 2004; 43(1):71–78.

46. Kobashi G, Shido K, Hata A, et al. Multivariate analysis of genetic and acquired factors; T235 variant of the angiotensinogen gene is a potent independent risk factor for preeclampsia. *Semin Thromb Hemost* 2001; 27(2):143–147.

47. Zhang X, Varner M, Dizon-Townson D, et al. A molecular variant of angiotensinogen is associated with idiopathic intrauterine growth restriction. *Obstet Gynecol* 2003; 101(2):237–242.

48. Hollenberg NK, Moore T, Shoback D, et al. Abnormal renal sodium handling in essential hypertension. Relation to failure of renal and adrenal modulation of responses to angiotensin II. *Am J Med* 1986; 81(3):412–418.

49. Hopkins PN, Hunt SC, Jeunemaitre X, et al. Angiotensinogen genotype affects renal and adrenal responses to angiotensin II in essential hypertension. *Circulation* 2002; 105(16):1921–1927.

50. Bernstein IM, Ziegler W, Stirewalt WS, et al. Angiotensinogen genotype and plasma volume in nulligravid women. *Obstet Gynecol* 1998; 92(2):171–173.

51. Chapman AB, Abraham WT, Zamudio S, et al. Temporal relationships between hormonal and hemodynamic changes in early human pregnancy. *Kidney Int* 1998; 54(6):2056–2063.

52. Robson SC, Hunter S, Boys RJ, Dunlop W. Serial study of factors influencing changes in cardiac output during human pregnancy. *Am J Physiol* 1989; 256(4 Pt 2):H1060–H1065.

53. Bayliss C, Davison JM. The urinary system. In: Chamberlain G, Broughton Pipkin F, eds. *Clinical physiology in obstetrics, 3rd edn.* Oxford: Blackwell Science; 1998:263–307.

54. Brown MA, Zammit VC, Mitar DM. Extracellular fluid volumes in pregnancy-induced hypertension. *J Hypertens* 1992; 10(1):61–68.

55. Ganzevoort W, Rep A, Bonsel GJ, et al. Plasma volume and blood pressure regulation in hypertensive pregnancy. *J Hypertens* 2004; 22(7):1235–1242.

56. Aardenburg R, Spaanderman ME, Ekhart TH, et al. Low plasma volume following pregnancy complicated by pre-eclampsia predisposes for hypertensive disease in a next pregnancy. *Br J Obstet Gynaecol* 2003; 110(11):1001–1006.

57. Brown MA, Gallery ED, Ross MR, Esber RP. Sodium excretion in normal and hypertensive pregnancy: a prospective study. *Am J Obstet Gynecol* 1988; 159(2):297–307.

58. Morgan L, Crawshaw S, Baker PN, et al. Functional and genetic studies of the angiotensin II type 1 receptor in pre-eclamptic and normotensive pregnant women. *J Hypertens* 1997; 15(12 Part 1):1389–1396.

59. Roberts CB, Rom L, Moodley J, Pegoraro RJ. Hypertension-related gene polymorphisms in pre-eclampsia, eclampsia and gestational hypertension in Black South African women. *J Hypertens* 2004; 22(5):945–948.

60. Bouba I, Makrydimas G, Kalaitzidis R, et al. Interaction between the polymorphisms of the renin-angiotensin system in preeclampsia. *Eur J Obstet Gynecol Reprod Biol* 2003; 110(1):8–11.

61. Plummer S, Tower C, Alonso P, et al. Haplotypes of the angiotensin II receptor genes AGTR1 and AGTR2 in women with normotensive pregnancy and women with preeclampsia. *Hum Mutat* 2004; 24(1):14–20.

62. Kurland L, Melhus H, Sarabi M, et al. Polymorphisms in the renin-angiotensin system and endothelium-dependent vasodilation in normotensive subjects. *Clin Physiol* 2001; 21(3):343–349.

63. Volpe M, Musumeci B, De Paolis P, et al. Angiotensin II AT2 receptor subtype: an uprising frontier in cardiovascular disease? *J Hypertens* 2003; 21(8):1429–1443.

64. Oats JN, Broughton Pipkin F, Symonds EM, Craven DJ. A prospective study of plasma angiotensin-converting enzyme in normotensive primigravidae and their infants. *Br J Obstet Gynaecol* 1981; 88(12):1204–1210.

65. Rasmussen AB, Pedersen EB, Romer FK, et al. The influence of normotensive pregnancy and pre-eclampsia on angiotensin-converting enzyme. *Acta Obstet Gynecol Scand* 1983; 62(4):341–344.

66. Goldkrand JW, Fuentes AM. The relation of angiotensin-converting enzyme to the pregnancy-induced hypertension-preeclampsia syndrome. *Am J Obstet Gynecol* 1986; 154(4):792–800.

67. Paul M, Wagner J, Dzau VJ. Gene expression of the renin-angiotensin system in human tissues. Quantitative analysis by the polymerase chain reaction. *J Clin Invest* 1993; 91(5):2058–2064.

68. Pinet F, Corvol M, Bourguignon J, Corvol P. Isolation and characterization of renin-producing human chorionic cells in culture. *J Clin Endocrinol Metab* 1988; 67(6):1211–1220.

69. Rigat B, Hubert C, Alhenc-Gelas F, et al. An insertion/deletion polymorphism in the angiotensin I-converting enzyme gene accounting for half the variance of serum enzyme levels. *J Clin Invest* 1990; 86(4):1343–1346.

70. Tamura T, Johanning GL, Goldenberg RL, et al. Effect of angiotensin-converting enzyme gene polymorphism on pregnancy outcome, enzyme activity, and zinc concentration. *Obstet Gynecol* 1996; 88(4 Part 1):497–502.

71. Morgan L, Foster F, Hayman R, et al. Angiotensin-converting enzyme insertion-deletion polymorphism in normotensive and pre-eclamptic pregnancies. *J Hypertens* 1999; 17(6):765–768.

72. Mello G, Parretti E, Gensini F, et al. Maternal–fetal flow, negative events, and preeclampsia: role of ACE I/D polymorphism. *Hypertension* 2003; 41(4):932–937.

73. Ness RB, Roberts JM. Epidemiology of hypertension. In: Lindheimer M, Roberts JM, Cunningham FG, eds. *Chesley's hypertensive disorders in pregnancy, 2nd edn.* Stamford, CT: Appleton & Lange; 1999:43–65.

74. Shojaati K, Causevic M, Kadereit B, et al. Evidence for compromised aldosterone synthase enzyme activity in preeclampsia. *Kidney Int* 2004; 66(6):2322–2328.

75. Myatt L, Rosenfield RB, Eis AL, et al. Nitrotyrosine residues in placenta. Evidence of peroxynitrite formation and action. *Hypertension* 1996; 28(3).

76. Many A, Hubel CA, Fisher SJ, et al. Invasive cytotrophoblasts manifest evidence of oxidative stress in preeclampsia. *Am J Pathol* 2000; 156(1):321–331.

77. Tanus-Santos JE, Desai M, Flockhart DA. Effects of ethnicity on the distribution of clinically relevant endothelial nitric oxide variants. *Pharmacogenetics* 2001; 11(8):719–725.

78. Wang XL, Sim AS, Wang MX, et al. Genotype dependent and cigarette specific effects on endothelial nitric oxide synthase gene expression and enzyme activity. *FEBS Lett* 2000; 471(1):45–50.

79. Arngrimsson R, Hayward C, Nadaud S, et al. Evidence for a familial pregnancy-induced hypertension locus in the eNOS gene region. *Am J Hum Genet* 1997; 61(2):354–362.

80. Savvidou MD, Vallance PJ, Nicolaides KH, Hingorani AD. Endothelial nitric oxide synthase gene polymorphism and maternal vascular adaptation to pregnancy. *Hypertension* 2001; 38(6):1289–1293.

81. Yoshimura T, Yoshimura M, Tabata A, et al. Association of the missense Glu298Asp variant of the endothelial nitric oxide synthase gene with severe preeclampsia. *J Soc Gynecol Investig* 2000; 7(4):238–241.

82. Serrano NC, Casas JP, Diaz LA, et al. Endothelial NO synthase genotype and risk of preeclampsia: a multicenter case-control study. *Hypertension* 2004; 44(5):702–707.

83. Tempfer CB, Jirecek S, Riener EK, et al. Polymorphisms of thrombophilic and vasoactive genes and severe preeclampsia: a pilot study. *J Soc Gynecol Investig* 2004; 11(4):227–231.

84. Landau R, Xie HG, Dishy V, et al. No association of the Asp298 variant of the endothelial nitric oxide synthase gene with preeclampsia. *Am J Hypertens* 2004; 17(5 Part 1):391–394.

85. Yoshimura T, Chowdhury FA, Yoshimura M, Okamura H. Genetic and environmental contributions to severe preeclampsia: lack of association with the endothelial nitric oxide synthase Glu298Asp variant in a developing country. *Gynecol Obstet Invest* 2003; 56(1):10–13.

86. Tempfer CB, Dorman K, Deter RL, et al. An endothelial nitric oxide synthase gene polymorphism is associated with preeclampsia. *Hypertens Pregnancy* 2001; 20(1):107–118.

87. Fitzgerald D, Entman S, Mulloy K, FitzGerald G. Decreased prostacyclin biosynthesis preceding the clinical manifestation of pregnancy-induced hypertension. *Circulation* 1987; 75(5):956–963.

88. Siffert W. G protein polymorphisms in hypertension, atherosclerosis, and diabetes. *Annu Rev Med* 2005; 56:17–28.

89. Jansen MW, Bertina RM, Vos HL, et al. C825T polymorphism in the human G protein beta 3 subunit gene and preeclampsia; a case control study. *Hypertens Pregnancy* 2004; 23(2):211–218.

90. Foidart J, Hustin J, Dubois M, Schaaps J. The human placenta becomes haemochorial at the 13th week of pregnancy. *Int J Dev Biol* 1992; 36(3):451–453.

91. Jauniaux E, Watson A, Hempstock J, et al. Onset of maternal arterial blood flow and placental oxidative stress. A possible factor in human early pregnancy failure. *Am J Pathol* 2000; 157(6):2111–2122.

92. Wickens D, Wilkins MH, Lunec J, et al. Free radical oxidation (peroxidation)products in plasma in normal and abnormal pregnancy. *Ann Clin Biochem* 1981; 18(3):158–162.

93. Raijmakers MT, Dechend R, Poston L. Oxidative stress and preeclampsia: rationale for antioxidant clinical trials. *Hypertension* 2004; 44(4):374–380.

94. Zusterzeel PL, Peters WH, De Bruyn MA, et al. Glutathione *S*-transferase isoenzymes in decidua and placenta of preeclamptic pregnancies. *Obstet Gynecol* 1999; 94(6):1033–1038.

95. Zusterzeel P, Visser W, Peters WH, et al. Polymorphism in the glutathione *S*-transferase P1 gene and risk for preeclampsia. *Obstet Gynecol* 2000; 96(1):50–54.

96. Cahilly C, Ballantyne CM, Lim DS, et al. A variant of p22(phox), involved in generation of reactive oxygen species in the vessel wall, is associated with progression of coronary atherosclerosis. *Circ Res* 2000; 86(4):391–395.

97. Raijmakers MT, Roes EM, Steegers EA, Peters WH. The C242T-polymorphism of the NADPH/NADH oxidase gene p22phox subunit is not associated with pre-eclampsia. *J Hum Hypertens* 2002; 16(6):423–425.

98. Brenner B. Thrombophilia and pregnancy loss. *Thromb Res* 2002; 108(4):197–202.

99. Schjetlein R, Haugen G, Wisloff F. Markers of intravascular coagulation and fibrinolysis in preeclampsia: association with intrauterine growth retardation. *Acta Obstet Gynecol Scand* 1997; 76(6):541–546.

100. Shaarawy M, Didy HE. Thrombomodulin, plasminogen activator inhibitor type 1 (PAI-1) and fibronectin as biomarkers of endothelial damage in preeclampsia and eclampsia. *Int J Gynaecol Obstet* 1996; 55(2):135–139.

101. Andersson A, Hultberg B, Brattstrom L, Isaksson A. Decreased serum homocysteine in pregnancy. *Eur J Clin Chem Clin Biochem* 1992; 30(6):377–379.

102. Raijmakers MT, Zusterzeel PL, Steegers EA, Peters WH. Hyperhomocysteinaemia: a risk factor for preeclampsia? *Eur J Obstet Gynecol Reprod Biol* 2001; 95(2):226–228.

103. Frosst P, Blom H, Milos R, et al. A candidate genetic risk factor for vascular disease: a common mutation in methylenetetrahydrofolate reductase. *Nat Genet* 1995; 10(1):111–113.

104. Weisberg I, Tran P, Christensen B, et al. A second genetic polymorphism in methylenetetrahydrofolate reductase (MTHFR) associated with decreased enzyme activity. *Mol Genet Metab* 1998; 64(3):169–172.

105. Harmon DL, Woodside JV, Yarnell JW, et al. The common 'thermolabile' variant of methylene tetrahydrofolate reductase is a major determinant of mild hyperhomocysteinaemia. *Quart J Med* 1996; 89(8):571–577.

106. Prasmusinto D, Skrablin S, Hofstaetter C, et al. The methylenetetrahydrofolate reductase 677 C→T polymorphism and preeclampsia in two populations. *Obstet Gynecol* 2002; 99(6):1085–1092.

107. Williams MA, Sanchez SE, Zhang C, Bazul V. Methylenetetrahydrofolate reductase 677 C→T polymorphism and plasma folate in relation to pre-eclampsia risk among Peruvian women. *J Mat Fetal Neonatal Med* 2004; 15(5):337–344.

108. Sohda S, Arinami T, Hamada H, et al. Methylenetetrahydrofolate reductase polymorphism and pre-eclampsia. *J Med Genet* 1997; 34(6):525–526.

109. Grandone E, Margaglione M, Colaizzo D, et al. Factor V Leiden, C > T MTHFR polymorphism and genetic susceptibility to preeclampsia. *Thromb Haemost* 1997; 77(6):1052–1054.

110. Kosmas IP, Tatsioni A, Ioannidis JP. Association of C677T polymorphism in the methylenetetrahydrofolate reductase gene with hypertension in pregnancy and pre-eclampsia: a meta-analysis. *J Hypertens* 2004; 22(9):1655–1662.

111. Lin J, August P. Genetic thrombophilias and preeclampsia: a meta-analysis. *Obstet Gynecol* 2005; 105(1):182–192.

112. Kim YJ, Williamson RA, Murray JC, et al. Genetic susceptibility to preeclampsia: roles of cytosineto-thymine substitution at nucleotide 677 of the gene for methylenetetrahydrofolate reductase, 68-base pair insertion at nucleotide 844 of the gene for cystathionine beta-synthase, and factor V Leiden mutation. *Am J Obstet Gynecol* 2001; 184(6):1211–1217.

113. Chesley LC, Cosgrove RE. The remote prognosis of preeclamptic women: sixth periodic report. *Am J Obstet Gynecol* 1976; 124:446–459.

114. Ness RB, Roberts JM. Heterogeneous causes constituting the single syndrome of preeclampsia: a hypothesis and its implications. *Am J Obstet Gynecol* 1996; 175(5):1365–1370.

115. Livingston JC, Barton JR, Park V, et al. Maternal and fetal inherited thrombophilias are not related to the development of severe preeclampsia. *Am J Obstet Gynecol* 2001; 185(1):153–157.

116. Zusterzeel PL, Visser W, Blom HJ, et al. Methylenetetrahydrofolate reductase polymorphisms in preeclampsia and the HELLP syndrome. *Hypertens Pregnancy* 2000; 19(3):299–307.

117. Kaiser T, Brennecke SP, Moses EK. Neither the A1298C polymorphism alone nor a combination of both polymorphisms showed an association with PE/E in our population of Australian women. *Gynecol Obstet Invest* 2000; 50(2):100–102.

118. Bertina RM, Koeleman BP, Koster T, et al. Mutation in blood coagulation factor V associated with resistance to activated protein C. *Nature* 1994; 369:364–367.

119. Rees DC, Cox M, Clegg JB. World distribution of factor V Leiden. *Lancet* 1995; 346(8983):1133–1134.

120. de Groot CJ, Bloemenkamp KW, Duvekot EJ, et al. Preeclampsia and genetic risk factors for thrombosis: a case-control study. *Am J Obstet Gynecol* 1999; 181(4):975–980.

121. Murphy RP, Donoghue C, Nallen RJ, et al. Prospective evaluation of the risk conferred by factor V Leiden and thermolabile methylenetetrahydrofolate reductase polymorphisms in pregnancy. *Arterioscler Thromb Vasc Biol* 2000; 20(1):266–270.

122. de Maat MP, Jansen MW, Hille ET, et al. Preeclampsia and its interaction with common variants in thrombophilia genes. *J Thromb Haemost* 2004; 2(9):1588–1593.

123. Poort SR, Rosendaal FR, Reitsma PH, Bertina RM. A common genetic variation in the 3′-untranslated region of the prothrombin gene is associated with elevated plasma prothrombin levels and an increase in venous thrombosis. *Blood* 1996; 88(10):3698–3703.

124. Rosendaal FR, Doggen CJ, Zivelin A, et al. Geographic distribution of the 20210 G to A prothrombin variant. *Thromb Haemost* 1998; 79(4):706–708.

125. O'Shaughnessy KM, Fu B, Downing S, Morris NH. Thrombophilic polymorphisms in preeclampsia: altered frequency of the functional 98C→T polymorphism of glycoprotein IIIa. *J Med Genet* 2001; 38(11):775–777.

126. Morrison ER, Miedzybrodzka ZH, Campbell DM, et al. Prothrombotic genotypes are not associated with pre-eclampsia and gestational hypertension: results from a large population-based study and systematic review. *Thromb Haemost* 2002; 87(5):779–785.

127. Zhou Y, Fisher SJ, Janatpour M, et al. Human cytotrophoblasts adopt a vascular phenotype as they differentiate. A strategy for successful endovascular invasion? *J Clin Invest* 1997; 99(9):2139–2151.

128. Zhou Y, Damsky CH, Fisher SJ. Preeclampsia is associated with failure of human cytotrophoblasts to mimic a vascular adhesion phenotype. One cause of defective endovascular invasion in this syndrome? *J Clin Invest* 1997; 99(9):2152–2164.

129. Pegoraro RJ, Hira B, Rom L, Moodley J. Plasminogen activator inhibitor type 1 (PAI1) and platelet glycoprotein IIIa (PGIIIa) polymorphisms in Black South Africans with pre-eclampsia. *Acta Obstet Gynecol Scand* 2003; 82(4):313–317.

130. Chappell LC, Seed PT, Briley A, et al. A longitudinal study of biochemical variables in women at risk of preeclampsia. *Am J Obstet Gynecol* 2002; 187(1):127–136.

131. He S, Bremme K, Blomback M. Increased blood flow resistance in placental circulation and levels of plasminogen activator inhibitors types 1 and 2 in severe preeclampsia. *Blood Coagul Fibrinol* 1995; 6(8):703–708.

132. Kohler HP, Grant PJ. Plasminogen-activator inhibitor type 1 and coronary artery disease. *N Engl J Med* 2000; 342(24):1793–1801.

133. Humphries SE, Lane A, Dawson S, Green FR. The study of gene-environment interactions that influence thrombosis and fibrinolysis. Genetic variation at the loci for factor VII and plasminogen activator inhibitor-1. *Arch Pathol Lab Med* 1992; 116(12):1322–1329.

134. Yamada N, Arinami T, Yamakawa-Kobayashi K, et al. The 4G/5G polymorphism of the plasminogen activator inhibitor-1 gene is associated with severe preeclampsia. *J Hum Genet* 2000; 45(3):138–141.

135. Hakli T, Romppanen EL, Hiltunen M, et al. Plasminogen activator inhibitor-1 polymorphism in women with pre-eclampsia. *Genet Test* 2003; 7(3):265–268.

136. Zidane M, de Visser MC, ten Wolde M, et al. Frequency of the TAFI −438 G/A and factor XIIIa Val34Leu polymorphisms in patients with objectively proven pulmonary embolism. *Thromb Haemost* 2003; 90(3):439–445.

137. Endler G, Mannhalter C. Polymorphisms in coagulation factor genes and their impact on arterial and venous thrombosis. *Clin Chim Acta* 2003; 330(1-2):31–55.

138. Redman CW, Sargent I. Preeclampsia and the systemic inflammatory response. *Semin Nephrol* 2004; 24(6):565–570.
139. Kilpatrick DC. Influence of human leukocyte antigen and tumour necrosis factor genes on the development of pre-eclampsia. *Hum Reprod Update* 1999; 5(2):94–102.
140. Bouma G, Crusius JB, Oudkerk Pool M, et al. Secretion of tumour necrosis factor alpha and lymphotoxin alpha in relation to polymorphisms in the TNF genes and HLA-DR alleles. Relevance for inflammatory bowel disease. *Scand J Immunol* 1996; 43(4):456–463.
141. Chen G, Wilson R, Wang SH, et al. Tumour necrosis factor-alpha (TNF-alpha) gene polymorphism and expression in pre-eclampsia. *Clin Exp Immunol* 1996; 104(1):154–159.
142. Dizon-Townson DS, Major H, Ward K. A promoter mutation in the tumor necrosis factor alpha gene is not associated with preeclampsia. *J Reprod Immunol* 1998; 38(1):55–61.
143. Lachmeijer AM, Crusius JB, Pals G, et al. Polymorphisms in the tumor necrosis factor and lymphotoxin-alpha gene region and preeclampsia. *Obstet Gynecol* 2001; 98(4):612–619.
144. Kaiser T, Grehan M, Brennecke SP, Moses EK. Association of the TNF2 allele with eclampsia. *Gynecol Obstet Invest* 2004; 57(4):204–209.
145. Gallery ED, Campbell S, Arkell J, et al. Preeclamptic decidual microvascular endothelial cells express lower levels of matrix metalloproteinase-1 than normals. *Microvasc Res* 1999; 57(3):340–346.
146. Merchant SJ, Narumiya H, Zhang Y, et al. The effects of preeclampsia and oxygen environment on endothelial release of matrix metalloproteinase-2. *Hypertens Pregnancy* 2004; 23(1):47–60.
147. Jurajda M, Kankova K, Muzik J, et al. Lack of an association of a single nucleotide polymorphism in the promoter of the matrix metalloproteinase-1 gene in Czech women with pregnancy-induced hypertension. *Gynecol Obstet Invest* 2001; 52(2):124–127.
148. Lachmeijer AM, Nosti-Escanilla MP, Bastiaans EB, et al. Linkage and association studies of IL1B and IL1RN gene polymorphisms in preeclampsia. *Hypertens Pregnancy* 2002; 21(1):23–38.
149. Hefler LA, Tempfer CB, Gregg AR. Polymorphisms within the interleukin-1 beta gene cluster and preeclampsia. *Obstet Gynecol* 2001; 97(5 Part 1):664–668.
150. Faisel F, Romppanen EL, Hiltunen M, et al. Polymorphism in the interleukin 1 receptor antagonist gene in women with preeclampsia. *J Reprod Immunol* 2003; 60(1):61–70.
151. Robillard P, Hulsey TC, Perianin J, et al. Association of pregnancy-induced hypertension with duration of sexual cohabitation before conception. *Lancet* 1994; 344(8928):973–975.
152. Salha O, Sharma V, Dada T, et al. The influence of donated gametes on the incidence of hypertensive disorders of pregnancy. *Hum Reprod* 1999; 14(9):2268–2273.
153. Goldman-Wohl DS, Ariel I, Greenfield C, et al. Lack of human leukocyte antigen-G expression in extravillous trophoblasts is associated with pre-eclampsia. *Mol Hum Reprod* 2000; 6(1):88–95.
154. Maejima M, Fujii T, Kozuma S, et al. Presence of HLA-G-expressing cells modulates the ability of peripheral blood mononuclear cells to release cytokines. *Am J Reprod Immunol* 1997; 38(2):79–82.
155. Humphrey KE, Harrison GA, Cooper DW, et al. HLA-G deletion polymorphism and pre-eclampsia/eclampsia. *Br J Obstet Gynaecol* 1995; 102(9):707–710.
156. Aldrich C, Verp MS, Walker MA, Ober C. A null mutation in HLA-G is not associated with preeclampsia or intrauterine growth retardation. *J Reprod Immunol* 2000; 47(1):41–48.
157. Hylenius S, Andersen AM, Melbye M, Hviid TV. Association between HLA-G genotype and risk of pre-eclampsia: a case-control study using family triads. *Mol Hum Reprod* 2004; 10(4):237–246.
158. O'Brien M, McCarthy T, Jenkins D, et al. Altered HLA-G transcription in pre-eclampsia is associated with allele specific inheritance: possible role of the HLA-G gene in susceptibility to the disease. *Cell Mol Life Sci* 2001; 58(12–13):1943–1949.
159. King A, Burrows TD, Hiby SE, et al. Surface expression of HLA-C antigen by human extravillous trophoblast. *Placenta* 2000; 21(4):376–387.
160. Uhrberg M, Valiante NM, Shum BP, et al. Human diversity in killer cell inhibitory receptor genes. *Immunity* 1997; 7:753–763.
161. Hiby SE, Walker JJ, O'Shaughnessy KM, et al. Combinations of maternal KIR and fetal HLA-C genes influence the risk of preeclampsia and reproductive success. *J Exp Med* 2004; 200(8):957–965.
162. Roth I, Fisher SJ. IL-10 is an autocrine inhibitor of human placental cytotrophoblast MMP-9 production and invasion. *Dev Biol* 1999; 205(1):194–204.
163. Westendorp RG, van Dunne FM, Kirkwood TB, et al. Optimizing human fertility and survival. *Nat Med* 2001; 7(8):873.
164. de Groot CJ, Jansen MW, Bertina RM, et al. Interleukin 10-2849AA genotype protects against pre-eclampsia. *Genes Immun* 2004; 5(4):313–314.
165. Basso O, Weinberg CR, Baird DD, et al; Danish National Birth Cohort. Subfecundity as a correlate of preeclampsia: a study within the Danish National Birth Cohort. *Am J Epidemiol* 2003;157(3):195–202.

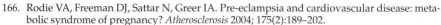

166. Rodie VA, Freeman DJ, Sattar N, Greer IA. Pre-eclampsia and cardiovascular disease: meta-bolic syndrome of pregnancy? *Atherosclerosis* 2004; 175(2):189–202.

167. Eskenazi B, Fenster L, Sidney S. A multivariate analysis of risk factors for preeclampsia. *JAMA* 1991; 266(2):237–241.

168. Laivuori H, Kaaja R, Koistinen H, et al. Leptin during and after preeclamptic or normal preg-nancy: its relation to serum insulin and insulin sensitivity. *Metabolism* 2000; 49(2):259–263.

169. Williams MA, Havel PJ, Schwartz MW, et al. Pre-eclampsia disrupts the normal relationship between serum leptin concentrations and adiposity in pregnant women. *Paediatr Perinat Epidemiol* 1999; 13(2):190–204.

170. Shintani M, Ikegami H, Fujisawa T, et al. Leptin gene polymorphism is associated with hypertension independent of obesity. *J Clin Endocrinol Metab* 2002; 87(6):2909–2912.

171. Muy-Rivera M, Ning Y, Frederic IO, et al. Leptin, soluble leptin receptor and leptin gene polymorphism in relation to preeclampsia risk. *Physiol Res* 2004; E-pub ahead of print.

172. Fisher RM, Humphries SE, Talmud PJ. Common variation in the lipoprotein lipase gene: effects on plasma lipids and risk of atherosclerosis. *Atherosclerosis* 1997; 135(2):145–159.

173. Hubel CA, Roberts JM, Ferrell RE. Association of pre-eclampsia with common coding sequence variations in the lipoprotein lipase gene. *Clin Genet* 1999; 56(4):289–296.

174. Keavney B, Palmer A, Parish S, et al. Lipid-related genes and myocardial infarction in 4685 cases and 3460 controls: discrepancies between genotype, blood lipid concentrations, and coronary disease risk. *Int J Epidemiol* 2004; 33(5):1002–1013.

175. Belo L, Gaffney D, Caslake M, et al. Apolipoprotein E and cholesteryl ester transfer protein polymorphisms in normal and preeclamptic pregnancies. *Eur J Obstet Gynecol Reprod Biol* 2004; 112(1):9–15.

176. Law A, Wallis SC, Powell LM, et al. Common DNA polymorphism within coding sequence of apolipoprotein B gene associated with altered lipid levels. *Lancet* 1986; 1(8493):1301–1303.

177. Miettinen TA. Impact of apo E phenotype on the regulation of cholesterol metabolism. *Ann Med* 1991; 23(2):181–186.

178. Nagy B, Rigo J Jr, Fintor L, et al. Apolipoprotein E alleles in women with severe pre-eclamp-sia. *J Clin Pathol* 1998; 51(4):324–325.

179. Makkonen N, Heinonen S, Hiltunen M, et al. Apolipoprotein E alleles in women with pre-eclampsia. *J Clin Pathol* 2001; 54(8):652–654.

180. Widen E, Lehto M, Kanninen T, et al. Association of a polymorphism in the beta 3-adrenergic-receptor gene with features of the insulin resistance syndrome in Finns. *New Engl J Med* 1995; 333(6):348–351.

181. Malina AN, Laivuori HM, Agatisa PK, et al. The Trp64Arg polymorphism of the [beta] 3-adrenergic receptor is not increased in women with preeclampsia. *Am J Obstet Gynecol* 2004; 190(3):779–783.

7 | Meta-analyses in genetics: methodological considerations with a focus on the renin–angiotensin system

Bernard Keavney

INTRODUCTION

Rapid developments in the tools available to investigate the contribution of human genetic variation to complex disease susceptibility are in progress. At the time of writing, a total of ~6 million out of the predicted 11 million single nucleotide polymorphisms (SNPs) with minor allele frequency > 0.01 genome wide have been discovered. The international Haplotype Map project has genotyped over 1 million common SNPs in 270 individuals drawn from four populations (Utah residents with Northern and Western European ancestry; Yoruba people in Ibadan, Nigeria; Japanese individuals in Tokyo, Japan; and Han Chinese people in Beijing, China) or one SNP every 5 kilobases (kb) throughout the human genome. Relationships between neighboring SNPs have been defined to facilitate both comprehensive candidate gene studies and, potentially, genome-wide studies to examine association between common genetic polymorphisms and common diseases (see http://www.hapmap.org). Genotyping technology has advanced with great rapidity, such that the highest-throughput laboratories can now generate over 500 000 genotypes per week. However, collection of suitable population resources in which to apply these tools has lagged behind significantly. Mathematical genetics theory suggests that the genetic effects that are most likely to be present in complex diseases (relative risks of disease in general between 1.2 and 1.5) will in the main be undetectable using family-based linkage methods (typically, in pairs of siblings affected with the disease of interest) because unfeasibly large studies would be required.[1] It therefore seems likely that the majority of new studies will continue to be of the population-based, case-control association design, either prospectively or retrospectively ascertained. There are evident close parallels between this study design and the classical observational epidemiological study or clinical trial, and it is therefore not unexpected that the technique of meta-analysis has been increasingly applied in the genetics literature in recent years.

Meta-analysis attempts to combine data from all available qualifiying studies of a research question by weighting the results of each individual study according to its size, and combining these results to arrive at an optimally accurate estimate of the effect in question. Initially, meta-analysis was developed to investigate the effects of interventions in randomized controlled clinical trials. Although methodology for the meta-analysis of randomized trials is well established, meta-analysis of observational epidemiological studies remains an area of some controversy because of the potential for spurious results resulting from study design differences, insufficient adjustment for confounders and publication bias. It can be argued, however, that because of the random allocation of alleles at any particular locus at conception ('Mendelian randomization'), genetic association studies are more analogous to randomized trials than observational studies and might be less susceptible to confounding.[2] This chapter discusses the principal issues influencing the application of meta-analysis to genetics, focusing on examples where polymorphisms of the genes involved in the renin–angiotensin system have been investigated.

REPRODUCIBILITY OF GENETIC ASSOCIATION STUDIES

Larger and more rigorous studies

The number of genetic association studies published is increasing rapidly year on year. Unfortunately, the speed with which the field has advanced our understanding of the genetic contribution to complex disease susceptibility does not match the publication rate. Case-control genetic association studies have a deserved reputation of yielding nonreproducible results, and this is very likely to be due to the reporting of 'positive' findings in underpowered samples with inappropriately lax levels of statistical significance.

There is a clear need for far larger and more rigorous studies than have thus far been usual. Zondervan & Cardon have shown that to detect relative risks (RR) of 1.2–1.5, samples of between 2000 and 10 000 cases of disease (and an equivalent or greater number of controls) are required, even in the best-case scenario where the allele frequencies of the marker variant typed and the unobserved disease-causing variants match.[3] Very few individual studies in any disease area have involved even 1000 cases of disease and the conduct of appropriately large-scale studies, initially to reliably confirm or refute the many hypothesized associations described so far, is the most pressing requirement in this field. This is likely to involve extensive collaboration between groups.

With respect to statistical significance levels, the prior probability that any randomly selected genetic polymorphism is causally associated with the risk of a complex disease, while not formally calculable, seems likely to be very small; in this context, association between such a polymorphism and disease at the level $P < 0.05$ does not represent strong evidence. Even for more carefully selected polymorphisms, such as those of candidate genes supported by physiology that is of importance in the disease process, this level of stringency is likely to be insufficient. The absolute level of significance cannot be arbitrarily defined, although Colhoun and colleagues constructed a Bayesian argument to illustrate how much more stringent it might have to be to make the literature more reliable.[4] These authors pointed out that the proportion of reports in the literature that are true positives is influenced not only by study power and significance levels, but by the proportion of cases in which the null hypothesis (i.e. that of no association) is true. They showed that to obtain 20 : 1 posterior odds that a reported association was true (and thus to give a reasonable expectation that

95% of reports in the literature would subsequently be confirmed) then if the prior odds of an association were 1 : 50 a level of $P < 0.00005$ would be required. Even if the prior odds of association were as good as 1 : 20 – perhaps a more reasonable estimate when a physiologically relevant polymorphism of a strong candidate gene is typed – then a significance level of $P < 0.0001$ would be required. Power calculations based on these figures show that even quite large effects (RR of 1.5 to the heterozygote and 2.25 to the homozygote) could not be detected in samples of greater than 10 000 cases and 10 000 controls for common polymorphisms (alleles of 10% frequency) under all conditions, so it seems likely that some compromise of this extreme level of statistical stringency dependent on other features of the study (e.g. the presence of complete characterization of all the common variation in a candidate gene or region, the typing of polymorphisms of known physiological function, or the replication of the association in independent populations) will be required in practice. In their meta-analysis of 25 genetic associations, Lohmueller and colleagues noted that the presence of one report (other than the first positive study) with $P < 0.001$, or two studies with $P < 0.01$, was strongly predictive of further replication.[5] However, the majority of association studies continue to achieve publication with P values in the range 0.01–0.05.

Overviews of genetic association studies

The degree of replication between association studies was qualitatively assessed by Hirschhorn and colleagues, who reviewed studies of 166 proposed genetic associations spanning all areas of disease, and found that only six of these associations were replicated in > 75% of studies.[6] Subsequent studies have approached this issue in a more quantitative fashion. An overview of 36 published meta-analyses conducted by Ioannidis and colleagues showed that significant heterogeneity in effect estimate between contributing studies in meta-analyses is frequent, that the results of the first published study often correlate poorly with subsequent studies of the same association, and that the first study often suggests a stronger genetic effect than that found by subsequent studies.[7] In a more extensive study of 55 meta-analyses, these authors found that the magnitude of the genetic effect differed significantly in large versus small studies in 20–40% of meta-analyses depending on the heterogeneity test used.[8] Larger studies tended to provide more conservative estimates of the magnitude of associations than did smaller ones. These findings suggest that publication bias (a tendency for small positive studies to achieve publication whereas small negative studies do not do so), time-lag bias (a tendency for negative studies to be published later than positive ones) or both are significant factors in the published literature potentially influencing the validity of meta-analyses. Overall, Ioannidis et al found significant between-study heterogeneity in 47% of studies and showed that only nine (16%) of the associations showed replicable significance without any evidence of heterogeneity or bias among the contributing studies. Lohmueller and colleagues conducted meta-analyses of 301 studies of 25 associations, half of which were randomly selected from the literature and half of which related to diseases of specific interest to the authors.[5] Using statistical techniques that attempt to estimate the number of unpublished studies that must be present for particular associations to be due to publication bias, they robustly rejected the hypothesis that all the associations observed arose as a result of publication bias. However, the evidence for association was concentrated in

11 of the 25 associations studied, and pooled analyses of follow-up studies replicated the first report in just eight of these cases. Thus, even among selected associations, less than 50% were supported by the totality of the available evidence. If the results of these overviews are generalizable, it appears that between one-sixth and one-third of the genetic associations in the published literature are likely to be true, although very few of these are established robustly at present.

The overviews conducted by both these groups also identified evidence that novel associations, detected in underpowered samples, disproportionately influence the subsequent literature. Ioannidis and colleagues found that first studies tended to overestimate genetic effects, particularly if the studies were of small size, and showed that the greater the number of studies in the meta-analysis, the greater this tendency was.[7,8] Lohmueller and colleagues also observed the phenomenon of more extreme associations being reported in first studies, and invoked the 'winner's curse' phenomenon as a possible alternative explanation to publication bias.[5] Simply put, this phenomenon might arise because of upward bias in the estimate of the strength of a genetic association conditional upon the 'winning' study being the first to achieve statistical significance and be published. These observations suggest that journal editors should take care to set the standard for papers that describe new associations particularly high, specifically with regard to the need for positive results to be obtained either in one large population consisting of thousands of cases and controls or in more than one smaller population, which together provide a total number of cases in the thousands. The quality and size of initial investigations are particularly important since overoptimistic early findings can lead to subsequent studies being seriously underpowered as the 'benchmark' effect for detection is assumed to be inappropriately large. Conversely, it has been shown that if first studies (most of which were seriously underpowered) are negative, fewer subsequent studies tend to be performed, resulting in inadequate investigation of potential real associations.[5]

STUDY SIZE AND PUBLICATION BIAS

Example: angiotensin-converting enzyme gene

The literature examining the association between the angiotensin-converting enzyme (ACE) insertion/deletion (I/D) polymorphism and cardiovascular endpoints is particularly instructive with respect to the issues of study size and publication bias. In 1992, Cambien and colleagues presented evidence in a study of 610 myocardial infarction (MI) patients and 733 controls that people homozygous for the deletion allele (DD genotype) had a significantly higher risk of MI – odds ratio (OR) 1.34; 95% confidence interval (CI) 1.05–1.70 – than those of the other two genotypes (ID and II).[9] It should be appreciated that by the standards of the time this represented a very large association study, and even at the time of writing, the majority of genetic association studies that have been published in cardiovascular disease continue to involve fewer cases than did this important cohort. This paper is the most cited in the entire cardiovascular genetics literature, with over 450 citations to date. Between 1992 and 2000, 49 subsequent studies investigated the association, although 35 of these studies involved fewer than 200 cases of MI and it was not until 1998 that a study involving a larger number of cases than the original investigation was published. In 2000, investigation of the large International Studies of Infarct Survival (ISIS) genetic study of 5000 cases and 5000 controls showed that there was no significant evidence for association between the polymorphism and MI (OR 1.10; 95% CI 1.00–1.21).[10] A meta-analysis of the 50 studies, involving 15 070 cases of MI, conducted by the ISIS group showed clear evidence that smaller studies that had examined the association gave more extreme ORs than larger studies (Fig. 7.1), raising the strong possibility that publication bias could in large part account for the enduring uncertainty about this association up to that point. In anecdotal support of this view, the ISIS group had also obtained personally communicated data from investigators known to have cohorts who had not published on this question, which supported the notion that some negative findings, even in relatively large cohorts, were not made publicly available. When all the larger studies were jointly analyzed, there was no evidence of association between the polymorphism and MI risk (risk ratio for DD versus other genotypes of 1.02; 95% CI 0.95–1.11).

The ACE I/D polymorphism has also been investigated for association with restenosis after coronary angioplasty. A 2002 meta-analysis of 16 studies involving 4631 angioplasty patients showed a combined OR for restenosis with the DD genotype of 1.23 (99% CI 1.03–1.46) among all studies.[11] However, there was significant heterogeneity between larger and smaller studies: the OR for restenosis in people with the DD genotype was 1.94 (99% CI 1.39–2.71) for studies with less than 100 cases, 1.33 (99% CI 0.92–1.93) for studies with 100–200 cases, and 0.92 (99% CI 0.72–1.18) for studies with more than 200 cases (trend $P = 0.02$; Fig. 7.2). This meta-analysis also investigated the impact of quality-control issues in the genotyping process by obtaining laboratory practice details through correspondence with authors. When studies were grouped by genotyping procedures, significantly larger ORs were found in the studies that did not conceal disease status from laboratory staff carrying out the genotyping. Additionally, the deletion (D)

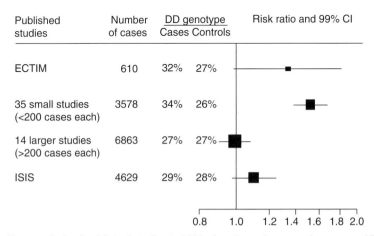

Fig. 7.1 Meta-analysis of published studies to 2000 of angiotensin-converting enzyme I/D polymorphism and myocardial infarction. Risk ratios in each study or group of studies are represented by squares (area proportional to the amount of statistical information) with horizontal lines denoting 99% confidence intervals (CIs). The hypothesis-generating study (ECTIM) and the single largest study (ISIS) are shown separately.

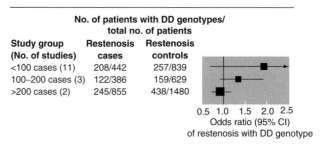

	No. of patients with DD genotypes/ total no. of patients		
Study group (No. of studies)	Restenosis cases	Restenosis controls	
<100 cases (11)	208/442	257/839	
100–200 cases (3)	122/386	159/629	
>200 cases (2)	245/855	438/1480	

0.5 1.0 1.5 2.0 2.5
Odds ratio (95% CI)
of restenosis with DD genotype

Fig. 7.2 Meta-analysis of studies of angiotensin-converting enzyme I/D polymorphism and restenosis after percutaneous coronary intervention grouped by size. Conventions as in Fig. 7.1.

allele of the polymorphism is known to be preferentially amplified by the polymerase chain reaction (PCR), and a second PCR method to check heterozygote genotypes is routinely used in the majority of studies typing this polymorphism. The studies that did not use a second PCR assay to reduce genetic mistyping tended to have larger ORs in favor of association. These results suggested that publication or detection bias could have an equally large effect as the small genetic effects being sought in such investigations.

METHODOLOGICAL ISSUES IN META-ANALYSIS

Quality of contributing studies

Apart from study size, other issues regarding the quality of individual contributing studies potentially affect the validity of meta-analyses of genetic associations. Although a number of 'checklists' have been suggested to ensure the quality of gene–disease association studies (perhaps the most comprehensive being that put forward by Little and colleagues based on a Human Genome Epidemiology workshop[12]) there is no universally accepted standard to which authors, reviewers, editors and meta-analysts can refer with respect to study quality. Although measurement error and the generation of subtle biases by study design flaws are issues very familiar to classical epidemiologists, they tend to be less comprehensively addressed in genotyping experiments. Study characteristics such as recruitment methods for cases and controls, participation rates in different groups, success rates for DNA extraction (and any differences in these rates between cases and controls), and consideration of the similarity or otherwise in sociodemographic characteristics of those successfully genotyped and those not successfully genotyped are rarely reported in detail, but could potentially generate substantial biases. Similarly, genotyping error rates are not always estimated and reported. Duplicate genotyping of a randomly selected subset of DNA samples should be routine in all association studies, and any study with less than 95% reproducibility of genotypes should be viewed with extreme caution. Genotyping should be carried out by laboratory staff 'blinded' to disease status, and cases and controls should be allocated to genotyping plates in a nonsystematic manner; nonobservance of these laboratory practices has been associated with more extreme ORs in some meta-analyses.[11] Contributing studies in a meta-analysis might differ very substantially with respect to the amount of information regarding genotyping methodology present in their methods sections; wherever possible, additional information should be sought from authors by meta-analysts regarding these issues.

Issues specific to genetic meta-analyses

'Traditional' meta-analyses in epidemiology have benefited from guidelines regarding their conduct; certain minimum standards such as stating databases and search terms, explicit inclusion and exclusion criteria for studies, the use of appropriate statistical methodology in data pooling, and exploration for heterogeneity and publication bias, are generally agreed.[13] However, in a review of 37 genetic meta-analyses, Attia and colleagues noted frequent deficiencies in the application of 'traditional' methodology, and highlighted two additional problems specific to genetic meta-analyses that were generally inadequately explored.[14]

First, there was a widespread failure to test studies included in meta-analyses for Hardy–Weinberg equilibrium. The Hardy–Weinberg law relates the expected genotype frequencies seen in an idealized population to the observed allele frequencies: if two alleles A and a with the frequencies p and q are in equilibrium, then the proportions of individuals with genotypes AA, Aa and aa will be p^2, $2pq$ and q^2, respectively. Deviation from Hardy–Weinberg equilibrium (HWE) might occur for many reasons but genotyping error is probably the most frequent, i.e. when common polymorphisms have been typed in case-control studies recruited from general populations. Certainly, it would seem prudent to expect individual studies observing genotype frequencies in control individuals that are not in HWE to check the data using an alternative genotyping method, although this is rarely performed. Although there is currently no consensus on whether studies showing departure from HWE should be included in a meta-analysis, it is appropriate at the very least to carry out sensitivity (subgroup) analyses both including and excluding such studies.

Second, Attia and colleagues commented that meta-analyses did not always pool data in a way that reflected the biology of gene effects. Comparison between genotypes can be done in a variety of ways: by comparing allele frequencies in case and control groups, by testing a specific genetic model (dominant, recessive or codominant), or by multiple pairwise comparisons between genotypes. Evidently the testing of a variety of models raises issues of multiple comparisons, but the mode of inheritance of complex disorders is generally unknown. In a subsequent paper, these authors proposed a method that allowed the pooled data to 'dictate' the best genetic model to apply in a meta-analysis to overcome this difficulty.[15] Although this approach might be appropriate for polymorphisms where no biological information is available, incorporation of such biological information where available, and the *a priori* testing of the genetic model it suggests, might be preferable. A potential problem for testing alternative genetic models in meta-analyses to those explored in contributing studies is that the presentation of data in individual studies does not always permit derivation of the numbers of individuals in each genotype group.

Heterogeneity

Significant between-study heterogeneity in effect estimates has been observed in about half of the published associations between genes and disease that have been the subject of meta-analyses.[8] Adequate consideration of heterogeneity, investigation of the reasons for its presence and application of the appropriate statistical model to account for it, are key issues in genetic meta-analysis. Some examples of sources of heterogeneity identified in meta-analyses have been discussed above (study size, genotyping conducted 'blind' to disease status) and others are considered below. Two statistical models can be used to combine the estimates of effect size derived from studies contributing to a meta-analysis: a fixed-effect or random-effect model. These test two different hypotheses: the *fixed-effects model* assumes that all the study samples are drawn from a single population with a common effect size, and so differences between the estimates in the contributing studies are due to sampling error alone. By contrast, the *random-effects model* assumes that the samples included in the meta-analysis are drawn from a distribution of populations, each one of which could have a different size of effect. Thus, the fixed and random-effects models do not ask the same scientific question: the fixed-effects model asks what the best estimate of the population effect size is, whereas the random-effects model asks what the range and distribution of population effect sizes is (allowing for the possibility that in different populations the effects may vary widely in size, and even be in opposite directions). The assumed homogeneity of the populations involved in the fixed-effect model means that if significantly heterogeneous studies are erroneously pooled under this model, there is a high risk of type 1 error (i.e. false-positive findings). Conversely, the incorporation of between-study heterogeneity as an additional source of variation in the random-effects model results in wider confidence intervals around the effect size of the weighted average. However, if the genetic effect in all contributing populations is in reality similar, and the heterogeneity identified results from sources of bias, this model will produce inaccurate estimates. It should also be noted that one of the assumptions of the random-effects model is that the studies included in the meta-analysis represent a random selection of studies that could have been conducted in a research domain, and this is probably never true in practice. Also, the substitution of a random-effects analysis for a fixed-effects analysis changes the nature of the question asked, as outlined above; this should be borne in mind when random-effects models are used.[16]

Typically, heterogeneity is assessed using Cochran's Q statistic, which is computed by summing the squared deviations of each study's estimate from the overall meta-analytic estimate, weighting each study's contribution in the same manner as the meta-analysis. This statistic follows a chi-square distribution with degrees of freedom equal to the number of studies minus one, and enables some estimation of whether the variation in effects observed is larger than that which might be expected due to chance alone.[17] But, as pointed out by Higgins and colleagues, this test is known to be poor at detecting true heterogeneity among studies, and this is a particular problem when the contributing number of studies is small.[18] These authors developed an alternative approach quantifying the effect of heterogeneity by an index (I^2), which describes the percentage of variation across studies due to heterogeneity rather than chance:

$$I^2 = 100\% \times (Q - df)/Q$$

where Q is the heterogeneity statistic and df is the degrees of freedom. It was suggested that I^2 values of 25%, 50% and 75% would indicate low, moderate and high levels of heterogeneity. Originally discussed with respect to epidemiological meta-analyses, the I^2 value has been used by Ioannidis and colleagues to quantify heterogeneity between different ethnic groups included in genetic meta-analyses (see below) and can be a useful quantitative guide to the degree of heterogeneity present in such studies.[19]

It is standard practice for heterogeneity, once identified, to be further explored. If the sources of heterogeneity can be identified then they can be incorporated in the analysis; if not, then there is a degree of subjectivity regarding whether studies should be pooled using a random-effects model or not pooled at all. Lohmueller and colleagues in their analysis of 25 associations adopted the approach of reviewing the methods sections of studies exhibiting heterogeneity for flaws or evident differences with other studies and removing such studies; if significant heterogeneity remained, this was followed by successive removal of studies with the greatest contributions to heterogeneity until homogeneity was achieved.[5] This seems a logically consistent and practical approach.

There are many potential clinical sources of heterogeneity relating to case and control selection strategy. For a number of conditions, twin studies have shown that the genetic contribution to risk is larger in people developing the disease at younger ages, and therefore the effects of particular genetic polymorphisms on risk might be larger at younger ages. Thus, if some contributing studies have selected younger cases whereas others have selected older cases, there might be heterogeneity between the studies that appropriately reflects the biological mechanisms. Genetic risks can also differ by sex – an important practical consideration since many of the clinical trial populations that have been adapted for use as genetic cohorts collected only males or females.

To maximize power to detect genetic influences on quantitative traits, it is crucial to select individuals from the extremes of the distribution. For example, with respect to blood pressure, 'case' individuals selected from the upper 5% – or better – 1% of the distribution will yield far greater power than an equivalent number of cases selected from the top 20–25%. However, estimates of risk derived from such extremely selected populations are likely to be greater than those estimated in less selected populations. Where different disease endpoints are used in studies contributing to a meta-analysis, this can contribute to heterogeneity. For example, in a meta-analysis of studies of paraoxonase polymorphisms and coronary heart disease conducted by Wheeler and colleagues, endpoints included coronary artery stenosis defined as at least 20% in one study, 50% in 17 studies, 70% in three studies and 75% in two studies.[20]

If a particular polymorphism is strongly related to the risk of a fatal event, ORs in prospective studies and retrospectively ascertained case-control studies can differ due to survival bias. For example, in Song and colleagues' meta-analysis of apolipoprotein E (apo E) genotypes and risk of coronary heart disease (CHD), significant heterogeneity between prospective and retrospective studies was shown. It was noted that the apo E ε4 allele (which is related to CHD risk) was strongly associated with CHD death in four prospective studies.[21]

Unintended features of the individual study populations can give rise to heterogeneity, for example, population stratification. This occurs when within an apparently homogeneous population under investigation there are in fact two or more subpopulations, which differ in both their genetic makeup and their rates of disease. This combination leads to undetected differences in the genetic makeup of the case and control groups ascertained from such a population. In such a case, differences in allele frequencies observed between cases and controls would not entirely reflect causal associations with disease, but rather wholly or partly the baseline differences in allele frequencies between the genetically inhomogeneous case and control groups (Fig. 7.3). Stratification artifact is a classically cited cause of false positive findings, although it can also lead to failure to detect true associations.[22] The importance of stratification artifact has been widely debated and opposing views have been strongly held despite a paucity of data. Recently, however, Marchini and colleagues typed 15 000 genome-wide SNPs in three population groups (European–Americans, African–Americans and Asians), quantified the extent of population stratification within and between the populations, and assessed the potential impact of stratification on large association studies.[23] This study showed that even small amounts of stratification could undermine the findings of an association study and lead to false-positive results, and that these adverse effects increased markedly with sample size. For the size of study required to detect small effects (many thousands of cases and controls), even the relatively small amounts of stratification present within a population were shown to have important effects. The typing of a large number of anonymous markers not related to disease status (and which therefore should have similar frequencies in genetically homogeneous case and control populations – a technique referred to as 'genomic control') is a method to detect and account for population stratification in association studies, but it has been seldom used in studies so far.[24,25] When, despite consideration of the most commonly found sources of heterogeneity, considerable heterogeneity remains among studies in a meta-analysis, stratification remains a potential contributor that is impossible to exclude in most studies published to date.

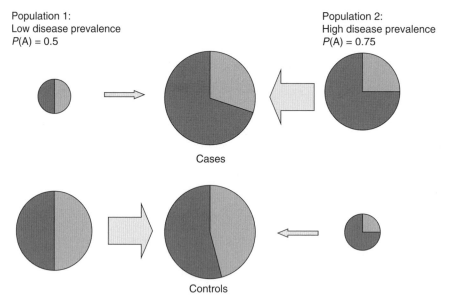

Population 1:
Low disease prevalence
$P(A) = 0.5$

Population 2:
High disease prevalence
$P(A) = 0.75$

Cases

Controls

Fig. 7.3 Effects of population stratification at a single nucleotide polymorphism (SNP) locus. Allele frequencies in each population are represented by the shaded proportions within the circles, and the sizes of the populations represented by the areas of the circles. The population of cases and controls consists of two subpopulations that differ genetically and in their disease prevalence. Population 1 will tend to contribute more to the control group, whose allele frequency will be similar to that population, whereas population 2 will contribute more to the case group. Here, allele A (represented in light gray) would appear to be associated with disease, but this signal would not reflect causal association.

Genomic sources of heterogeneity include differences in the degree of allelic association (linkage disequilibrium; LD) between the typed polymorphism and the unobserved putative causative variant in the gene, differences in allele frequencies at either variant, and differences in the level of risk associated with particular alleles between populations. Available data suggest that LD is relatively homogeneous within ethnic groups but that there are substantial differences between populations, in particular a much lower level of LD in populations of African origin.[26] Allele frequencies at many polymorphisms differ substantially between different ethnic groups, although the risks associated with those alleles might not. Ioannidis and colleagues screened 134 meta-analyses and showed that large heterogeneity in allele frequencies between ethnic groups ($I^2 > 75\%$) was present in 58% of 43 gene–disease associations, although there was large heterogeneity in the ORs of disease between ethnic groups in only 14% of cases.[19] The consistency of the genetic effects across ethnic groups suggests common biological effects of the polymorphisms studied. Indeed, in many of the studies evaluated by Ioannidis and colleagues, polymorphisms with probable functional effects were typed. Although ORs for disease conferred by particular alleles might be similar, differences in allele frequency between populations will mean that population attributable risks for some such alleles may differ substantially in different ethnicities.

Gene–environment interaction might be an important source of heterogeneity between contributing studies in a meta-analysis. A potential example was provided by Klerk and colleagues, who assessed the relationship between the MTHFR C677T polymorphism and the risk of CHD by conducting a meta-analysis of 40 studies involving 11 162 cases and 12 758 controls.[27] The T allele of MTHFR C677T is associated with higher plasma homocysteine levels. Among studies conducted in Europe, the OR of CHD for TT versus CC genotype was 1.14 (95% CI 1.01–1.28), whereas among studies conducted in North America, the OR was 0.87 (95% CI 0.73–1.04). There was significant heterogeneity between the European and American studies ($P = 0.01$). Previous studies had shown that the TT genotype is only associated with high homocysteine levels in the setting of low folate status. Plasma levels of homocysteine were higher in the European than the American studies and it was suggested that effect modification by dietary intake of folate could account for at least some of the differences between these ORs. Folate fortification of breakfast cereals had been undertaken some time before the North American studies were recruited and the average use of vitamin supplementation in North America is considerably higher than that in Europe. The positive result in the European population (comprising 6207 cases and 8343 controls) remains statistically borderline and results from further large-scale studies of Europeans would be required to confirm or refute the presence of this possible gene–environment interaction.

When study design (prospective versus retrospective; population versus hospital-based controls), study size, population origins and ethnicity, difference in endpoints, allele frequency and presence of HWE, genotyping methods and potentially relevant gene–environment interaction have all been explored as potential sources of heterogeneity, substantial heterogeneity might still remain. For example, in Wheeler and colleagues' meta-analysis of 45 studies of paraoxonase polymorphisms and CHD risk, the above study characteristics explained little of the overall heterogeneity.[20] Other potentially highly relevant factors, such as age and the presence of other risk factors, are difficult to explore unless individual participant data is available for review. Such an approach has been successfully implemented in a number of recent meta-analyses (see below).

Meta-analysis of linkage studies

Although the overwhelming majority of individual studies and meta-analyses have been conducted using a case-control association design, statistical methods have also been developed to combine data from genome-wide linkage studies for complex diseases. In such studies, allele-sharing at around 500 highly polymorphic microsatellite markers distributed throughout the genome is assessed in pairs of relatives, most usually affected siblings. Advantages of this study design include the feasibility of an unbiased 'hypothesis-free' assessment of the evidence for determination of the phenotype by genes anywhere in the genome, and the small number of markers that need to be typed to obtain genome-wide coverage (for comparison, genome-wide association studies would require hundreds of thousands of markers). The principal disadvantage of this study design when compared with case-control association is lack of power. Small genetic effects will not be detected even in the largest feasible studies. However, if certain loci contribute disproportionately, they might be detected, and the 'genome-screening' approach has yielded positive results that have led to gene identification in a variety of conditions (although not hypertension as yet). Statistical methods have recently been developed to allow combination of datasets in which nonidentical markers have been typed, potentially widening the applicability of the technique if authors are willing to share data.[28,29] Genome screens for hypertension or blood-pressure regulation had been reported in 14 cohorts to October 2004.[30,31] Six of these cohorts had reported results that met the criteria for genome-wide statistical significance, although there was no replication of the conventionally significant loci between studies. Pooled analysis of the data from the four multicentre networks making up the National Heart, Lung and Blood Institute (NHLBI) Family Blood Pressure Program, including over 6000 individuals, was carried out by Province and colleagues using Fisher's method (which is applicable where the same markers have been typed).[32] Liu and colleagues used the Genome Search Meta-Analysis (GSMA) method, which can be applied when nonidentical markers are typed, to combine the results of six further datasets, including over 8000 individuals.[33] No region showed evidence of significant linkage to hypertension in either meta-analysis. However, as neither of these two meta-analyses have included all available studies, it remains possible that a pooled analysis of all available genome screens may prove useful in the future.

THE ANGIOTENSINOGEN GENE AND BLOOD PRESSURE

Sethi and colleagues conducted a meta-analysis of 63 studies involving 45 267 individuals examining the association of angiotensinogen gene polymorphisms with a variety of cardiovascular endpoints.[34] This meta-analysis illustrates several of the issues discussed above. The principal angiotensinogen polymorphism that has been studied is the M235T variant. Individuals with TT genotype were originally found by Jeunemaitre and colleagues in 1992 to have a 20% higher level of plasma angiotensinogen and an OR for hypertension of 1.95

when compared with MM homozygotes.[35] The meta-analysis found highly significant evidence for a stepwise increase of 5% in plasma angiotensinogen levels per T allele, and ORs for hypertension in white subjects of 1.08 (95% CI 1.01–1.15) in MT subjects and 1.19 (95% CI 1.10–1.30) in TT subjects relative to the MM genotype. In Asian populations the aggregated OR for hypertension was 1.29 (95% CI 0.96–1.71) in MT subjects and 1.60 (95% CI 1.19–2.15) in TT homozygotes. M235T genotype did not predict systolic or diastolic blood pressure in those studies that had investigated BP as a quantitative trait, nor was it related to risk of CHD or MI in either ethnic group. Although 127 studies were found by the meta-analysis search strategy, 36 studies had to be excluded from analysis for reasons such as failure to report genotype frequencies in each genotype group or to give the numbers in case and control groups. As with most literature-based meta-analyses, only studies in English were included. The authors noted that included studies were not homogeneous with respect to selection and characterization of hypertensive cases and controls, and that important risk factors for hypertension, such as age and BMI, could not be adjusted for in the analysis; these are issues that will undoubtedly continue to prove particularly difficult in genetic meta-analyses of hypertension in the future. There was significant heterogeneity between the studies in white subjects ($P = 0.006$). All studies were nonetheless pooled and both fixed-effects and random-effects models were applied; under the random-effects model the OR for TT versus MM genotype was 1.29 (95% CI 1.10–1.50); no heterogeneity was reported between the studies in Asians. Funnel plots were used to assess the presence of publication bias, and none was evident; however, formal statistical tests to explore the influence of other sources of heterogeneity in the studies of white subjects were not performed. In both ethnicities, the ratio of hypertensive cases to controls was approximately 1 : 1. Despite this careful meta-analysis of a large number of studies, there remains some uncertainty about the relationship of this polymorphism to the risk of hypertension. In white subjects, there was only one large study involving nearly 9000 of the 18 000 or so subjects studied for hypertension, and that study, which was well-conducted in a representative population sample, was negative. There was also residual unexplained heterogeneity between studies in white subjects pooled in the meta-analysis. In Asian subjects, despite the lack of heterogeneity between studies and the statistically highly significant result, a total of only around 5000 subjects had been studied and the largest study involved just 838 hypertensive subjects. There is a clear need for further large studies, particularly in Asian subjects, to confirm or refute this suggestive meta-analysis result definitively.

RELATIONSHIPS BETWEEN META-ANALYSES AND LARGE STUDIES

Where small genetic effects on rare diseases are being sought, it is possible that no single investigator will be able to collect the thousands of cases necessary to achieve statistical precision. In these cases, meta-analysis might prove to be the only method of achieving sufficient power to address the question. For common diseases, however, large collaborative projects (such as the MRC British Genetics of Hypertension Study in the UK)[36] or national-level resources such as the proposed UK Biobank study (see http://www.ukbiobank.ac.uk), should achieve sufficient numbers of carefully phenotyped individuals to be able to test genetic hypotheses reliably. In these cases, meta-analyses could fulfill an important role by identifying and prioritizing particular associations to be studied.

Wheeler and colleagues showed that regularly updated review of the available data on the association between paraoxonase-1 polymorphisms and CHD could have been helpful in addressing some of the problems associated with the proliferation of underpowered studies on the subject.[20] For both the Q192R and L55M polymorphisms of paraoxonase-1, point estimates and confidence intervals were very similar when studies conducted up to the year 2000 or up to the year 2003 were included (Fig. 7.4). Between the years 2000 and 2003, some 4000 additional cases and 6000 additional controls were genotyped, mostly in underpowered studies, with minimal effect on the overall estimate of the association. A timely meta-analysis (in 2000) could have shown that such small studies were unlikely to contribute much to the precision with which the association was quantified at that time, and possibly saved resources and effort.

It is encouraging that the findings of genetic meta-analyses have been subsequently confirmed by large-scale studies in a number of cases, for example with respect to the apo E ε2/ε3/ε4 polymorphism and MI risk,[37,38] and the peroxisome proliferator-activated receptor gamma (PPARG) Pro12Ala polymorphism and type 2 diabetes.[39,40] However, in other cases, the results of meta-analyses and large studies have been discrepant. For example, Jellema and colleagues carried out a meta-analysis of 27 studies including 3408 cases and 5419 controls that had

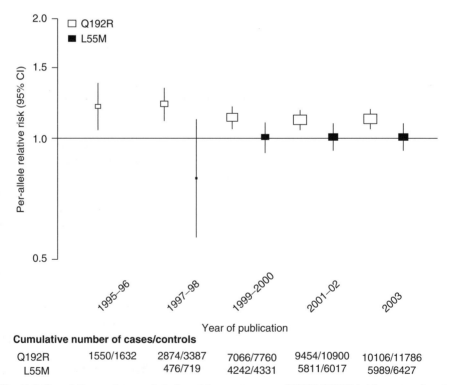

Fig. 7.4 Cumulative syntheses of studies of the paraoxonase (PON1) Q192R (white squares) and L55M (black squares) polymorphisms and coronary heart disease. The vertical axis is plotted on a log-doubling scale.

examined the association between the Gly972Arg variant in the insulin receptor substrate-1 gene and type 2 diabetes.[41] The summary risk ratio was 1.25 (95% CI 1.05–1.48). The largest study included just 321 cases and 992 controls. The meta-analysts noted heterogeneity dependent on type of study (clinic versus population based), diagnostic test used to exclude diabetes in control subjects, and age of the case subjects. Florez and colleagues subsequently tested this variant in 4279 cases of diabetes, 3532 controls and 1189 siblings discordant for type 2 diabetes.[40] This sample size was estimated to have > 95% power at $P < 0.05$ to detect the OR of 1.25 that emerged from the meta-analysis. In this study, the Gly972Arg variant was not associated with diabetes (OR 0.96; 95% CI 0.84–1.10; $P = 0.60$). By contrast, two well-documented associations between other genetic polymorphisms (PPARG Pro12Ala and Kir6.2 E23K) and type 2 diabetes were robustly observed in these samples. Such 'validated' polymorphisms, when available, can potentially act as 'positive controls' of the power of large study cohorts to detect association.

There are several possible reasons for the discrepancy between the meta-analysis and the large-scale study of IRS-1 Gly972Arg, but perhaps most likely is that the meta-analysis result was a statistical fluctuation: the meta-analysis result was not highly statistically significant, the number of patients included was below 5000, and significant between-study heterogeneity, which could not be completely accounted for, was present. Thus, meta-analyses, even when reasonably large (several thousands) numbers of patients are included, should not be considered as substitutes for adequately powered studies where these are possible.

META-ANALYSES OF INDIVIDUAL PARTICIPANT DATA

Meta-analysis of individual participant data is an alternative strategy to literature-based meta-analysis that – as yet – has been applied to relatively few research questions, probably because of its far more labor-intensive nature. In classical epidemiology, this approach has produced striking and authoritative results, for example the Prospective Studies Collaboration report on the relationship between usual levels of blood pressure and the risks of stroke and MI.[42] In genetic epidemiology, Ioannidis and colleagues were among the first to use individual participant data in this way, investigating host genetic effects in human immunodeficiency virus type 1 (HIV-1) disease progression.[43] The approach involves contacting primary investigators to submit their raw data, which is then 'cleaned' and harmonized with other studies; this has the potential to reduce between-study heterogeneity and increase the precision of analysis in a number of important ways. Because not all studies are published, and for those reports that are published not all potentially relevant data (e.g. information regarding other risk factors) are presented, this approach is likely to increase the completeness of information available. Standardized definitions of disease affection status can be applied consistently across studies. Synthesis of time-to-event information, where relevant, is facilitated. More extensive adjustment for covariates is possible, and knowledge of individuals' genotypes enables a consistent statistical treatment of loci that are in linkage disequilibrium. As some published studies do not report genotype frequencies in all genotype groups, testing of alternative genetic models to that used in the original report is sometimes impossible in literature-based meta-analysis; availability of raw data clearly overcomes this potentially important problem. Finally, availability of individual participant data may enable more thorough evaluation of remaining sources of heterogeneity.

Using this approach, Ioannidis and colleagues were able to confirm with greater precision the findings of an earlier literature-based meta-analysis of the same question for one polymorphism influencing progression to AIDS in HIV-1 positive patients, and to make conclusive inferences regarding the effects of a further two polymorphisms which could not be accurately quantified based on the data from the literature-based meta-analysis.

As another recent example, the GENOMOS investigators carried out a meta-analysis of individual participant data in 18 917 individuals to resolve the hitherto unclear issue (despite over 40 published studies) of whether polymorphisms in the estrogen receptor alpha (ESR1) gene confer susceptibility to osteoporotic fracture.[44] This study represented a further methodological step forward in that the genotyping methods in the participating centers were standardized, and blinded genotyping of the same 50 randomly selected samples was conducted in each center to ensure genotyping accuracy. The authors made the important point that a meta-analysis involving prospectively performed genotyping should be immune to the problems of publication bias.

The potential disadvantages of meta-analysis of individual participant data include unwillingness of particular groups to make their data available for collaborative analysis, achieving consensus among collaborators with respect to data interpretation, and the very substantial increase in cost and time required to conduct the analyses. These considerations mean that meta-analysis of individual participant data will probably be reserved for particularly pressing and difficult to resolve questions: in that regard the field of hypertension, where robust associations have been very difficult to establish, may well benefit from such an approach.

CONCLUSIONS

There is increasing evidence that common genetic polymorphisms make small but potentially important contributions to the risk of a number of common diseases. Although it is debatable whether any such polymorphism has yet been identified for hypertension, conditions of a similar order of heritability, such as type 2 diabetes and CHD, now have at least one robustly supported association. Meta-analysis has contributed significantly to the conclusive identification of such associations. The challenges of incomplete reporting and publication bias are perhaps the most difficult for meta-analysis to overcome; in this regard, consensus standards for the reporting, presentation and analysis of results of genetic association studies would be a considerable advance. Web-based depositories for detailed results of all studies, including negative findings, in a standardized format, could be particularly useful to combat publication bias. A useful first step towards this goal has been taken by the Genetic Association Database (see: http://geneticassociationdb.nih.gov), which has the ultimate aim of collecting, standardizing and archiving genetic association data and making it easily accessible to the scientific community. The database currently contains over 5000 studies. Perhaps the most important contribution of meta-analysis in areas where adequately powered cohorts currently exist, or are being assembled, will be in evaluating the currently available associations to prioritize hypotheses for testing in very large studies. For those conditions where it is impractical to assemble studies consisting of many thousands of cases and controls, meta-analysis, particularly of individual participant data, may have the capacity to provide sufficiently robust conclusions to commence functional genetic investigations of particular polymorphisms.

References

1. Risch N, Merikangas K. The future of genetic studies of complex human diseases. *Science* 1996; 273(5281):516–517.
2. Davey Smith G, Ebrahim S. 'Mendelian randomization': can genetic epidemiology contribute to understanding environmental determinants of disease? *Int J Epidemiol* 2003; 32:1–22.
3. Zondervan KT, Cardon LR. The complex interplay among factors that influence allelic association. *Nat Rev Genet* 2004; 5:29–100.
4. Colhoun HM, McKeigue PM, Davey Smith G. Problems of reporting genetic associations with complex outcomes. *Lancet* 2003; 361(9360):865–872.
5. Lohmueller KE, Pearce CL, Pike M, et al. Meta-analysis of genetic association studies supports a contribution of common variants to susceptibility to common disease. *Nat Genet* 2003; 33(2):177–182.
6. Hirschhorn JN, Lohmueller K, Byrne E, Hirschhorn K. A comprehensive review of genetic association studies. *Genet Med* 2002; 4(2):45–61.
7. Ioannidis JP, Ntzani EE, Trikalinos TA, Contopoulos-Ioannidis DG. Replication validity of genetic association studies. *Nat Genet* 2001; 29(3):306–309.
8. Ioannidis JP, Trikalinos TA, Ntzani EE, Contopoulos-Ioannidis DG. Genetic associations in large versus small studies: an empirical assessment. *Lancet* 2003; 361(9357):567–571.
9. Cambien F, Poirier O, Lecerf L, et al. Deletion polymorphism in the gene for angiotensin-converting enzyme is a potent risk factor for myocardial infarction. *Nature* 1992; 359(6396):641–644.
10. Keavney B, McKenzie C, Parish S, et al. Large-scale test of hypothesised associations between the angiotensin-converting-enzyme insertion/deletion polymorphism and myocardial infarction in about 5000 cases and 6000 controls. International Studies of Infarct Survival (ISIS) Collaborators. *Lancet* 2000; 355(9202):434–442.
11. Bonnici F, Keavney B, Collins R, Danesh J. Angiotensin converting enzyme insertion or deletion polymorphism and coronary restenosis: meta-analysis of 16 studies. *Br Med J* 2002; 325(7363):517–520.
12. Little J, Bradley L, Bray MS, et al. Reporting, appraising, and integrating data on genotype prevalence and gene-disease associations. *Am J Epidemiol* 2002; 156(4):300–310.
13. Stroup DF, Berlin JA, Morton SC, et al. Meta-analysis of observational studies in epidemiology: a proposal for reporting. Meta-analysis of Observational Studies in Epidemiology (MOOSE) group. *JAMA* 2000; 283(15):2008–2012.
14. Attia J, Thakkinstian A, D'Este C. Meta-analyses of molecular association studies: methodologic lessons for genetic epidemiology. *J Clin Epidemiol* 2003; 56(4):297–303.
15. Thakkinstian A, McElduff P, D'Este C, et al. A method for meta-analysis of molecular association studies. *Stat Med* 2005; 24(9):1291–1306.
16. Cohn LD, Becker BJ. How meta-analysis increases statistical power. *Psychol Methods* 2003; 8(3):243–253.
17. Salanti G, Sanderson S, Higgins JP. Obstacles and opportunities in meta-analysis of genetic association studies. *Genet Med* 2005; 7(1):13–20.
18. Higgins JP, Thompson SG, Deeks JJ, Altman DG. Measuring inconsistency in meta-analyses. *Br Med J* 2003; 327(7414):557–560.
19. Ioannidis JP, Ntzani EE, Trikalinos TA. 'Racial' differences in genetic effects for complex diseases. *Nat Genet* 2004; 36(12):1312–1318.
20. Wheeler JG, Keavney BD, Watkins H, et al. Four paraoxonase gene polymorphisms in 11212 cases of coronary heart disease and 12786 controls: meta-analysis of 43 studies. *Lancet* 2004; 363(9410):689–695.
21. Song Y, Stampfer MJ, Liu S. Meta-analysis: apolipoprotein E genotypes and risk for coronary heart disease. *Ann Intern Med* 2004; 141(2):137–147.
22. Pritchard JK, Donnelly P. Case-control studies of association in structured or admixed populations. *Theor Popul Biol* 2001; 60(3):227–237.
23. Marchini J, Cardon LR, Phillips MS, Donnelly P. The effects of human population structure on large genetic association studies. *Nat Genet* 2004; 36(5):512–517.

24. Pritchard JK, Stephens M, Donnelly P. Inference of population structure using multilocus genotype data. *Genetics* 2000; 155(2):945–959.

25. Pritchard JK, Stephens M, Rosenberg NA, Donnelly P. Association mapping in structured populations. *Am J Hum Genet* 2000; 67(1):170–181.

26. Stephens JC, Schneider JA, Tanguay DA, et al. Haplotype variation and linkage disequilibrium in 313 human genes. *Science* 2001; 293(5529):489–493.

27. Klerk M, Verhoef P, Clarke R, et al. MTHFR 677C→T polymorphism and risk of coronary heart disease: a meta-analysis. *JAMA* 2002; 288(16):2023–2031.

28. Levinson DF, Levinson MD, Segurado R, Lewis CM. Genome scan meta-analysis of schizophrenia and bipolar disorder, part I: Methods and power analysis. *Am J Hum Genet* 2003; 73(1):17–33.

29. Wise LH, Lanchbury JS, Lewis CM. Meta-analysis of genome searches. *Ann Hum Genet* 1999; 63(Pt 3):263–272.

30. Samani NJ. Genome scans for hypertension and blood pressure regulation. *Am J Hypertens* 2003; 16(2):167–171.

31. Dominiczak AF, Graham D, McBride MW, et al. Corcoran lecture. Cardiovascular genomics and oxidative stress. *Hypertension* 2005; 45(4):636–642.

32. Province MA, Kardia SL, Ranade K, et al. A meta-analysis of genome-wide linkage scans for hypertension: the National Heart, Lung and Blood Institute Family Blood Pressure Program. *Am J Hypertens* 2003; 16(2):144–147.

33. Liu W, Zhao W, Chase GA. Genome scan meta-analysis for hypertension. *Am J Hypertens* 2004; 17(12 Pt 1):1100–1106.

34. Sethi AA, Nordestgaard BG, Tybjaerg-Hansen A. Angiotensinogen gene polymorphism, plasma angiotensinogen, and risk of hypertension and ischemic heart disease: a meta-analysis. *Arterioscler Thromb Vasc Biol* 2003; 23(7):1269–1275.

35. Jeunemaitre X, Soubrier F, Kotelevtsev YV, et al. Molecular basis of human hypertension: role of angiotensinogen. *Cell* 1992; 71(1):169–180.

36. Caulfield M, Munroe P, Pembroke J, et al. Genome-wide mapping of human loci for essential hypertension. *Lancet* 2003; 361(9375):2118–2123.

37. Wilson PW, Schaefer EJ, Larson MG, Ordovas JM. Apolipoprotein E alleles and risk of coronary disease. A meta-analysis. *Arterioscler Thromb Vasc Biol* 1996; 16(10):1250–1255.

38. Keavney B, Parish S, Palmer A, et al. Large-scale evidence that the cardiotoxicity of smoking is not significantly modified by the apolipoprotein E epsilon2/epsilon3/epsilon4 genotype. *Lancet* 2003; 361(9355):396–398.

39. Altshuler D, Hirschhorn JN, Klannemark M, et al. The common PPARgamma Pro12Ala polymorphism is associated with decreased risk of type 2 diabetes. *Nat Genet* 2000; 26(1):76–80.

40. Florez JC, Sjogren M, Burtt N, et al. Association testing in 9,000 people fails to confirm the association of the insulin receptor substrate-1 G972R polymorphism with type 2 diabetes. *Diabetes* 2004; 53(12):3313–3318.

41. Jellema A, Zeegers MP, Feskens EJ, et al. Gly972Arg variant in the insulin receptor substrate-1 gene and association with type 2 diabetes: a meta-analysis of 27 studies. *Diabetologia* 2003; 46(7):990–995.

42. Lewington S, Clarke R, Qizilbash N, et al. Age-specific relevance of usual blood pressure to vascular mortality: a meta-analysis of individual data for one million adults in 61 prospective studies. *Lancet* 2002; 360(9349):1903–1913.

43. Ioannidis JP, Rosenberg PS, Goedert JJ, et al. Effects of CCR5-Delta32, CCR2-64I, and SDF-1 3′ A alleles on HIV-1 disease progression: an international meta-analysis of individual-patient data. *Ann Intern Med* 2001; 135(9):782–795.

44. Ioannidis JP, Ralston SH, Bennett ST, et al. Differential genetic effects of ESR1 gene polymorphisms on osteoporosis outcomes. *JAMA* 2004; 292(17):2105–2114.

8 | Genetics and genomics: impact on drug discovery and development

Klaus Lindpaintner

This communication represents the author's personal views and not necessarily those of any of his institutional or corporate affiliations, including F. Hoffmann-La Roche.

INTRODUCTION

Genetics and genomics are today widely proclaimed as about to revolutionize the face of medicine. In a more measured assessment, their use provides significant opportunities, based on a more fundamental understanding of cell biology and molecular disease pathology, but also raises significant challenges with regard to work yet to be done. The implementation of molecular genetics and biology will continue to provide us, as it has done already, with better ways to diagnose and treat illnesses, but it will do so at a stepwise and evolutionary pace, based on an improved understanding of the nature of disease, allowing more specific treatments, better risk prediction and the implementation of preventive strategies. As such, future progress in biomedicine will travel the same well-trodden paths of improved differential diagnosis and risk prediction along which it has advanced for the last decades and centuries. So, while meaningful biomedical research today, by and large, depends on the use of the newly developed tools of genetics and genomics, and the insights we gain through them, it is unlikely to fundamentally change the direction of medical progress.

Advances made over the last 30 years in molecular biology, molecular genetics and genomics, and in the development and refinement of associated methods and technologies, have had a major impact on our understanding of biology, including the action of drugs and other biologically active xenobiotics. The tools that have been developed to allow these advances, and the knowledge of fundamental principles underlying cellular function thus derived, have become quintessential and indeed indispensable for almost any kind and field of biological research, including future progress in biomedicine and health care.

One aspect in particular of the broad scope across which progress in biology has been achieved – namely our understanding of genetics and, in particular, our sequencing of the human genome – has uniquely captured the imagination of both scientists and the public. Given the austere beauty of Mendel's laws of inheritance, the compelling aesthetics of the double helix structure and the awe-inspiring accomplishment of cataloguing billions of base pairs, and – last but not least – a public relations campaign unprecedented in its scope in the history of scientific achievement, this reaction is quite understandable. However, the high expectations raised regarding the degree and timeframe of impact that these technologies will have on the practice of health care are almost certainly unrealistic. Situated at the interface between pharmacology and genetics/genomics, 'pharmacogenetics and pharmacogenomics' (usually without any further definition of what these terms mean) are commonly touted as heralding a 'revolution' in medicine.

It is important to realize that, with regard to pharmacology and drug discovery, accomplishments in basic biology – starting sometime in the last third or quarter of the twentieth century – have indeed already led to what could well be considered a rather fundamental – perhaps paradigmatic – shift from the 'chemical paradigm' to a 'biological paradigm': historically, drug discovery was driven by medicinal chemistry, with biology serving an almost secondary, ancillary role that examined new molecules for biological function. The ability to comprehend cell biology and function based on a newly developed set of tools to investigate the physiological effects of biomolecules and pathways on their basic, molecular level, has reversed this directionality: the biologist is now driving the process, requesting from the chemist compounds that modulate the function of these biomolecules or pathways, with the expectation of a more predictable impact on physiological function and the correction of its pathological derailments. Indeed, as pointed out above, the major change in how we discover drugs – from the chemical to the biological paradigm – occurred some time ago. What the current advances, in due time, promise to allow us to do is to move from a physiology-based to a (molecular) pathology-based approach towards drug discovery, promising the advancement from a largely palliative to a more cause/contribution targeting pharmacopoeia.

This chapter provides a – necessarily somewhat subjective – view of what the disciplines of genetics and genomics stand to contribute, and how they have actually contributed for many years, to drug discovery and development and – more broadly – to the practice of health care. Particular emphasis is placed on examining the role of genetics – acquired or inherited variations at the level of DNA-encoded information – in 'real life', i.e. with regard to common complex disease; a realistic understanding of this role is absolutely essential for a balanced assessment of the impact of 'genetics' on health care in the future. Definitions of some of the terms that are in wide and often unreflective use today – almost always sorely missing from both academic and public policy-related documents on the topic – will be provided, with an understanding that much of the field is still in flux and they might well change.

With regard to the actual opportunities and challenges genetics and genomics provide in the field of health care, a perspective staged by time-frames is helpful. Thus:

- The aspect that holds the greatest promise – successfully targeting newly recognized, causally relevant targets with innovative drugs based on a more fundamental and functional understanding of disease causation or contribution on the molecular level – is also the one that lies farthest in the future, and commensurately little can be said about it lest we lose ourselves in pure speculation.

- The more mid-term impact of these technologies, applicable to the earlier stages of drug discovery, will be covered in some detail, as here, too, the true relevance of various applications of genomic technologies has yet to be fully established.
- The most imminent application to medicines that are either on the market or in clinical trials, i.e. pharmacogenetics, will receive the major emphasis for the obvious reason that these applications are in part already being implemented today in clinical trials. Here, a more systematic classification than generally found will be attempted.

It is important to remain mindful that what will be discussed is - to a large extent - still uncharted territory, so by necessity many of the positions taken, reasoned on today's understanding and knowledge, must be viewed as somewhat tentative in nature. Where appropriate and possible, select examples will be provided, although it should be pointed out that much of the literature in the area of genetic epidemiology and pharmacogenetics lacks the stringent standards normally applied to peer-reviewed research, and replicate data are generally absent.

DEFINITION OF TERMS

There is widespread indiscriminate use of, and thus confusion about, the terms 'pharmacogenetics' and 'pharmacogenomics'. No universally accepted definition exists but there is an emerging consensus on the differential meaning and use of the two terms:

- Pharmacogenetics:
  - differential effects of a drug – *in vivo* – in different patients, dependent on the presence of inherited gene variants
  - assessed primarily by genetic (single nucleotide polymorphisms; SNP) and genomic (expression) approaches
  - a concept to provide more patient/disease-specific health care
  - one drug, many genomes (i.e. different patients)
  - focus: patient variability
- Pharmacogenomics:
  - differential effects of compounds – *in vivo* or *in vitro* – on gene expression, among the entirety of expressed genes
  - assessed by expression profiling
  - a tool for compound selection/drug discovery
  - many 'drugs' (i.e. early-stage compounds), one genome [i.e. 'normative' genome (database, technology platform)]
  - focus: compound variability.

Pharmacogenetics

The term '—genetics' relates etymologically to the presence of individual properties, and interindividual differences in these properties, as a consequence of having inherited (or acquired) them. Thus, the term 'pharmacogenetics' describes the interactions between a drug and an individual's (or perhaps more accurately: groups of individuals') characteristics as they relate to differences in the DNA-based information. Pharmacogenetics, therefore, refers to the assessment of clinical efficacy and/or the safety and tolerability profile – the pharmacological, or reponse phenotype – of a drug in groups of individuals that differ with regard to certain DNA-encoded characteristics and tests the hypothesis that these differences, if indeed associated with a differential response-phenotype, will allow prediction of individual drug response. The DNA-encoded characteristics are most commonly assessed based on the presence or absence of polymorphisms at the level of the nuclear DNA, but could also be assessed at different levels where such DNA variation translates into different characteristics, such as differential mRNA expression – splicing, protein levels or functional characteristics, or even physiological phenotypes – all of which would be seen as surrogate, or more integrated, markers of the underlying genetic variant. (It should be noted that some authors continue to subsume all applications of expression profiling under the term 'pharmacogenomics' in a definition of the terms that is more driven by the technology used than by functional context.)

Pharmacogenomics

By contrast, the terms 'pharmacogenomics' and its close relative 'toxicogenomics' are etymologically linked to 'genomics', the study of the genome and of the entirety of expressed and nonexpressed genes in any given physiologic state. These two fields of study are concerned with a comprehensive, genome-wide assessment of the effects of pharmacological agents, including toxins/toxicants on gene expression patterns. Pharmacogenomic studies are thus used to evaluate the differential effects of a number of chemical compounds (in the process of drug discovery this is commonly applied to lead selection) with regard to inducing or suppressing the expression of transcription of genes in an experimental setting. Except for situations in which pharmacogenetic considerations are 'front-loaded' into the discovery process, interindividual variations in gene sequence are not usually taken into account in this process. Unlike pharmacogenetics, pharmacogenomics therefore does not focus on differences among individuals with regard to the drug's effects, but rather examines differences among several (prospective) drugs or compounds with regard to their biological effects using a 'generic' set of expressed or nonexpressed genes. The basis of comparison is quantitative measures of expression, using a number of more or less comprehensive gene-expression-profiling methods, commonly based on microarray formats. By extrapolation from the experimental results to – theoretically – desirable patterns of activation or inactivation of expression of genes in the setting of integrative pathophysiology it is hoped this approach will provide a faster, more comprehensive and perhaps even more reliable way to assess the likelihood of finding an ultimately successful drug than previously available schemes involving mostly *in vivo* animal experimentation.

Thus, although both pharmacogenetics and pharmacogenomics refer to the evaluation of drug effects using (primarily) nucleic acid markers and technology, the directionalities of their approaches are distinctly different:

- pharmacogenetics represents the study of differences among a number of individuals with regard to clinical response to a particular drug ('one drug, many genomes')
- pharmacogenomics represents the study of differences among a number of compounds with regard to gene expression response in a single (normative) genome/expressome ('many drugs, one genome')

Accordingly, the fields of intended use are distinct: the former will help in the clinical setting to find the medicine most likely to be optimal for a patient (or the patients most likely to respond to a drug), the latter will aid in the setting of pharmaceutical research to find the 'best' drug candidate from a given series of compounds under evaluation.

LONG-TERM TIMEFRAME: CAUSATIVE TARGETS – ADDRESSING DERANGED FUNCTION DIRECTLY

Palliative and causative acting drugs

The largest fraction by far of today's pharmacopoeia does not target disease at its cause – because these causes are largely unknown – but modulates a pathway that affects the disease-relevant phenotype or function. We refer to such drugs as symptomatic or palliative agents. The pathways they target are known from more than a century of physiological, biochemical and pharmacological research. The pathways they modulate are disease-phenotype-relevant (albeit not disease-cause-relevant) and although they are not dysfunctional, their modulation can effectively be used to counterbalance the effect of a dysfunctional, disease-causing pathway. Thus signs and symptoms of the disease can be alleviated, often with striking success, notwithstanding the fact that the real cause of the disease remains untouched. A classic example of such an approach is the acute treatment of thyro-toxicity with beta-adrenergic blocking agents: even though the sympathetic nervous system does not in this case contribute causally to tachycardia and hyper-tension, dampening even its baseline tonus using this class of rapidly acting drugs can quickly and successfully relieve the cardiovascular symptoms and signs of this condition, and might well prevent a heart attack if the patient has underlying coronary disease, before the causal treatment (in this case available through partial chemical ablation of the hyperactive thyroid gland) can take effect.

The twofold challenge of common complex disease

It stands to reason that a drug that addresses the actual cause of the disease should provide superior treatment. However, finding these 'deranged functions' is not easy, even with the aid of all the molecular biological, genetic and genomic tools that we have at our command today.

There is an emerging consensus that all common complex diseases, i.e. the health problems that are by far the main contributors to society's disease burden as well as to public and private health spending, are 'multifactorial' in nature, i.e. that they are brought about by the coincidence of certain intrinsic (inborn or acquired) predispositions and susceptibilities on the one hand, and extrinsic, envi-ronment-derived influences on the other, with the relative importance of these two influences varying across a broad spectrum. In some diseases, external factors appear to be more important, while in others intrinsic predispositions prevail.

However, it is important to note – as it is commonly neglected in discussions on this topic – that, in the majority of common complex diseases, genetic factors are less important than environmental and lifestyle factors, as exemplified by heritability coefficients – generally of between 02 and 0.5 – for these conditions. Thus, it must be recognized from the outset that by targeting the genetic aspects of these diseases we can at best hope to make a minor contribution to curing or preventing them.

The complex nature of these diseases renders the discovery of genetic variants that contribute causally to any of them a major challenge. The complexity confronted occurs on two levels: several inherent predisposing susceptibility traits, and generally more than one environmental or lifestyle risk factor, coincide in any one individual for the disease to occur; thus any of the genetic variants present provides only a modest contribution to overall disease causation, and thus investigational hurdles of discovering it. This intraindividual complexity is further accentuated by interindividual diversity based on the fact that any one clinical diagnosis is bound to be etiologically heterogeneous at the level of molecular pathology. Thus, consensus exists that the same 'conventional' clinical diagnosis given to different individuals is quite likely to reflect the outcome of different constellations of inborn susceptibility factors and/or of environmental and lifestyle-related risks. So we would expect that – both on the level of an individual patient and even more so on the population level, where all relevant genetic–epidemiological studies need to be conducted – the disease-causing (or, better, disease-contributing) effect of any one intrinsic, genetically encoded characteristic will, by and large, be quite modest and probably drowned out by noise, unless very large (and very expensive) studies are conducted. Carrying out such studies, which will attach function and clinical outcomes to the human genome sequence and its variations, is a huge task that looms many times larger than the sequencing effort itself; however, it is the *sine qua non* without which the whole genome sequencing effort will essentially remain inconsequential.

Now that large-scale efforts based primarily on the sibpair linkage study design have failed – with a few exceptions – to yield disease–gene variants in common complex disease, it appears that populations with large, genealogically well-characterized families and a certain degree of 'genetic isolation' could provide the most likely successful approach towards characterization of these disease susceptibility gene variants. Not many such populations exist; examples are the Utah Mormons, the Icelandic nation, and the French settlers in Northern Quebec, where initial work has proved promising. Results obtained in such isolated populations will need to be validated in other, more 'mainstream' populations if the new target is to be pursued strictly as a causative target.

Common, complex diseases – and thus the vast majority of what is to be 'clinically applied genetics' – behave almost fundamentally differently from rare, classic, monogenic, 'Mendelian' diseases. Whereas in the latter the impact of the genetic variant is typically categorical in nature (i.e. deterministic), in the former case the presence of a disease-associated genetic variant is merely of probabilistic value, raising (or lowering) the likelihood of disease occurrence to some extent but never predicting it in a black-and-white fashion.

Communicating this difference to a public that has long been misled into a perception of everything 'genetic' being of deterministic, Mendelian quality, represents a second, no less important and difficult challenge. Unless we engage in a true dialogue with all stakeholders, and succeed in providing the basis for informed discourse and sensible decision-making on the societal level, the full potential of our deepening understanding of biology and of these technological advances will not be recognized.

Applicability of 'genetic' targets/medicines

Will such newly discovered causative targets, and the medicines that might eventually be developed to modulate them, indeed be applicable only to that fraction of the population with the clinical diagnosis in whom the targeted mechanism contributes materially to the disease? It is too early to tell. It is perhaps not unreasonable to expect that, in the latter group, such medicines will be particularly effective, and sometimes they will be exclusively effective in these patients. However, by uncovering what essentially will commonly be a new, previously unrecognized mechanistic pathway, such drugs could also be of value as palliative medicines in those individuals in whom the mechanism in question is actually not dysfunctional. The former case is illustrated by Herceptin (see below); an example for the latter is the finding that glucokinase activators, which correct the molecular defect in the rare mature onset diabetes of the young (MODY) type 2 patients in whom the enzyme is dysfunctional, can raise the activity of normal glucokinase and thus lower glucose in just about everyone.

Acceleration of drug discovery/development through 'better' targets?

Hopes have been nurtured by some that the implementation of genetics and genomics would 'smarten' up the drug discovery process and thus potentially accelerate it and reduce its cost. Quite the contrary: it appears that the opposite is happening. Latencies from the inception of a project to the launch of a new drug have lengthened to almost 15 years, and the average cost per successful launch has gone up to almost US $900 million.[1] Interestingly, about two-thirds of the costs incurred now seem to be spent in the preclinical phase.[1] Although it is unclear to what extent these data truly reflect reality, it does stand to reason that the preclinical phase, in particular, would be more lengthy and expensive if it was tackling a completely novel target about which – other than the association with disease that the genetic approach provides us with – virtually nothing is known. This would be complicated by the fact that such targets might not belong to the few, classic 'drug-gable' target families. Indeed, such a target might not be chemically tractable at all, or might encounter additional hurdles due to the bias of most chemical libraries in favor of 'conventional' target families. These formidable challenges are somewhat counterbalanced by the expectation that targets selected based on causative disease contribution might, overall, have a somewhat higher likelihood of success. Thus, if today's attrition rate of nine out of ten compounds that are introduced into clinical testing could be reduced by as little as to eight out of ten, this would translate – over time – to a doubling of productivity.

MIDTERM TIMEFRAME: PHARMACOGENOMICS/ TOXICOGENOMICS – FINDING NEW MEDICINES MORE QUICKLY AND MORE EFFICIENTLY

Once a screen (assay) has been set up in a drug discovery project and lead compounds are identified, the major task becomes the identification of an optimized clinical candidate molecule among the many compounds synthesized by medicinal chemists. Conventionally, such compounds are screened in a number of animal or cell models for efficacy and toxicity, experiments that – while having the advantage of being conducted in the *in vivo* setting – commonly take significant amounts of time and depend entirely on the similarity between the experimental animal condition/setting and its human counterpart, i.e. the validity of the model.

Although such experiments will never be entirely replaced by expression profiling on either the nucleic acid (genomics) or the protein (proteomics) level, these techniques offer powerful advantages and complementary information. First, the efficacy and profile of induced changes can be assessed in a comprehensive fashion (within the limitations – primarily sensitivity and completeness of transcript representation – of the technology platform used). Second, these assessments of differential efficacy can be carried out much more expeditiously than in conventionally used (patho-)physiology-based animal models. Third, the complex pattern of expression changes revealed by such experiments will provide new insights into possible biological interactions between the actual drug target and other biomolecules, and thus reveal new elements, or branch-points of a biological pathway that might be useful as surrogate markers, novel diagnostic analytes or as additional drug targets. Fourth – and increasingly important – these tools serve to determine specificity of action among members of gene families that might be highly important for both efficacy and safety of a new drug. It must be borne in mind that any and all such experiments are limited by the coefficient of correlation with which the expression patterns determined are linked to the desired *in vivo* physiological action of the compound.

A word of caution regarding microarray-based expression profiling would appear to be in order: the power of comprehensive (almost) genome-wide assessment of expression patterns has led to what can justly be described as somewhat of an infatuation with this technology that at times leaves a certain degree of critical skepticism to be desired. In particular, the pair-wise comparison algorithms used in much of this work (competition staining of a case and a control sample on the same physical array) raise a number of questions regarding selection bias, which take on particular significance when the overall sample sizes are commonly (very) small. Biostatistical analytical approaches are commonly less than sophisticated, if used at all. Additionally, it is important to remain aware of the fact that all microarray expression data are of an associative character, and must be interpreted with this limitation in mind.

As a subcategory of this approach, toxicogenomics is increasingly evolving as a powerful adjuvant to classic toxicological testing. As pertinent databases are being created from experiments with known toxicants, revealing expression patterns that might be predictive of longer-term toxic liabilities of compounds, future drug discovery efforts should benefit by insights allowing earlier 'killing' of compounds likely to cause such complications.

When using these approaches in drug discovery – even if implemented with proper biostatistics and analytical rigor – it is imperative to understand the probabilistic nature of such experiments: a promising profile on pharmacogenomic and toxicogenomic screens will enhance the likelihood of having selected an ultimately successful compound, and will achieve this goal quicker than conventional animal experimentation, but will do so only with a certain likelihood of success. The less reductionist approach of the animal experiment will still be needed. It is to be anticipated, however, that such approaches will constitute an important, time- and resource-saving first evaluation or screening step that will help to focus and reduce the number of animal experiments that will ultimately need to be conducted.

SHORT-TERM TIMEFRAME: PHARMACOGENETICS – MORE TARGETED, MORE EFFECTIVE MEDICINES

Genes and environment

It is common knowledge that today's pharmacopoeia, in as much as it represents enormous progress compared with what was available to physicians only 15 or 20 years ago, is far from perfect. Many patients respond only partially, or fail to respond altogether, to the drugs they are given, and others suffer adverse events that range from unpleasant to serious and life-threatening.

If we regard a pharmacological agent as one of the extrinsic, environmental factors in a common complex disease scenario, with a potential to affect the health status of the individual to whom it is administered, then individually differing responses to such an agent would – under the multifactorial and heterogeneous paradigm of common complex disease elaborated upon earlier – be regarded as the expression of differences in the 'intrinsic' characteristics of these patients (as long as we can exclude variation in the exposure to the drug: this is important, as in clinical practice nonadherence to prescribed regimens of administration, or drug–drug interactions interfering with bioavailability of the drug, are by far the most likely culprits when such differences in response phenotype are observed). The influence of such intrinsic variation on drug response can be predicted to be more easily recognizable and more relevant the steeper the dose–response curve of a given drug is.

The argument for the particular likelihood of observing environmental-factor–gene interactions with drugs among all other 'environmental influences' goes along the same lines. Among all these 'environmental factors' that we are exposed to, drugs might be particularly likely to 'interact' specifically and selectively with the genetic properties of a given individual, as their potency and – compared, say, to foodstuffs – narrow therapeutic window makes interactions with innate individual susceptibilities that affect the interaction with drugs more likely.

Clearly, a better, more fundamental and mechanistic understanding of the molecular pathology of disease in general and of the role of intrinsic, biological properties regarding the predisposition to contract such diseases, as well as of drug action on the molecular level, will be essential for future progress in health care. Current progress in molecular biology and genetics has indeed provided us with some of the prerequisite tools that should help us reach the goal of such a more refined understanding.

An attempt at a systematic classification of pharmacogenetics

Two conceptually quite different scenarios of interindividually differential drug response can be distinguished on the basis of the underlying biological variance:

- 'Classical' pharmacogenetics:
  - Pharmacokinetics:
    - absorption
    - metabolism:
      - activation of prodrugs
      - deactivation
      - generation of biologically active metabolites
    - distribution
    - elimination
  - Pharmacodynamics:
    - palliative drug action (modulation of disease-symptoms or disease-signs by targeting physiologically relevant systems, without addressing those mechanisms that cause or causally contribute to the disease)
- 'Molecular differential-diagnosis-related' pharmacogenetics:
  - Causative drug action (modulation of actual causative or contributory mechanisms.

In the first case ('classical pharmacogenetics'), the underlying biological variation is not, in itself, disease-causing or disease-contributing, and becomes clinically relevant *only* in response to the exposure to the drug in question.

In the second case ('disease-mechanism-related pharmacogenetics'), the biological variation is directly disease-related, is – *per se* – of pathological importance, and represents a subgroup of the overall clinical disease/diagnostic entity. The differential response to a drug is thus related to how well this drug addresses, or is matched to, the presence or relative importance of the pathomechanism it targets, in different patients, i.e. the 'molecular differential diagnosis' of the patient.

Although these two scenarios are conceptually rather different, they result in similar practical consequences with regard to the administration of a drug, namely stratification based on a particular, DNA-encoded marker. It seems therefore legitimate to subsume both under the umbrella of 'pharmacogenetics'.

Classical pharmacogenetics

This category includes differential pharmacokinetics and pharmacodynamics. Pharmacokinetic effects are due to interindividual differences in absorption, distribution, metabolism (with regard to activation of prodrugs, inactivation of the active molecule and generation of derivative molecules with biological activity) or excretion of the drug. In any of these cases, differential effects observed are due to the presence at the intended site of action either of inappropriate concentrations of the pharmaceutical agent, or of inappropriate metabolites, or of both, resulting either in lack of efficacy or toxic effects.

Pharmacogenetics, as it relates to pharmacokinetics, has been recognized as an entity for more than 100 years, going back to the observation, commonly credited to Archibald Garrod, that a subset of psychiatric patients treated with the hypnotic, sulphonal, developed porphyria. We have since then come to understand the underlying genetic causes for many of the previously known differences in enzymatic activity, most prominently with regard to the P450 enzyme family, and these have been the subject of recent reviews[2,3] (Tables 8.1 and 8.2). However, such pharmacokinetic effects are also seen with membrane transporters, such as in the

Table 8.1 Pharmacogenetics chronology

Pharmacogenetic phenotype	Described	Underlying gene/mutation	Identified
Sulphonal porphyria	ca. 1890	Porphobilinogen-deaminase?	1985
Suxamethonium hypersensitivity	1957–60	Pseudocholinesterase	1990–92
Primaquin hypersensitivity; favism	1958	Glucose-6-phosphate dehydrogenase	1988
Long QT syndrome	1957–60	*Herg*, etc	1991–97
Isoniazid slow/fast acetylation	1959–60	*N*-acetyltranferase	1989–93
Malignant hyperthermia	1960–62	Ryanodine receptor	1991–97
Fructose intolerance	1963	Aldolase B	1988–95
Vasopressin insensitivity	1969	Vasopressin receptor2	1992
Alcohol susceptibility	1969	Aldehyde dehydrogenase	1988
Debrisoquine hypersensitivity	1977	CYP2D6	1988–93
Retinoic acid resistance	1970	PML-RARA fusion gene	1991–93
6-Mercaptopurin toxicity	1980	Thiopurine-methyltransferase	1995
Mephenytoin resistance	1984	CYP2C19	1993–94
Insulin insensitivity	1988	Insulin receptor	1988–93

case of differential activity of genetic variants of MDR-1 that affects the effective intracellular concentration of antiretrovirals,[4] or of the purine-analog-metabolizing enzyme, thiomethyl-purine-transferase.[5]

Notably, despite the widespread recognition of isoenzymes with differential metabolizing potential since the middle of the twentieth century, the practical application and implementation of this knowledge has been minimal so far. This might be the consequence, on one hand, of the irrelevance of such differences in the presence of relatively flat dose–effect curves (i.e. a sufficiently wide

Table 8.2 Pharmacogenetics systematics

Enzyme	Testing substance
Phase I enzyme	
Aldehyde dehydrogenase	Acetaldehyde
Alcohol dehydrogenase	Ethanol
CYP1A2	Caffeine
CYP2A6	Nicotine, coumarin
CYP2C9	Warfarin
CYP2C19	Mephenytoin, omeprazole
CYP2D6	Dextromethorphan, D-brisoquine, sparteine
CYP2E1	Chloroxazone, caffeine
CYP3A4	Erythromycin
CYP3A5	Midazolam
Serum cholinesterase	Benzoylcholine, butrylcholine
Paraoxonase/arylesterase	Paraoxon
Phase II enzyme	
Acetyltransferase (NAT1)	*para*-aminosalizyl
Acetyltransferase (NAT2)	Isoniazid, sulfamethazine, caffeine
Dihydropyrimidin-dehydrogenase	5-fluorouracil
Glutathione transferase (GST-M 1)	Trans-stilbene-oxid
Thiomethyltransferase	2-mercaptoethanol, D-penicillamine, captopril
Thiopurine methyltransferase	6-mercaptopurine, 6-thioguanine, 8-azathioprine
UDP-glucuronosyl-transferase (UGT1A)	Bilirubin
UDP-glucuronosyl-transferase (UGT2B7)	Oxazepam, ketoprofen, estradiol, morphine

therapeutic window) as well as, on the other hand, the fact that many drugs are subject to complex, parallel metabolizing pathways, where – in the case of underperformance of one enzyme – another one might compensate. Such compensatory pathways might well have somewhat different substrate affinities but allow plasma levels to remain within therapeutic concentrations. Thus, the number of such polymorphisms that have found practical applicability is rather limited and, by and large, restricted to determinations of the presence of functionally deficient variants of the enzyme, thiopurine-methyl-tranferase, in patients prior to treatment with purine analog chemotherapeutics.

Pharmacodynamic effects, by contrast, might lead to interindividual differences in a drug's effects despite the presence of appropriate concentrations of the intended active (or activated) drug compound at the intended site of action. Here, DNA-based variation in how the target molecule or another (downstream) member of the target molecule's mechanistic pathway can respond to the medicine modulates the effects of the drug. This will apply primarily to palliatively working medicines, as discussed above.

Fig. 8.1 helps clarify these somewhat complex concepts. It presents a hypothetical case of a complex trait/disease in which excessive, dysregulated function of one of the trait-controlling/contributing pathways (Fig. 8.1A,B) causes symptomatic disease. The example used refers to blood pressure as the trait and hypertension as the disease in question (for the case of a defective or diminished function of a pathway, an analogous schematic could be constructed, and again for a deviant function). A palliative treatment would be one that addresses one of the pathways that – although not dysregulated – contributes to the overall deviant physiology (Fig. 8.1F), while the respective pharmacogenetic/pharmacodynamic scenario would occur if this particular pathway was, due to a genetic variant, not responsive to the drug chosen (Fig. 8.1G). A palliative treatment might also be ineffective if the particular mechanism targeted by the palliative drug – due to the presence of a molecular variant – provides less than the physiologically expected baseline contribution to the relevant phenotype (Fig. 8.1H). In such a case, modulating an *a priori* unimportant pathway in the disease scenario will not yield successful palliative treatment results (Fig. 8.1I,J).

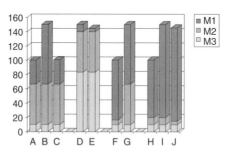

Fig. 8.1 A hypothetical case of a complex trait/disease: blood pressure is the trait and hypertension the disease in question. A, normal physiology, three molecular mechanisms (M1, M2, M3) contribute to a trait; B, diseased physiology D1, derailment (cause/contribution) of molecular mechanism 1 (M1); C, diseased physiology D1, causal treatment T1 (aimed at M1); D, diseased physiology D3, derailment (cause/contribution) of molecular mechanism 3 (M3); E, diseased physiology D3, treatment T1, treatment does not address cause; F, diseased physiology D1, palliative treatment T2 (aimed at M2); G, diseased physiology D1, palliative treatment T2, T2-refractory gene variant in M2; H, normal physiology variant, differential contribution of M1 and M2 to normal trait; I, diseased physiology D1-variant, derailment of mechanism M1; J, diseased physiology D1-variant: treatment with T2. Solid colors indicate normal function, stippling indicates pathologic dysfunction, hatching indicates therapeutic modulation.

Several of the most persuasive examples we have accumulated to date for such palliative drug-related pharmacogenetic effects have been observed in the field of asthma. The treatment of asthma relies on an array of drugs aimed at modulating different 'generic' pathways, thus mediating bronchodilation or anti-inflammatory effects, often without regard to the possible causative contribution of the targeted mechanism to the disease. One of the mainstays of the treatment of asthma is activation of the beta-2-adrenoceptor by specific agonists, which leads to relaxation of bronchial smooth muscles and, consequently, bronchodilation. Recently, several molecular variants of the beta-2-adrenoceptor have been shown associated with differential treatment response to such beta-2-agonists.[6,7] Individuals carrying one or two copies of a variant allele that contains a glycine in place of arginine in position 16 were found to have a 3- and 5-fold reduced response to the agonist, respectively.

This was shown, in both *in vitro*[8,9] and *in vivo*[9] studies, to correlate with an enhanced rate of agonist-induced receptor downregulation, but not with any difference in transcriptional or translational activity of the gene, or with agonist binding. In contrast, a second polymorphism affecting position 19 of the beta upstream peptide was shown to affect translation (but not transcription) of the receptor itself, with a 50% decrease in receptor numbers associated with the variant allele, which happens to be in strong linkage disequilibrium with a variant allele position 16 in the receptor. The simultaneous presence of both mutations would thus be predicted to result in low expression and enhanced downregulation of an otherwise functionally normal receptor, depriving patients carrying such alleles of the benefits of effective bronchodilation as a 'palliative' (i.e. noncausal) countermeasure to their pathological airway hyperreactivity. Importantly, there is no evidence that any of the allelic variants encountered are associated with the prevalence or incidence, and thus potentially the etiology of the underlying disease.[10,11] This would reflect the scenario depicted in Fig. 8.1H.

Inhibition of leukotriene synthesis, another palliative approach toward the treatment of asthma, proved clinically ineffective in a small fraction of patients who carried only non-wild-type alleles of the 5-lipoxygenase promoter region.[12] These allelic variants had previously been shown to be associated with decreased transcriptional activity of the gene.[13] It stands to reason – consistent with the clinical observations – that, in the presence of already reduced 5-lipoxygenase activity, pharmacological inhibition might be less effective (Fig. 8.1H,I,J). Of note: again, there is no evidence for a primary, disease-causing or disease-contributing role of any 5-lipoxygenase variants; all were observed at equal frequencies in disease-affected and nonaffected individuals.[13]

Pharmacogenetic effects might not only account for differential efficacy but might also contribute to differential occurrence of adverse effects. An example for this scenario is provided by the well-documented 'pharmacogenetic' association between molecular sequence variants of the 12S rRNA, a mitochondrion-encoded gene, and aminoglycoside-induced ototoxicity.[14] Intriguingly, the mutation that is associated with susceptibility to ototoxicity renders the sequence of the human 12S rRNA similar to that of the bacterial 12S rRNA gene, and thus effectively turns the human 12S rRNA into the (bacterial) target for aminoglycoside drug action – presumably mimicking the structure of the bacterial binding site of the drug.[15] As in the other examples, presence of the 12S rRNA mutation has no primary, drug-treatment-independent pathologic effect *per se*.

One can speculate that, analogously, such 'molecular mimicry' might occ[ur] within one species: adverse events would arise if the selectivity of a drug is [

because a gene that belongs to the same gene-family as the primary target, loses its 'identity' *vis-à-vis* the drug and attains – based on its structural similarity with the principal target – similar or at least increased affinity to the drug. Depending on the biological role of the 'imposter' molecule, adverse events might occur, even though the variant molecule, again, might be quite silent with regard to any contribution to disease causation. Although we currently have no obvious examples for this scenario, it is certainly imaginable for various classes of receptors and enzymes.

Pharmacogenetics as a consequence of molecular differential diagnosis

As alluded to earlier, there is general agreement today that any of the major clinical diagnoses in the field of common complex disease (such as diabetes, hypertension, or cancer) comprise a number of etiologically (i.e. at the molecular level) more or less distinct subentities. In the case of a causally acting drug this would imply that the agent will only be appropriate, or will work best, in that fraction of all the patients who carry the (all-inclusive and imprecise) clinical diagnosis in whom the dominant molecular etiology, or at least one of the contributing etiological factors, matches the biological mechanism of action that the drug in question modulates (Fig. 8.1C). If the mechanism of action of the drug addresses a pathway that is not disease relevant, perhaps already downregulated as an appropriate physiologic response to the disease, then the drug may – logically – be expected not to show efficacy (Fig. 8.1D,E).

Thus, unrecognized and undiagnosed disease heterogeneity – disclosed indirectly by the presence or absence of response to a drug targeting a mechanism that contributes to only one of several molecular subgroups of the disease – provides an important explanation for differential drug response and likely represents a substantial fraction of what we today somewhat indiscriminately subsume under the term 'pharmacogenetics.'

Currently, the most frequently cited example for this category of pharmacogenetics is trastuzamab (Herceptin®), a humanized monoclonal antibody directed against the *her-2* oncogene. This breast cancer treatment is prescribed based on the level of *her-2* oncogene expression in the patient's tumor tissue. Differential diagnosis at the molecular level not only provides an added level of diagnostic sophistication but also actually represents the prerequisite for choosing the appropriate therapy. Because tastuzamab specifically inhibits a 'gain-of-function' variant of the oncogene, it is ineffective in the two-thirds of patients who do not 'overexpress' the drug's target, whereas it significantly improves survival in the one-third of patients who constitute the 'subentity' of the broader diagnosis 'breast cancer' in whom the gene is expressed.[16] (Some have argued against this being an example of 'pharmacogenetics', because the parameter for patient stratification, i.e. for differential diagnosis, is the somatic gene expression level rather than particular 'genotype' data.[17] This is a difficult argument to follow because, in the case of a treatment-effect-modifying germline mutation it would obviously not be the nuclear gene variant *per se*, but also its specific impact on either structure/function or expression of the respective gene/gene product that would represent the actual physiological corollary underlying the differential drug action. Conversely, an *a priori* observed expression difference is highly likely to reflect a – potentially as yet undiscovered – sequence variant. Indeed, as pointed out earlier, there are a number of examples in the field of pharmacogenomics where the connection between genotypic variant and altered expression has already been demonstrated.[13,18])

Another example, although still hypothetical, of how proper molecular diagnosis of relevant pathomechanisms will significantly influence drug efficacy, is in the evolving class of anti-AIDS/HIV drugs that target the CCR5 cell-surface receptor.[19–21] These drugs would be predicted to be ineffective in those rare patients who carry the delta-32 variant but who have nevertheless contracted AIDS or test HIV positive (most likely due to infection with an SI-virus phenotype that utilizes CXCR4).[22,23]

It should be noted that the pharmacogenetically relevant molecular variant need not affect the primary drug target, but might equally well be located in another molecule belonging to the system or pathway in question, both up or downstream in the biological cascade with respect to the primary drug target.

Different classes of markers

Pharmacogenetic phenomena, as pointed out previously, need not be restricted to the observation of a direct association between allelic sequence variation and phenotype, but could extend to a broad variety of indirect manifestations of underlying, but often (as yet) unrecognized sequence variation. Thus, differential methylation of the promoter-region of O-6-methylguanine-DNA-methylase has recently been reported to be associated with differential efficacy of chemotherapy with alkylating agents. If methylation is present, expression of the enzyme that rapidly reverses alkylation and induces drug resistance is inhibited, and therapeutic efficacy is greatly enhanced.[24]

Complexity is to be expected

In the real world, it is likely that not only one of the scenarios depicted, but a combination of several, will affect how well a patient responds to a given treatment or how likely it is that he or she will suffer an adverse event. Thus, a fast-metabolizing patient with poor-responder pharmacodynamics will be particularly unlikely to gain any benefit from taking the drug in question; the slow-metabolizing status of another patient might counterbalance the same inopportune pharmacodynamics; whereas a third patient, who is a slow metabolizer and displaying normal pharmacodynamics, might be more likely to suffer adverse events. In all of these patients, both the pharmacokinetic and pharmacodynamic properties could result from the interaction of several of the mechanisms described above. In addition, we know that coadministration of other drugs, and even the consumption of certain foods, can affect and further complicate the picture for any given treatment.

INCORPORATING PHARMACOGENETICS INTO DRUG DEVELOPMENT STRATEGY

Diagnostics first, therapeutics second

It is important to note that, despite the public hyperbole and the high expectations surrounding the use of pharmacogenetics to provide 'personalized care', these approaches are likely to be applicable to only a fraction of medicines that are being developed. Further, if and when such approaches are used, they will represent no radical new direction or concept in drug development but simply a stratification strategy, as we have been using all along.

An increasingly sophisticated and precise diagnosis of disease, arising from a deeper, more differentiated understanding of pathology at the molecular level, that will increasingly subdivide today's clinical diagnoses into molecular subtypes, will foster medical advances that, if considered from the viewpoint of today's clinical diagnosis, will appear as 'pharmacogenetic' phenomena, as described above. However, the sequence of events that is today often presented as characteristic for a 'pharmacogenetic scenario' – namely, exposing patients to the drug, recognizing a differential [i.e. (quasi-)bimodal-] response pattern, discovering a marker that predicts this response and creating a diagnostic product to be comarketed with the drug henceforth – is likely to be reversed. Rather, in the case of 'pharmacogenetics' due to a match between drug action and dysregulation of a disease-contributing mechanism, we will likely search for a new drug specifically and, *a priori*, based on a new mechanistic understanding of disease causation or contribution (i.e. a newly found ability to diagnose a molecular subentity of a previously more encompassing, broader, and less precise clinical disease definition). Thus, pharmacogenetics will not be so much about finding the 'right medicine for the right patient' but about finding the 'right medicine for the disease (-subtype)', as we have aspired to do throughout the history of medical progress. This is, in fact, good news: the conventional 'pharmacogenetic scenario' would invariably present major challenges from both a regulatory and a business development and marketing standpoint, as it would confront development teams with a critical change in the drug's profile at a very late point during the development process. In addition, the timely development of an approvable diagnostic in this situation is difficult at best, and its marketing as an 'add-on' to the drug a less than attractive proposition to the diagnostics business. Thus, the 'practice' of pharmacogenetics will, in many instances, be marked by progress along the very same path that has been one of the main avenues of medical progress for the last several hundred years: differential diagnosis first, followed by the development of appropriate, more specific treatment modalities.

Thus, the sequence of events in this case might well involve the development of an *in vitro* diagnostic test as a standalone product that could be marketed on its own merits, allowing the physician to establish an accurate, state-of-the-art diagnosis of the molecular subtype of the patient's disease. Sometimes such a diagnostic will prove helpful even in the absence of specific therapy by guiding the choice of existing medicines and/or of nondrug treatment modalities such as specific changes in diet or lifestyle. The availability of such a diagnostic – as part of the more sophisticated understanding of disease – will undoubtedly foster and stimulate the search for new, more specific drugs; and once such drugs are found, availability of the specific diagnostic will be important for carrying out the appropriate clinical trials. This will allow a prospectively planned, much more systematic approach towards clinical and business development, with a commensurate greater chance of actual realization and success.

Probability, not certainty

In practice, some degree of guesswork will remain because of the nature of common complex disease. First, all diagnostic approaches – including those based on DNA analysis in common complex disease (as stressed above) – will ultimately provide a measure only of probability, not of certainty: thus, although the variances of drug response among patients who do (or do not) carry the drug-specific subdiagnosis will be smaller, there will still be a distribution of differential responses. Although – by and large – the drug will work better in the 'responder' group, some patients in this subgroup will respond less or not at all and, conversely, not everyone in the 'nonresponder' group will completely fail to respond, depending perhaps on the relative magnitude with which the particular mechanism contributes to the disease. It is important to bear in mind, therefore, that even cases of fairly obvious bimodality patient responses will still show distribution patterns, and that all predictions as to responder or nonresponder status will only have a certain likelihood of being accurate (Fig. 8.2). The terms 'responder' and 'nonresponder' as applied to groups of patients stratified based on a DNA marker represent, therefore, Mendelian-thinking-inspired misnomers that should be replaced by more appropriate terms that reflect the probabilistic nature of any such classification, e.g. 'likely (non)responder'.

In addition, based on our current understanding of the polygenic and heterogeneous nature of these disorders, we will – even in an ideal world where we would know about all possible susceptibility gene variants for a given disease and have treatments for them – only be able to exclude, in any one patient, those that do not appear to contribute to the disease, and therefore deselect certain treatments. We will, however, most likely find ourselves left with a small

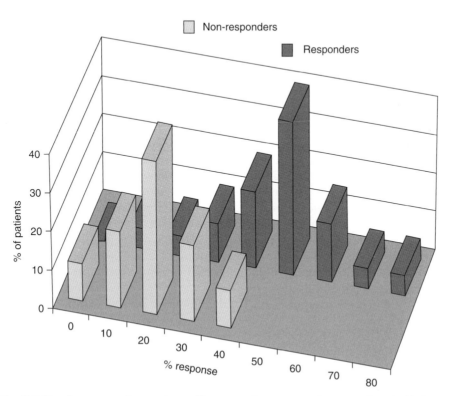

Fig. 8.2 Despite common, incorrect use of language, drug response is never categorical but always follows probabilistic distributions.

number – two to four, perhaps – of potentially disease-contributing gene variants whose relative contribution to the disease will be very difficult, if not impossible, to rank in an individual patient. It is likely, then, that trial and error, and that great intangible quantity 'physician experience', will still play an important role, albeit on a more limited and subselective basis.

The alternative scenario, where differential drug response and/or safety occurs as a consequence of a pathologically not relevant, purely drug-response-related pharmacogenetics scenario, is more likely to present greater difficulty in planning and executing a clinical development program because, presumably, it will be more difficult to anticipate or predict differential responses *a priori*. When such a differential response occurs, it will also potentially be more difficult to find the relevant marker(s), unless this happens to be among the 'obvious' candidate genes implicated in the disease physiopathology or in the mode of action of the treatment. Although screening for molecular variants of these genes, and testing for their possible associations with differential drug response, is a logical first step, if this is unsuccessful it might be necessary to embark on an unbiased genome-wide screen for such a marker or markers. Despite recent progress in high-throughput genotyping, the technical, data analysis and cost obstacles that will have to be overcome are formidable and will limit the deployment of such programs, at least for the foreseeable future, to select cases in which there are very solid indications for doing so, based on clinical data showing a near-categorical (e.g. bimodal) distribution of treatment outcomes. Even then, for every success (resulting from a favorably strong linkage disequilibrium across considerable genomic distance in the relevant chromosomal region) we should expect to encounter as many or more failures (in cases where the culpable gene variant cannot be found due to the higher recombination rate or other characteristics of the stretch of genome on which it is located).

REGULATORY ASPECTS

At the time of writing, regulatory agencies in both Europe and the US are beginning to show keen interest in the potential role that pharmacogenetic approaches can play in the development and clinical use of new drugs, and the potential challenges that such approaches present to the regulatory approval process. Although no formal guidelines have been issued, the pharmaceutical industry has already been reproached – albeit in a rather nonspecific manner – for not being more proactive in the use of pharmacogenetic markers. It is crucial for all concerned to engage in an intensive dialogue at the end of which – it is hoped – will emerge a joint understanding that stratification according to DNA-based markers is fundamentally nothing new, and no different from stratification according to any of the other clinical or demographic parameters that have been used all along.

Still, based on the (in the case of common complex diseases, scientifically unjustified) perception that DNA-based markers represent a different class of stratification parameters, a number of important questions will need to be addressed and answered – hopefully always in analogy to 'conventional' stratification parameters, including those referring to ethical aspects. Among the most important ones are questions concerning:

- The need and/or ethical justification (or lack thereof) to include likely nonresponders in a trial for the sake of meeting safety criteria, which, given the restricted indication of the drug, might indeed be excessively broad.
- The need to carry out conventional-sized safety trials in the disease stratum eligible for the drug (if the stratum represents a relatively small fraction of all patients with the clinical diagnosis, it might be difficult to amass sufficient numbers and/or discourage companies from pursuing such drugs to the disadvantage of patients).
- The need to use active controls if the patient/disease stratum is different from that in which the active control was originally tested.
- The strategies to develop and gain approval for the applicable first-generation diagnostic, as well as for the regulatory approval of subsequent generations of tests to be used to determine eligibility for prescription of the drug.
- A number of ethical–legal questions relating to the unique requirements regarding privacy and confidentiality for 'genetic testing' that may raise novel problems with regard to regulatory audits of patient data (see below).

A concerted effort to avoid what has been termed 'genetic exceptionalism' – the differential treatment of DNA-based markers as compared with other personal medical data – should be made so as not to further unnecessarily complicate the already very difficult process of obtaining regulatory approval. This seems justified, based on the recognized fact that in the field of common complex disease DNA-based markers are not at all different from 'conventional' medical data in all relevant aspects – namely specificity, sensitivity and predictive value.

PHARMACOGENETIC TESTING FOR DRUG EFFICACY VERSUS SAFETY

Greater efficacy: likely

In principle, pharmacogenetic approaches could be useful both to raise efficacy and to avoid adverse events, by stratifying patient eligibility for a drug according to appropriate markers. In both cases, clinical decisions and recommendations must be supported by data that have undergone rigorous biostatistical scrutiny. Based on the substantially different prerequisites and opportunities for acquiring such data, and applying them to clinical decision-making, we expect the use of pharmacogenetics for enhanced efficacy to be considerably more common than for the avoidance of adverse events.

The likelihood that adequate data on efficacy in a subgroup can be generated is reasonably high, given the fact that unless the drug is viable in a reasonably sizeable number of patients, it will probably not be developed for lack of a viable business case, or at least only under the protected environment of orphan drug guidelines. Implementation of pharmacogenetic testing to stratify for efficacy, provided that safety in the nonresponder group is not an issue, will primarily be a matter of physician preference and sophistication, and potentially of third-party payer directives, but would appear less likely to become a matter of regulatory mandate, unless a drug has been developed selectively in a particular stratum of the overall indication (in which case a contraindication label for other strata is likely to be issued). Indeed, an argument can be made against depriving those who carry the '"likely" nonresponder' genotype regarding eligibility for the drug, but who individually, of course, might respond to the drug with a certain, albeit lower probability. From a regulatory aspect, use of pharmacogenetics for efficacy, if adequate safety data exist, appears largely unproblematic: the worst-case scenario (a genotypically inappropriate patient receiving the drug) would result in treatment without expected beneficial effect, but with no increased odds to suffer adverse consequences, i.e. much of what one would expect under conventional paradigms.

Avoidance of serious adverse effects: less likely – with exceptions

The utility and clinical application of pharmacogenetic approaches towards improving safety, in particular with regard to serious adverse events, will meet with considerably greater hurdles and is therefore less likely to become reality. A number of reasons are cited for this: first, in the event of serious adverse events associated with the use of a widely prescribed medicine, withdrawal of the drug from the market is usually based almost entirely on anecdotal evidence from a rather small number of cases – in accordance with the Hippocratic mandate *primum non nocere*. If the sample size is insufficient to demonstrate a statistically significant association between drug exposure and event, as is typically the case, it will almost certainly be insufficient to allow meaningful testing for genotype–phenotype correlations; the biostatistical hurdles become progressively more difficult as many markers are tested and the number of degrees of freedom applicable to the analysis for association continues to rise. Therefore, the fraction of attributable risk shown to be associated with a given at-risk (combination of) genotype(s) would have to be very substantial for regulators to accept such data. Indeed, the low prior probability of the adverse event, by definition, can be expected to yield an equally low positive (or negative) predictive value. Second, the very nature of safety issues raises the hurdles substantially because in this situation the worst-case scenario – administration of the drug to the 'wrong' patient – will result in higher odds of harm to the patient.

Therefore, it is likely that the practical application of successfully investigating and applying pharmacogenetics towards limiting adverse events will be restricted to the more exceptional cases: of diseases with dire prognosis, where a high medical need exists, where the drug in question offers unique potential advantages (usually bearing the characteristics of a 'life-saving' drug), and where, therefore, the tolerance even for relatively severe side effects is much greater than for other drugs. This applies primarily to areas like oncology or HIV/AIDS, for which the recently reported highly specific and acceptably sensitive association between the major histocompatibility complex (MHC) gene variant, *HLA B5701*, and occurrence of a severe hypersensitivity reaction is a prime example.[25,26]

In most other indications, the sobering biostatistical and regulatory considerations discussed represent barriers that are unlikely to be overcome easily; and the proposed, conceptually highly attractive, routine deployment of pharmacogenetics as generalized drug surveillance or pharmacovigilance practice following the introduction of a new pharmaceutical agent[27] faces these scientific hurdles, as well as formidable economic ones.

CHALLENGE: GENETICS AND SOCIETY –
ETHICAL–LEGAL–SOCIETAL ISSUES

Data protection needs to be matched by 'person protection'

Whereas public attitudes towards genetics and genomics span a broad spectrum from enthusiastic approval to total rejection, it is fair to say that many of the most outspoken voices from the 'lay'-community are skeptical, critical, or outright negative about the pursuit of genetic research and the possible implementations of some of its outcomes in society. There is a widespread public fear of the consequences; this centers primarily on two issues: (1) genetic engineering and (2) the lack of control over one's private medical–genetic data. Both concerns are thoroughly understandable, if not always justified, as any new and powerful technology carries the innate risk of being abused by unscrupulous individuals to the detriment of others. In the following, as is appropriate for the scope of this discussion, we shall focus on the latter of these concerns regarding the fate of 'genetic information'.

Much of the discussion about ethical and legal issues relating to pharmacogenetics is centered on the issue of 'genetic testing', a topic that has recently also been the focus of a number of guidelines, advisories and White Papers issued by a number of committees in both Europe and the US. It is interesting to note that the one characteristic that virtually all these documents share is an almost studious avoidance of defining exactly what a 'genetic test' *is*. Where definitions *are* given, they tend to be very broad, including not only the analysis of DNA but also of transcription and translation products affected by inherited variation. In as much as the most sensible solution to this dilemma will ultimately – hopefully – be a consensus to treat all personal medical data in a similar fashion, regardless of the degree to which DNA-encoded information affects it (noting that there really aren't any medical data that are not to some extent affected by intrinsic patient properties), it might , for the time being, be helpful to let the definition of what constitutes 'genetic data' be guided by the public perception of 'genetic data' – in as much as the whole discussion of this topic is prompted by these public perceptions.

In the public eye, the term 'genetic test' is usually understood to mean either: (1) any kind of test that establishes the diagnosis of or predisposition for one of the classic monogenic, heritable disease; or (2) any kind of test based on structural nucleic acid analysis (sequence). This includes the (non-DNA-based) Guthrie test for phenylketonuria and forensic and paternity testing, as well as a DNA-based test for lipopolysaccharide A [Lp(a)], but not the plasma-protein-based test for the same marker (even though the information derived is identical). As monogenic disease is, in effect, excluded from this discussion, it stands to reason that the definition of 'genetic testing' should be restricted to the analysis of the (human) DNA sequence.

It is clear that DNA-based structural data ('genetic' data) must never be procured without the explicit permission and informed consent of the individual. It is equally clear that once such information is created, it should be guarded by the most reliable data-protection systems available, to prevent any of this information getting into the hands of third parties not intended to have access to it. At the same time, to provide the expected benefits in terms of guiding medical management, this information will need to be shared with a more or less extensive number of participants in the patient's health care – some of whom might use it in ways contrary to the patient's interests. This is true for any drug approved in conjunction with a DNA-based test: mere prescription of such a medicine discloses implicitly the outcome of the test to a wide number of stakeholders. Among these will almost certainly be the patient's health insurer, who will gain additional knowledge about the patient's future health risks from this information and take, accordingly, certain actions; whether these are scientifi-cally–actuarially justified is irrelevant in this discussion.

As data protection, in real life, is therefore always limited or compromised, additional measures are needed to protect the individual from disadvantages based on his or her data. Thus, 'personal protection', in addition to data protection, must be provided. This requires a framework of regulations or laws that govern the use of 'personal medical information' – the latter term is preferred to restricting such protection to DNA-derived data because many 'conventional' medical data carry similar or greater information content, particularly in the area of common complex disease. Such a framework can, in democratically governed systems, only arise as a consensus among all stakeholders involved – among them patients, physicians, insurers, employers – that represents the optimal compromise that maximizes the benefits for both the individual and society. Such a framework will define which uses of the information are endorsed by society as lawful and which are shunned as illegal. Given such a framework, much of the anxiety that abounds today with regard to the possible leakage of private medical data will be laid to rest, because it is primarily the potential (ab)use of information to their detriment that patients fear (this is not to trivialize the loss of autonomy, which is also of concern).

Public education and information

The essential requirement to reach such a consensus that will allow the use of genetics and genomics in the best interest of all concerned is an informed dialog among the various stakeholders. This can only begin to take place once (mis)per-ceptions are replaced by objective and neutral information as the basis to make informed opinions. Progress in the fields of genetic and genomics has been rapid and substantial over the last few decades and has been accompanied by a great deal of hyperbole in the popular press. Meanwhile, instead of making extra efforts to reach out to the public in a concerted educational campaign, geneticists have continued to cultivate an arcane and forbidding vernacular that only adds to the appearance of purposeful secrecy to which the public is reacting. As part of the Human Genome Project, substantial amounts of funding have been provided to work in the area of bioethics and much progress has been achieved there. Similar or even greater efforts need to be made in the area of public infor-mation and education, which will surely go a long way towards resolving some of the fears and unrealistic hopes the public currently associate with genetics and genomics. The author of this chapter and his colleagues have assembled an interactive CD-ROM-based educational program that is distributed free on request (see: http://www.rochegenetics.com).[28]

Ethical–societal aspects of pharmacogenetics

Based on the – perceived – particular sensitivity of 'genetic' data, institutional review boards commonly apply a specific set of rules to granting permission to test for DNA-based markers in the course of drug trials or other clinical research, including (variably): separate informed consent forms, the anonymization of samples and data, specific stipulations about the availability of genetic counseling, and provision to be able to withdraw samples at any time in the future.

Arguments have been advanced[27] that genotype determinations for pharmacogenetic characterization, in contrast to 'genetic' testing for primary disease risk assessment, are less likely to raise potentially sensitive issues with regard to patient confidentiality, the misuse of genotyping data or other nucleic-acid-derived information, and the possibility of stigmatization. While this is certainly true when pharmacogenetic testing is compared to predictive genotyping for highly penetrant Mendelian disorders, it is not apparent why in common complex disorders issues surrounding the predictors of primary disease risk would be any more or less sensitive than those pertaining to the predictors of likely treatment success/failure. Both can be expected to provide, in most cases, a modicum of better probabilistic assessment, based on the modest degree of sensitivity, specificity and positive/negative predictive value we are likely to see with tests for pharmacogenetic interactions. If – however misguided this would be given the anticipated quite limited information content of such tests – such information was to be used 'against' the patient, then two lines of reasoning might actually indicate an increased potential for ethical issues and complex confrontations among the various stakeholders to arise from pharmacogenetic data.

First, while access to genotyping and other nucleic-acid-derived data related to disease susceptibility can be strictly limited, the very nature of pharmacogenetic data calls for a rather more liberal position regarding use: if this information is to serve its intended purpose (i.e. improving the patient's chance for successful treatment) then it is essential that it is shared among a somewhat wider circle of participants in the healthcare process at least. Thus, the prescription for a drug that is limited to a group of patients with a particular genotype will inevitably disclose the receiving patient's genotype to any one of a large number of individuals involved in the patient's care at the medical and administrative level. The only way to limit this quasipublic disclosure of this patient's genotype data would be if he or she were to sacrifice the benefits of the indicated treatment for the sake of data confidentiality.

Second, patients profiled to carry a high disease probability along with a high likelihood for treatment response might be viewed from the standpoint of, say, insurance risk, as comparable to patients displaying the opposite profile (i.e. at a low risk of developing the disease but with a high likelihood not to respond to medical treatment if the disease indeed occurs). For any given disease risk, then, patients less likely to respond to treatment would be seen as a more unfavorable insurance risk, particularly if nonresponder status is associated with chronic, costly illness rather than with early mortality, the first case having much more far-reaching economic consequences. The pharmacogenetic profile might thus, under certain circumstances, become an even more important (financial) risk-assessment parameter than primary disease susceptibility, and would be expected – in as much as it represents but one stone in the complex disease mosaic – to be treated with similar weight, or lack thereof, as other genetic and environmental risk factors.

Practically speaking, the critical issue is not only, and perhaps not even predominantly, the real or perceived sensitive nature of the information and how it is, if at all, disseminated and disclosed, but how and to what end it is used. Obviously, generation and acquisition of personal medical information must always be contingent on the individual's free choice and consent, as must be all application of such data for specific purposes. Beyond this, however, there is now an urgent need for the requisite dialog and discourse among all stakeholders within society to develop and endorse a set of criteria by which the use of genetic – indeed of all personal medical information – should occur. It is crucial that society as a whole endorses, in an act of solidarity with those less fortunate (i.e. at higher risk of developing disease or less likely to respond to treatment), rules that guarantee the beneficial and legitimate use of the data in the patient's interest while at the same time prohibiting their use in ways that might harm the individual, personally, financially or in any other way. As long as we trust our political decision-making processes to reflect societal consensus, and as long as such consensus reflects the principles of justice and equality, the resulting set of principles should ensure such proper use of medical information. Indeed, both aspects – data protection and patient/subject protection – are seminal components of the mandates included in the World Health Organization's *Proposed international guidelines on ethical issues in medical genetics and genetic services*,[29] which mandate autonomy, beneficence, nonmaleficence and justice.

SUMMARY

Genetics and genomics, in their various implementations, represent an important new avenue towards understanding disease pathology and drug action, and offer new opportunities of stratifying patients to achieve better treatment success. As such, these approaches are a logical, consequent step in the history of medicine – evolutionary rather than revolutionary. The implementation of genetic approaches will take time, and will not apply to all diseases and all treatments equally. Pharmacogenetic information will be probabilistic and relative, not deterministic or absolute. Application of genetics and genomics to the drug discovery and development process, as well as to medical practice, will provide help but no simple solutions, and will not be a panacea. Importantly, society at large will need to find ways to sanction the proper use of private medical information, thus allowing and protecting its unencumbered use for the benefit of patients while safeguarding them from unintended use. Increased efforts to inform and educate the general public, leading to a more realistic assessment of the actual potential of genetic approaches to provide benefit or cause harm, will be key to quelling both the exalted hopes and exaggerated fears that are so often associated with the topic.

References

1. The Boston consulting Group. Online. Available: http://www.bcg.com/publications
2. Dickins M, Tucker G: Drug disposition: to phenotype or genotype. *Int J Pharm Med* 2001; 15:70–73. Also online. Available: http://www.imm.ki.se/CYPalleles/
3. Evans WE, Relling MV. Pharmacogenomics: translating functional genomics into rational therapies. *Science* 1999;206:487–491. Also online. Available: http://www.sciencemag.org/feature/data/1044449.shl/
4. Fellay J, Marzolini C, Meaden ER, et al. Response to antiretroviral treatment in HIV-1-infected individuals with allelic variants of the multidrug resistance transporter 1: a pharmacogenetics study. *Lancet* 2002; 359:30–36.

5. Dubinsky M, Lamothe S, Yang HY, et al. Pharmacogenomics and metabolite measurement for 6-mercaptopurine therapy in inflammatory bowel disease. *Gastroenterology* 2000; 118:705-713.

6. Martinez FD, Graves PE, Baldini M, et al. Association between genetic polymorphisms of the beta2-adrenoceptor and response to albuterol in children with and without a history of wheezing. *J Clin Invest* 1997; 100:3184–3188.

7. Tan S, Hall IP, Dewar J, et al. Association between beta 2-adrenoceptor polymorphism and susceptibility to bronchodilator desensitisation in moderately severe stable asthmatics. *Lancet* 1997; 350:995–999.

8. Green SA, Turki J, Innis M, Liggett SB. Amino-terminal polymorphisms of the human beta 2-adrenergic receptor impart distinct agonist-promoted regulatory properties. *Biochemistry* 1994; 33:9414–9419.

9. Green SA, Turki J, Bejarano P, et al. Influence of beta 2-adrenergic receptor genotypes on signal transduction in human airway smooth muscle cells. *Am J Respir Cell Mol Biol* 1995; 13:15–33.

10. Reihsaus E, Innis M, MacIntyre N, Liggett SB. Mutations in the gene encoding for the beta 2-adrenergic receptor in normal and asthmatic subjects. *Am J Respir Cell Mol Biol* 1993; 8:334–349.

11. Dewar JC, Wheatley AP, Venn A, et al. 2 adrenoceptor polymorphisms are in linkage disequilibrium, but are not associated with asthma in an adult population. *Clin Exp All* 1998; 28:442–448.

12. Drazen JM, Yandava CN, Dube L, et al. Pharmacogenetic association between ALOX5 promoter genotype and the response to anti-asthma treatment. *Nat Genet* 1999; 22:168–170.

13. Asano K, Beier D, Grobholz J, et al. Naturally occurring mutations in the human 5-lipoxygenase gene promoter that modify transcription factor binding and reporter gene transcription. *J Clin Invest* 1997; 99(5):1130–1137.

14. Fischel-Ghodsian N. Genetic factors in aminoglycoside toxicity. *Ann NY Acad Sci* 1999; 884:99–109.

15. Hutchin T, Cortopassi G. Proposed molecular and cellular mechanism for aminoglycoside ototoxicity. *Antimicrob Agents Chemother* 1994; 38:2517–2520.

16. Baselga J, Tripathy D, Mendelsohn J, et al. Phase II study of weekly intravenous recombinant humanized anti-p185(HER2) monoclonal antibody in patients with HER2/neu-overexpressing metastatic breast cancer. *J Clin Oncol* 1996; 14:737–744.

17. Haseltine WA. Not quite pharmacogenomics [letter; comment]. *Nat Biotechnol* 1998; 16:1295.

18. McGraw DW, Forbes SL, Kramer LA, Liggett SB. Polymorphisms of the 5′ leader cistron of the human beta2-adrenergic receptor regulate receptor expression. *J Clin Invest* 1998; 102:1927–1932.

19. Huang Y, Paxton WA, Wolinsky SM, et al. The role of a mutant CCR5 allele in HIV-1 transmission and disease progression. *Nat Med* 1996; 2:1240–1243.

20. Dean M, Carrington M, Winkler C, et al. Genetic restriction of HIV-1 infection and progression to AIDS by a deletion of the CKR5 structural gene. *Science* 1996; 273:1856–1862.

21. Samson M, Libert F, Doranz BJ, et al. Resistance to HIV-1 infection in Caucasian individuals bearing mutant alleles of the CCR-5 chemokine receptor gene. *Nature* 1996; 382:722–725.

22. O'Brien TR, Winkler C, Dean M, et al. HIV-1 infection in a man homozygous for CCR5 32. *Lancet* 1997; 349:1219.

23. Theodorou I, Meyer L, Magierowska M, et al and Seroco Study Group. HIV-1 infection in an individual homozygous for CCR5 32. *Lancet* 1997; 349:1219–1220.

24. Esteller M, Garcia-Foncillas J, Andion E, et al. Inactivation of the DNA-repair gene mgmt and the clinical response of gliomas to alkylating agents. *N Engl J Med* 2000; 343:1350–1354.

25. Mallal S, Nolan D, Witt C, et al. Association between presence of HLA-B*5701, HLA-DR7, and HLA-DQ3 and hypersensitivity to HIV-1 reverse-transcriptase inhibitor abacavir. *Lancet* 2002; 359:727–732.

26. Hetherington S, Hughes AR, Mosteller M, et al. Genetic variations in HLA-B region and hyper-sensitivity reactions to abacavir. *Lancet* 2002; 359:1121–1122.

27. Roses A. Pharmacogentics and future drug development and delivery. *Lancet* 2000; 355:1358–1361.

28. Roche Genetics Educational Program. Online. Available on request from: http://www.rochegenetics.com

29. World Health Organization. Proposed international guidelines on ethical issues in medical genetics and genetic services. Online. Available: http://www.who.int/ncd/hgn/hgnethic.htm.

9 | Adducin genes as a paradigm for functional studies

Grazia Tripodi, Lorena Citterio and Giuseppe Bianchi

INTRODUCTION

Functional variants in the heterodimeric cytoskeletal protein adducin both in humans and in the Milan hypertensive strain (MHS) genetic rat model are thought to be involved in the pathophysiology of primary hypertension through the regulation of tubular reabsorption of sodium. But why did we become interested in studying adducin genes (ADD) and how did we approach the impact of their molecular mechanism in the complex etiology of essential hypertension? In this chapter we discuss: (1) the long series of physiological studies, made in parallel in humans and in rats, that allowed the identification of adducin as a candidate in hypertension; (2) the complexity of the ADD gene structure and the pattern of expression of three ADD subunits (making the most of the recent data into the genome database); (3) our studies at the molecular level that identified genetic variants and associated pathway function in MHS and human hypertension; (4) a brief summary of linkage and association studies in humans that followed our first evidence of ADD involvement in hypertension, dealing mainly with the appropriateness of the methodological and strategic approaches used to assess the role of ADD in hypertension and its organ complications; (5) the pharmacogenomic approach and the development of a new antihypertensive compound able to correct the specific genetic molecular mechanism underlying the altered tubular sodium reabsorption; (6) the future directions needed to fully elucidate the real impact of ADD polymorphisms in human hypertension and related complications.

COMPARISON BETWEEN THE MHS RAT MODEL AND HUMANS PRONE TO OR WITH HYPERTENSION AT RENAL AND CELLULAR LEVELS

We started our studies in arterial hypertension by producing a renal artery constriction to a sole remaining kidney in a conscious dog. After 2–3 weeks of this manipulation, all the initial alterations in plasma renin, body fluids and cardiac

145

function that were responsible for the initial rise in blood pressure disappeared, and the hormonal and hemodynamic patterns were identical to those found in primary hypertension.[1-3] Thus, genetic mechanisms affecting renal function might also underlie primary forms of hypertension. Using this rationale, we performed a series of parallel empirical observations in spontaneous MHS rats and in human hypertensives[4] to discover whether: (1) the sequence of changes in hemodynamics, body fluid, renal function and hormones that occurs during the development of 'primary' hypertension in the two species was compatible with a renal origin of hypertension; (2) renal transplantation could produce long-term bloodpressure changes, implying that the genetic message travels with the kidney.

As the most relevant pathophysiological changes of the variables at point (1), above, occur at the transition from normotension to hypertension, we compared animals and humans prone to developing hypertension with their respective controls at this early stage. Although the definition of the prehypertensive stage is easy in animals, in humans we have to define it arbitrarily as a young normotensive with two hypertensive parents, compared with matched subjects with two normotensive parents.[5]

Table 9.1 shows how many physiological variables are similar in prehypertensives or early hypertensives of the two species when compared with their respective controls. Of course, because of the heterogeneity of the human conditions, such similarities can be applied only to a subset of patients; this is the weakest aspect of the comparison between human and animal model.

Based on the findings of renovascular hypertension mentioned above,[1-3] the hypothesis that the kidney, despite its normal morphological appearance, could be the carrier of the 'genetic message' for hypertension was tested by kidney crosstransplantation experiments carried out between MHS and its control Milan normotensive strain (MNS).[6,7] This study showed that hypertension could be 'transplanted' with the kidney. Similar findings were also obtained in humans by evaluating hypertension in kidney donors and the antihypertensive drug requirements of the donor recipients.[8,9]

These results prompted us to study the function of the whole kidney, the function of isolated renal tubules and the function of the ion transport mechanism

Table 9.1 Comparison of humans either prone to or at the early hypertensive stage with rats of the Milan strain

	Human essential	MHS rats
Pressor effect of kidney transplantation	↑	↑
Renal blood flow	*↑ = ↓	= or ↑ in isolated kidney
Glomerular filtration rate	*↑ = ↓	↑
Sodium excretion afterload	↑	↑
24-hour urinary output	↑	↑
Plasma renin	↓	↓
Urine kallikrein	↓	↓
Erythrocyte sodium content	*↓ = ↑	↓
Net erythrocyte membrane sodium transport	*↑ = ↓	↑

See ref. 21 and the text for explanation.
*In subsets of patients.
↑, higher; ↓, lower; =, or equal (in the hypertensive humans and rats compared to the appropriate controls).

between the renal membrane and the erythrocytes.[10,17] We found that a genetic message that altered cellular ion transport was also present in nonrenal cells, e.g. erythrocytes.[17] As shown in Table 9.1, MHS erythrocytes have characteristics similar to those of tubular cells with regard to Na ion transport and intracellular content. These features are present before the development of hypertension and persist throughout the lifespan.[18,19] These studies yielded data supporting the hypothesis that an alteration in cell membrane transport could be responsible for a constitutive increase in tubular sodium reabsorption that, in the long run, could facilitate the development of renal Na retention and hypertension. We demonstrated that such a cell membrane alteration was genetically determined in the stem cells and genetically associated to hypertension both by bone marrow transplantation and by genetic crosses between MHS and MNS.[20]

In humans, a subset of patients showing a greater diuretic response to furosemide was found to have a low erythrocyte intracellular Na content and increased Na–K cotransport,[21] suggesting that in these patients, as in MHS, a widespread alteration in cell membrane ion transport is responsible for the abnormal handling of sodium in the tubules. We then showed that the difference in ion transport between MHS and MNS disappeared after the removal of the cytoskeleton.[22] Crossimmunization experiments with cytoskeletal proteins of one strain into the other allowed us to detect an antibody towards a cytoskeletal protein that was subsequently identified as adducin.[23]

PROTEIN FUNCTION

Adducin is a heterodimeric membrane skeleton protein consisting of an α [relative molecular weight (Mr) 103 kDa], β (Mr 97 kDa) and γ (Mr 90 kDa) subunit that assemble either as α–β or α–γ oligomers in the different tissues.[24] The main function of adducin is to promote the organization of the spectrin–actin lattice by favoring spectrin–actin binding.[25] Adducin is an end-capping actin protein and controls the rate of actin polymerization.[26] Its function is dependent on Ca^{2+} and calmodulin[27] and it is phosphorylated by protein kinase A, protein kinase C, tyrosine kinase and rho kinase,[28] making it a member of the MARCKS proteins involved in the signal transduction pathway.[29] Its translocation from the cytosol to the cell membrane at the level of the cell–cell contact sites[27] is controlled by its phosphorylation status, and it has been found to be involved in the processes of cell migration[30] and lymphocyte activation.[31]

THE ADD GENE FAMILY

Adducin subunits are encoded by genes *ADD1*, *ADD2* and *ADD3*, which are mapped on different chromosomes in human and in rat (Fig. 9.1). *ADD* genes belong to the same gene family and show a similar gene structure, suggesting that they derive from a single gene that has undergone duplication and rearrangements during evolution. These mechanisms have led to their different chromosome location and quite different intronic length, although exons are well conserved both in structure and in length. Every gene displays a complex alternative splicing pattern leading to a variety of possible combinations of transcript variants encoding distinct isoforms.

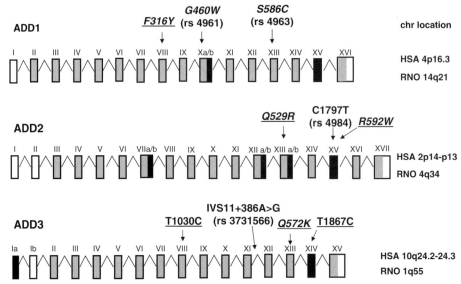

Fig. 9.1 *ADD1*, *ADD2*, *ADD3* gene structure and single nucleotide polymorphisms (SNPs) identi-fied in human and rat hypertension. The exon–intron structure of *ADD* genes is indicated by boxes and lines; closed and open boxes represent the exons for coding and noncoding regions of mRNA, respectively. Black-filled boxes indicate the alternatively spliced exons. Exons that contain alterna-tive donor or acceptor sites are presented as a/b (exon X for *ADD1*, exons VII, XII and XIII for *ADD2*). The position of human and rat (underlined) SNPs is indicated by the arrow. The SNP coordi-nate is based on the amino acid change (one letter code, italics) for missense mutation and nucleotide change for silent or intronic mutation. dbSNP ID for human SNP is reported in brackets. The human (HSA) and rat (RNO) chromosomal location is reported on the right.

The human *ADD1* gene is 86.2 Kb in size and composed of 16 exons, 15 of which code for the most common variant expressed in all the tissues. Two spliced variants are known: one results from an alternative use of the 5′ splice donor site for exon 10 with an in-frame 93 basepair (bp) insertion; the other vari-ant is a truncated protein following insertion of 34 bp comprising exon 15, fol-lowed by a premature stop codon.[32]

The human *ADD2* gene is 106 Kb in size and composed of 17 exons. *ADD2* is particularly expressed in neuronal and erythropoietic tissues but can be detected, at least at transcriptional level, in other tissues.[33] It shows the most complex alternative splicing pattern of expression. More than ten spliced vari-ants derived from the alternative use of the 5′ splice donor site for exons 7, 12, 13 result in the lack of internal exons and/or the use of a premature stop codon.[34] A further variant, named *ADD2-β4*, results in an out of frame insertion of exon 15, giving a truncated carboxy-terminus isoform with 63 novel amino acids.[35]

The human *ADD3* gene is 128.2 Kb in size and composed of 15 exons, 14 of them codifying for the most common variant expressed in all the tissues. One spliced variant, named *ADD3-γ2* results from an in-frame 96 bp insertion, corre-sponding to exon 14.[36] Detailed analysis of the *ADD3* alternative spliced tran-scripts reveals the presence of an alternative use of the 5′ splice donor site for exon 1 (Fig.9.1Ia,Ib) that could be the signal for the use of alternative promoters (unpublished data).

The similarity between human and rat *ADD* gene family can be easily obtained from the almost complete rat genome sequence in public databases (see http://www.ensembl.org/Rattus_norvegicus).[37] The three genes map to rat chromosomal regions that correspond to the human counterpart and genomic sequence alignments indicate a similar intron/exon structure between the two species. Each subunit shows more than 85% coding region similarity and more than 90% amino acid similarity. The most relevant alternative spliced variants are the results of a similar exon skipping in human and rats.[38–41] The similarity of *ADD* genes and transcript variants can be extended to mouse.[42] The high homology through the different species indicates a role in basic functional cell mechanisms.

MAPPING OF CHROMOSOMAL REGIONS SURROUNDING HUMAN AND RAT *ADD1* LOCI

The availability of the complete genome sequence, with the characterization of the pattern of linkage disequilibrium of the human genome and a paucity of haplotype diversity in 'linkage blocks' interspersed by apparent 'hot-spots' of recombination, enables us to better understand the studies of linkage and association analysis in the human population discussed above. Table 9.2 shows the fine mapping of the 2.64 Mb chromosomal region surrounding the *ADD1* locus, with all known genes and the main markers used in linkage studies involving the *ADD1* gene. This region was covered with 559 Tag single nucleotide polymorphisms (SNPs; genotyped in a Caucasian population) and a total of 45 haplotype blocks was found[43] (see: http://www.hapmap.org) with a number of haplotype blocks ranging from 3 to 16 in the regions between markers.

The rat genome sequence, unlike the human and mouse ones, is not completely reliable[37] and the generation of a dense polymorphism map for the most commonly used laboratory rat strains is still under construction. Recently, a different collection of candidate SNPs in gene-coding regions,[44–46] representing the first-generation SNP map for the rat genome, became available for mapping or association studies. Knowledge of the extent of these variations is crucial for refining maps in congenic strains and selecting substrains with the minimal resolvable region. Haplotype sharing analysis with a subset of cDNA-based SNP[44] and comparison with orthologous regions of mouse and human genome allowed us to define the minimal congenic region of 1.9 Mb for *Add1* reciprocal congenic strains.[47] The physical map in Table 9.3 shows that the congenic segment contains eleven rat genes beside *Add1* and sixteen genes with a mean amino acid identity of 83% and 94% in human and mouse, respectively. We have now identified 17 SNPs, with no evident functional significance, in nine of these genes.[47] This work aims to exclude *Add1* flanking loci as causal for blood pressure differences in MHS rats and to select congenic substrains whose limit of QTL localization is approximately 200 Kb.[48]

ADD IN HYPERTENSION OF MILAN RATS

The analysis of the full-length cDNA sequences in MHS and MNS revealed a missense mutation in *Add1* (F316Y), two missense mutations in *Add2* (Q529R,

Table 9.2 Physical map and haplotype blocks for 2.64 Mb of chr 4 surrounding the ADD1 locus. Map positions were taken from the human genome assembly

Gene/Marker	Start position (bp)	Gene description	Kb	Haploname type blocks
D4S3038	1083038			
SPON2	1150553	spondin 2, extracellular matrix protein.	134.7	3
CTBP1	1195091	C-terminal binding protein 1		
D4S115	1224698			
MAEA	1273509	macrophage erythroblast attacher		
Q15270	1386871	HPX-153 protein (Fragment)		
SLBP	1656166	Histone RNA hairpin-binding protein		
TACC3	1684903	Transforming acidic coiled-coil-containing protein 3		
FGFR3	1757262	Fibroblast growth factor receptor 3 precursor	1073	16
LETM1	1776399	leucine zipper-EF-hand containing transmembrane protein 1		
WHSC1	1856148	Wolf-Hirschhorn syndrome candidate 1		
WHSC2	1946096	Wolf-Hirschhorn syndrome candidate 2 protein		
POLN	2035284	polymerase (DNA directed)		
MXD4	2210799	Max-interacting transcriptional repressor MAD4		
D4S43	2298002			
RNF4	2432446	RING finger protein 4		
C4orf8	2658773	gene with multiple splice variants near HD locus on 4p16.3.	578.7	9
TNIP2	2775001	A20-binding inhibitor of NF-kappaB activation 2		
SH3BP2	2851954	SH3 domain-binding protein 2 (3BP-2)		
ADD1	2876998	Alpha adducin		
TETRAN	2963708	tetracycline transporter-like protein	30.5	5
D4S95	2993678			
GRK4	3017651	G protein-coupled receptor kinase GRK4		
HD	3107820	Huntingtin (Huntington's disease protein)	417.5	5
RGS12	3347251	Regulator of G-protein signaling 12		
D4S412	3412071			
HGFAC	3475103	Hepatocyte growth factor activator precursor		
LRPAP1	3545672	Alpha-2-macroglobulin receptor-associated protein precursor	311.4	7
D4S126	3723713			
D4S432	not mapped			

Haplotype blocks were retrieved from HapMap (www.hapmap.org).

R592W) and three mutations in *Add3* (Q572K, T1030C, T1867C), the exon positions of which are shown in Figure 9.1.[39,40,49] In the MHSxMNS F2 hybrid population the *Add1* mutation is genetically associated with blood pressure levels by accounting for the 43% of blood pressure difference between MHS and MNS.[49] The *Add2* and *Add3* mutations that are not associated with hypertension epistatically interact with *Add1* to determine the blood pressure level of the F2 hybrids.[50] The recent successful bilateral transfer of blood pressure QTL with *Add1* locus in reciprocal congenic strains, within the fine mapping of the 1.9 Mb minimal congenic segment, as shown in Table 9.3, strongly supports the role of the *Add1* locus in blood-pressure regulation in Milan rats.[47]

Table 9.3 Physical map for 1.9 Mb of chr 14 surrounding Add1 locus and homoloy with human and mouse genome. Map positions were taken from the rat genome sequence assembly (Rnor3.1)

Rat ID	Human ID	R.H%	Mouse ID	R.M%	SNPs	Start position (bp)	Gene description
Acox3	ACOX3	74	Acox3	88	1	80771847	acyl-coenzyme A oxidase 3
	NP_689757	75	NM030208	90		80818318	
Cpz	CPZ	82	Cpz	89		80859762	carboxypeptidase Z
	HMX1	72				80998300	homeo box (H6 family) 1
A2ac	ADRA2A	58	Adra2c	99		81110535	alpha-2C adrenoceptor
Lrpap1	LRPAP1	75	Lrpap1	96	3	81295085	alpha2-macroglobulin receptor-associated protein precursor
	NP_775931	79	NM_172708	95		81311076	
Hgfac	HGFAC	80	Hgfac	91		81350742	hepatocyte growth factor activator precursor
Rgs12	RGS12	84	Rgs12	95		81365933	regulator of G-protein signaling 12
		89	NM207277	98		81479652	
Hd	HD	91	Hdh	97		81493478	Huntingtin (Huntington's disease protein)
NM022928	GRK4	75	Gprk2l	90	3	81650394	G protein-coupled receptor kinase 2, groucho gene related
	C4orf9	82	NM029278	93	1	81725593	
	NP_001111	81	NM026660	94		81748388	
Add1	ADD1	92	Add1	98	1	81754256	alpha adducin
	SH3BP2	85	Sh3bp2	92	2	81822157	SH3 domain-binding protein 2 (3BP-2)
	TNIP2	74	Tnip2	92		81873428	A20-binding inhibitor of NF-kappaB activation 2
	C4orf8	87	Q8CGI1	95		81921150	
Rnf4	RNF4	89	Rnf4	91		82094523	RING finger protein 4
	ZY28	96	Q8CG84	98		82242683	
	MXD4	91	Mxd4	99		82255888	Max-interacting transcriptional repressor MAD4
	C4orf15	79				82275123	
	POLN	76	Poln	91		82343190	polymerase (DNA directed)
	NP_848652	100	Q8K065	100	2	82454774	
Whsc2	WHSC2	95	Whsc2	99	3	82505290	Wolf-Hirschhorn syndrome candidate 2 protein
			Whsc1	97	1	82532261	Wolf-Hirschhorn syndrome candidate 1 protein
	WHSC1	85				82571764	Wolf-Hirschhorn syndrome candidate 1 protein
Letm1	LETM1	84	Letm1	94	1	82644977	leucine zipper-EF-hand containing transmembrane protein 1

R-H%, rat-human identity; R-M%, rat-mouse identity; SNPs, number of SNPs identified between MHS-MNS as previously reported in ref. 47.

The molecular mechanism that links the *Add1* polymorphism to cell alterations responsible for the abnormal sodium handling and hypertension has been investigated in cell culture and in cell-free system studies. In renal cells, transfection with the *Add1* hypertensive variant increases Na–K pump expression and activity, and causes a rearrangement of the actin cytoskeleton compared with cells transfected with the respective wild-type variant.[51] In *in vitro* cell-free systems, mutated adducin favors a faster process of actin polymerization[51] and directly binds and activates the Na–K pump with higher affinity than the respective normal protein.[52] A unifying interpretation for both the increased cellular expression and activity of the Na–K pump and the alterations in the actin cytoskeleton caused by the expression of the *Add1* mutated variant has been furnished by recent studies[53,54] on the dynamics of the endocytotic processes in transfected cells. In fact, the *Add1* hypertensive variant increases the residual time of the Na–K pump on the cell membrane as a result of an impaired removal of the protein through the endocytotic pathways, through the increment of the phosphorylation state of intermediate protein.[54] The actin cytoskeleton is involved in each step of this process and might ultimately provide a physical barrier to the free diffusion of the endocytotic vesicles into the cytosol. In this respect, it has been reported that a rigid cortical actin cytoskeleton has an inhibitory effect on membrane traffic.[55] It could be speculated that a more rigid actin cytoskeleton, as observed in the presence of the mutated *Add1*, affects both the constitutive[53] and stimulated[54] processes of membrane protein internalization, and in particular those controlling the Na–K pump surface expression.

The molecular basis through which *Add2* and *Add3* polymorphisms are involved in hypertension in the Milan rat is still under investigation. The reciprocal congenic strains for *Add2* and *Add3* allow us to exclude a direct involvement of these loci in blood-pressure modulation[47] but provide evidence of a direct involvement in susceptibility to organ damage, e.g. cardiac hypertrophy and renal failure.[56] However, *Add2* and *Add3* epistatically interact with *Add1* in the regulation of blood-pressure levels in the F2 population;[49,50] the biochemical features of the protein promote this interaction. In fact, adducin acts within cells as either α–γ and α–β heterodimers in the tissues most relevant for the control of blood pressure (kidney, brain, heart and blood vessels). The physiological characterization of double congenic strains for *Add* subunits will shed light on the complex pattern of genetic effects of *Add* genes expressed as heterodimers.

The Q572K polymorphism of *Add3* has been found both in MHS and spontaneously hypertensive rats (SHR).[40] Yang et al[57,58] have provided very interesting data on the possible mechanisms through which *Add3* regulates blood pressure in SHR. They show a 33% decrease of *Add3* expression in the SHR neurons compared to Wistar Kyoto (WKY), associated with a more consistent reduction (60%) in the protein level. Similar reductions are present in the hypothalamus and brainstem of adult SHR. The inhibition of *Add3* with intracellular delivery of its specific antibodies increases the neuronal firing rate to the same extent as angiotensin II but the effects of these two maneuvers are not additive. Angiotensin II administration, and other maneuvers that increase blood pressure, reduce the brainstem content of *Add3*.[58] Therefore, it has been proposed that *Add3* reduction might favor, or mediate, the augmented basal neuronal firing rate in the cardiovascular regulatory brain areas of the SHR.[58] Similar *Add3* mRNA reduction has also been found in the same brain areas of MHS (unpublished data), indicating that the same missense mutation in *Add3* might be associated with similar alterations in protein expression and neuronal firing rate in MHS and SHR rats.

Gilligan et al[59] and Muro et al[60] independently selected an *Add2* null mice strain with concordant results that related the lack of the *Add2* gene with red blood cell spherocytosis, but only Muro found increased blood pressure.[61] We are currently investigating the *Add2* null mice strain selected by Gilligan et al and no clear evidence of blood pressure modulation has been observed (unpublished data).

ADD IN HUMAN HYPERTENSION

The renal and cellular analogies between rat and human, and the high degree of protein homology between the two species, lead us to suggest the presence of polymorphisms in the human *ADD1* locus that could account for the primary cell dysfunction responsible for essential hypertension, at least in a subgroup of patients. A case-control linkage analysis with marker D4S95 showed a significant association with blood pressure[62] (see also Table 9.2) and stimulated us to sequence *ADD1* cDNA in selected subjects. We found two mutations, G460W and S586C (see Fig. 9.1), in strong linkage disequilibrium and associated with hypertension in sibpair and case-control analyses.[63] Moreover, the carriers of the *ADD1* 460W allele, when compared with homozygotes for the *ADD1* 460G allele, showed a greater sensitivity to changes in Na balance,[63] decreased erythrocyte Na content and a faster Na–K cotransport.[64] Subsequently, polymorphisms in *ADD2* and *ADD3* (see Fig. 9.1) were also taken into account in association studies that investigated their effect alone or in interaction with the *ADD1* locus.

At a molecular level, the *ADD1* G460W polymorphism mirrors the effect of the rat *Add1* F316Y polymorphism, despite the difference in amino acid change. In fact, in an *in vitro* cell-free system, the hypertensive variant activates the Na–K pump with greater affinity than the normotensive variant and, in transfected cells, increases the residual time of the Na–K pump on the cell membrane.[52–54]

Since these first reports,[62,63] several studies have tried to assess the role of the *ADD1* polymorphism [alone or in interaction with *ADD2*, *ADD3* and angiotensin-converting enzyme (ACE)] in hypertension and its cardiovascular complications. Of 64 studies, five report results obtained in Italian populations, 13 concern populations studied in different centers and blindly genotyped in Milan and 46 describe results obtained by other groups in European, White–American, African–American, Chinese and Japanese populations (summarized in a recent review).[65] As for any candidate gene, the variable results obtained could reflect altered environmental, genetic and biological contexts.[65] We report here a brief summary of all these studies.

In four family-based association studies, *ADD* gene SNPs were associated with blood pressure alone, in reciprocal association or with salt intake. In family-based linkage studies, two positive results were obtained with the marker D4S95 closest to the *ADD1* locus whereas four negative results were obtained with markers D4S3038, D4S43, D4S412, D4S126, and D4S432 mapping at a distance greater than 450 Kb from the *ADD1* locus (as shown in Table 9.2). The increasing number of linkage blocks and relative 'hot-spots' of recombination within the distance from the *ADD1* locus, calls into question the validity of linkage studies with markers at such a distance from the candidate locus. Positive results were also obtained in 18 out of 20 studies that, with blood pressure, investigated variables that reflected body Na composition or the renin–angiotensin system. Some negative case-control studies or studies in predominantly normotensive populations did not consider the abovementioned variables.

Four out of five studies showed a selective beneficial effect of diuretics in carriers of the mutated *ADD1*. Twelve out of 16 studies found that the *ADD1* polymorphism alone or in combination with the ACE gene I/D polymorphism was positively associated with stroke, coronary heart disease or renal and vascular dysfunction. Taken together, these findings strongly support the clinical impact of *ADD* on hypertension and related disorders.[65]

RELATION BETWEEN ADD AND ENDOGENOUS OUABAIN: A COMMON GENETIC MECHANISM AS A PHARMACOLOGICAL TARGET FOR A NEW ANTIHYPERTENSIVE COMPOUND

Our group's interest in endogenous ouabain (EO) was triggered by the observation that, during the development of hypertension in MHS, the rise of blood pressure was associated to a reduction of a previously increased renal interstitial pressure.[4] These opposite changes in hydrostatic pressure and blood pressure could be explained by postulating the secretion of endogenous substances that, in keeping with the hypothesis of Blaustein,[66] limit the increase in tubular Na reabsorption (hence reducing renal interstitial pressure) and simultaneously facilitate vasoconstriction through inhibition of the Na–K pump. Indeed, the levels of EO are higher in the plasma, urine and hypothalamus of MHS than in MNS.[67]

In the congenic normotensive rats carrying the MHS *Add1*, the low-salt diet increases the plasma EO level; this maneuver does not produce any variation in the control MNS strain.[68] In isolated tubular cells, long-term incubation with subnanomolar concentrations of ouabain increases the surface expression of the Na–K pump;[69] this also occurs when the same cells are transfected with the mutated MHS *Add1*.[51] This intriguing parallelism between mutated *Add1* and EO has not yet been fully elucidated. In a predominantly normotensive population, the plasma levels of EO are increased in a dose-dependent manner by the presence of the *ADD1* 460W allele.[70] Moreover, the relationship between EO and blood pressure is dependent on Na intake.[70] At low salt intakes, subjects with plasma EO above the population median value tend to have higher blood pressures than the subjects with the plasma EO below this median value;[70] the opposite occurs at high sodium intake.[70] Also, in subjects placed on a low-salt diet or on diuretic therapy, plasma EO tends to increase.[71] Taken together, these observations are consistent with the hypothesis that, depending on the amount of Na intake, EO can either increase or decrease blood pressure. The mechanisms by which adducin affects this relationship remain unknown.

A drug that can interfere with the cellular and molecular alterations caused by the mutated *ADD1* and/or increased EO, namely the upregulation of the renal Na–K pump, represents appropriate antihypertensive therapy for patients in whom these mechanisms are at work. The prototype of such a drug is PST-2238.[69,72] In cultured renal cells, nanomolar concentrations of this compound normalize the Na–K pump upregulation caused by transfection of mutated *Add1*[73] or by long-term incubation with nanomolar concentrations of ouabain.[69] Similarly, in MHS rats and in rats made hypertensive by chronic ouabain infusion (OS rats), PST-2238 lowers blood pressure and normalizes the renal Na–K pump at oral doses of 0.1–5 µg/kg.[69,73] PST-2238 lacks any effect in normotensive animals and on normal cells, and its specificity of action is reinforced by the lack of interaction with other receptors or hormones involved in blood pressure regulation.[69] Furthermore, PST-2238 lacks a classic diuretic activity because it does not affect H_2O and Na excretion after either acute or chronic administration in rats.[74] More importantly, it neither activates the renin–angiotensin–aldosterone system nor affects carbohydrate or lipid metabolism, which is in keeping with the profile of a drug able to cure a primary genetic defect without influencing counter-regulatory responses like a traditional diuretic.[74] PST-2238 is currently under evaluation in hypertensive patients, taking into account both the *ADD1* polymorphism and EO levels.

FUTURE DIRECTIONS

Many important issues are currently under investigation: the complex signal transduction pathway underlying the differential cell effects on Na–K pump endocytosis of rat and human adducin variants; the interaction of adducin with hormones regulating body Na and, in particular, the interaction with EO that affects the Na–K pump; the relevance of *ADD2* and *ADD3* polymorphisms in the modulation of expression levels of these subunits and their impact on the protein function. As adducin functions within cells as α–β or α–γ heterodimers, we need to elucidate this complex multiway interaction at molecular, cellular, renal and blood pressure levels.

In rats, we are characterizing at different levels of biological complexity reciprocal congenic strains for all the possible combinations of *Add* subunits; in parallel, we are selecting substrains with the minimal resolvable region introgressed and, in humans, we are taking into account block-specific haplotypes in association studies of the three *ADD* loci, aimed both to the identification of *ADD2* and *ADD3* functional variants and to investigate interactions among *ADD* loci and other candidate genes.

References

1. Bianchi G, Tenconi LT, Lucca R. Effect in the conscious dog of constriction of the renal artery to a sole remaining kidney on haemodynamics, sodium balance, body fluid volume, plasma renin concentration and pressor responsiveness to angiotensin. *Clin Sci* 1970; 38:741–766.
2. Bianchi G, Baldoli E, Lucca E, et al. Pathogenesis of arterial hypertension after the constriction of the renal artery leaving the opposite kidney intact both in the anesthetized and in the conscious dog. *Clin Sci* 1972; 42:651–664.

3. Caravaggi AM, Bianchi G, Brown JJ, et al. Blood pressure and plasma angiotensin II concentration after renal artery constriction and angiotensin infusion in the dog. (5-Isoleucine) angiotensin II and its breakdown fragments in dog blood. *Circ Res* 1976; 38:315–321.

4. Ferrari P, Bianchi G. Lessons from experimental genetic hypertension. In: Laragh JH, Brenner BM, eds. *Hypertension: pathophysiology, diagnosis, and management. 2nd edn.* New York: Raven Press; 1995:1261–1279.

5. Ayman D. Heredity in arteriolar (essential) hypertension. A clinical study of blood pressure of 1524 members of 277 families. *Arch Intern Med* 1934; 53:792–802.

6. Bianchi G, Fox U, Di Francesco GF, et al. The hypertensive role of the kidney in spontaneously hypertensive rats. *Clin Sci Mol Med* 1973; 45:135s–139s.

7. Bianchi G, Fox U, Di Francesco GF, et al. Blood pressure changes produced by kidney cross-transplantation between spontaneously hypertensive rats and normotensive rats. *Clin Sci Mol Med* 1974; 47:435–448.

8. Guidi E, Bianchi G, Rivolta E, et al. Hypertension in man with a kidney transplant: role of familial versus other factors. *Nephron* 1985; 41:14–21.

9. Guidi E, Menghetti D, Milani S, et al. Hypertension may be transplanted with the kidney in humans: a long-term historical prospective follow-up of recipients grafted with kidneys coming from donors with or without hypertension in their families. *J Am Soc Nephrol* 1996; 7:1131–1138.

10. Bianchi G, Cusi D, Gatti M, et al. A renal abnormality as a possible cause of 'essential' hypertension. *Lancet* 1979; 1:173–177.

11. Bianchi G, Cusi D, Barlassina C, et al. Renal dysfunction as a possible cause of essential hypertension in predisposed subjects. *Kidney Int* 1983; 23:870–875.

12. Bianchi G, Baer PG, Fox U, et al. Changes in renin, water balance, and sodium balance during development of high blood pressure in genetically hypertensive rats. *Circ Res* 1975; 36:153–161.

13. Baer PG, Bianchi G, Duzzi L. Renal micropuncture study of normotensive and Milan hypertensive rats before and after development of hypertension. *Kidney Int* 1978; 13:452–466.

14. Persson AE, Bianchi G, Boberg U. Tubuloglomerular feedback in hypertensive rats of the Milan strain. *Acta Physiol Scand* 1985; 123:139–146.

15. Parenti P, Hanozet G, Bianchi G. Sodium and glucose transport across renal brush-border membranes of Milan hypertensive rats. *Hypertension* 1986; 8:932–939.

16. Bianchi G, Ferrari P. Renal factors involved in the pathogenesis of genetic forms of hypertension. In: J Sassard ed. *Genetic hypertension, vol 218.* France: Colloque INSERM/John Libbey Eurotext Ltd; 1992:447–458.

17. Bianchi G, Ferrari P, Trizio D, et al. Red blood cell abnormalities and spontaneous hypertension in the rat: a genetically determined link. *Hypertension* 1985; 7:319–325.

18. Ferrari P, Ferrandi M, Torielli L, et al. Relationship between erythrocyte volume and sodium transport in the Milan hypertensive rat and age-dependent changes. *J Hypertens* 1987; 5:199–206.

19. Ferrari P, Bianchi G. Pathophysiology of hypertension. Membrane ion transports in hypertension. In: Birkenhager WH, Reid JL, eds. *Handbook of hypertension.* London: Elsevier; 1997: 935–974.

20. Bianchi G, Ferrari P, Trizio D, et al. Red blood cell abnormalities and spontaneous hypertension in the rat: a genetically determined link. *Hypertension* 1985; 7:319–325.

21. Cusi D, Niutta E, Barlassina C, et al. Erythrocyte Na^+, K^+, Cl^- cotransport and kidney function in essential hypertension. *J Hypertens* 1993; 11:805–813.

22. Ferrari P, Torielli L, Cirillo M, et al. Sodium transport kinetics in erythrocytes and inside-out vesicles from Milan rats. *J Hypertens* 1991; 9:703–711.

23. Salardi S, Saccardo B, Borsani G, et al. Erythrocyte adducin differential properties in normotensive and hypertensive rats of the Milan strain (characterization of spleen adducin m-RNA). *Am J Hypertens* 1989; 2:229–237.

24. Matsuoka Y, Li X, Bennett V. Adducin: structure, function and regulation. *Cell Mol Life Sci* 2000; 57:884–895.

25. Hughes CA, Bennett V. Adducin: a physical model with implications for function in assembly of spectrin–actin complexes. *J Biol Chem* 1995; 270:18990–18996.

26. Kuhlman PA, Hughes CA, Bennett V, et al. A new function for adducin. Calcium/calmodulin-regulated capping of the barbed ends of actin filaments. *J Biol Chem* 1996; 271:7986–7991.

27. Kaiser HW, O'Keefe E, Bennett V. Adducin: Ca^{2+} dependent association with sites of cell–cell contact. *J Cell Biol* 1989; 109:557-569.

28. Matsuoka Y, Li X, Bennett V. Adducin is an in vivo substrate for protein kinase C: phosphorylation in the MARCKS-related domain inhibits activity in promoting spectrin–actin complexes and occurs in many cells, including dendritic spines of neurons. *J Cell Biol* 1998; 142:485–497.

29. Aderem A. The MARCKS brothers: a family of protein kinase C substrates. *Cell* 1992; 71:713–716.

30. Fukata Y, Oshiro N, Kinoshita N, et al. Phosphorylation of adducin by Rho-kinase plays a crucial role in cell motility. *J Cell Biol* 1999; 145:347–361.

31. Lu Q, Liu X, Trama J, et al. Identification of the cytoskeletal regulatory protein alpha-adducin as a target of T cell receptor signaling. *Mol Immunol* 2004; 41:435–447.

32. Lin B, Nasir J, McDonald H, et al. Genomic organization of the human alpha-adducin gene and its alternatively spliced isoforms. *Genomics* 1995; 25: 93–99.

33. Citterio L, Tizzoni L, Catalano M,, et al. Expression analysis of the human adducin gene family and evidence of ADD2 beta4 splicing variants. *Biochem Biophys Res Commun* 2003; 309:359–367.

34. Gilligan DM, Lozovatsky L, Silberfein A. Organization of the human beta-adducin gene (ADD2). *Genomics* 1997; 43:141–148.

35. Sinard JH, Stewart GW, Stabach PR, et al. Utilization of an 86 bp exon generates a novel adducin isoform (β4) lacking the MARCKS homology domain. *Biochim Biophys Acta* 1998; 1396:57–66.

36. Citterio L, Azzani T, Duga S, et al. Genomic organization of the human gamma adducin gene. *Biochem Biophys Res Commun* 1999; 266:110–114.

37. Rat Genome Sequencing Consortium. Genome sequence of the Brown Norway rat yields insights into mammalian evolution, *Nature* 2004; 428:493–521.

38. Tripodi G, Casari G, Tisminetsky S, et al. Characterization and chromosomal localisation of the rat alpha- and beta-adducin-encoding genes. *Gene* 1995; 166:307–311.

39. Tripodi G, Piscone A, Borsani G, et al. Molecular cloning of an adducin-like protein: evidence of a polymorphism in the normotensive and hypertensive rats of the Milan strain. *Biochem Biophys Res Commun* 1991; 177:939–947.

40. Tripodi G, Szpirer C, Reina C, et al. Polymorphism of gamma-adducin gene in genetic hypertension and mapping of the gene to rat chromosome 1q55. *Biochem Biophys Res Commun* 1997; 237:685–689.

41. Tripodi G, Modica R, Reina C, et al. Tissue-specific modulation of beta adducin transcripts in Milan hypertensive rats. *Biochem Biophys Res Commun* 2003; 303:230–237.

42. Suriyapperuma SP, Lozovatsky L, Ciciotte SL, et al. The mouse adducin gene family: alternative splicing and chromosomal localization. *Mammal Genome* 1999; 11:16–23.

43. The international HapMap Consortium. The International HapMap Project. *Nature* 2003; 426:789–796.

44. Zimdahl H, Nyakatura G, Brandt P, et al. A SNP map of the rat genome generated from cDNA sequences. *Science* 2004; 303:807.

45. Guryev V, Berezikov E, Malik R, et al. Single nucleotide polymorphism associated with rat expressed sequences. *Genome Res* 2004; 14:1438–1443.

46. Smits BM, van Zutphen BF, Plasterk RH, et al. Genetic variation in coding regions between and within commonly used inbred rat strains. *Genome Res* 2004; 14:1285–1290.

47. Tripodi G, Florio M, Ferrandi M, et al. Effect of Add1 gene transfer on blood pressure in reciprocal congenic strains of Milan rats. *Biochem Biophys Res Comm* 2004; 324:562–568.

48. Garrett MR, Rapp JP. Defining the blood pressure QTL on chromosome 7 in Dahl rats by a 177-kb congenic segment containing Cyp11b1. *Mamm Genome* 2003; 14:268–273.

49. Bianchi G, Tripodi MG, Casari G, et al. Two point mutations within the adducin genes are involved in blood pressure variation. *Proc Natl Acad Sci U S A* 1994; 91:3999–4003.

50. Zagato L, Modica R, Florio M, et al. Genetic mapping of blood pressure quantitative trait loci in Milan hypertensive rats. *Hypertension* 2000; 36:734–739.

51. Tripodi MG, Valtorta F, Torielli L, et al. Hypertension-associated point mutations in the adducin α and β subunits affect actin cytoskeleton and ion transport. *J Clin Invest* 1996; 97:2815–2822.

52. Ferrandi M, Salardi S, Tripodi MG, et al. Evidence for an interaction between adducin and Na, K-ATPase:relation to genetic hypertension. *Am J Physiol* 1999; 277:1338–1349.

53. Torielli L, Padoani G, Tarsini P, et al. Adducin may affect the residential time of the Na/K pump on the plasmamembrane. *Eur J Cell Biol* 2000; 79(suppl. 52):164.

54. Efendiev R, Kmar T, Ogimoto G, et al. Hypertension-linked mutation in the adducin alpha-subunit leads to higher AP2-u2 phosphorylation and impaired Na^+, K^+-ATPase trafficking in response to GPCR signals and intracellular sodium. *Circ Res* 2004; 95:1100–1108.

55. Trifarò JM, Vitale ML. Cytoskeleton dynamics during neurotransmitter release. *Trends Neurosci* 1993; 16:466–472.

56. Ferrandi M, Tripodi G, Barassi P, et al. Functional role of beta adducin in the progression of proteinuria in congenic rats from the Milan strain and in beta adducin null mice. *J Hypertens* 2003; S110 (abstract).

57. Yang H, Francis SC, Sellers K, et al. Hypertension-linked decrease in the expression of brain γ-adducin. *Circ Res* 2002; 91:633–639.

58. Yang H, Reaves PY, Katovich MJ, et al. Decrease in hypothalamic gamma adducin in rat models of hypertension. *Hypertension* 2004; 43:324–328.

59. Gilligan DM, Lozovatsky L, Gwynn B, et al. Targeted disruption of the beta adducin gene (Add2) causes red blood cell spherocytosis in mice. *Proc Natl Acad Sci U S A* 1999; 96:10717–10722.
60. Muro AF, Marro ML, Gajovic S, et al. Mild spherocytic hereditary elliptocytosis and altered levels of alpha- and gamma-adducins in beta-adducin-deficient mice. *Blood* 2000; 95:3978–3985.
61. Marro ML, Scremin OU, Jordan MC, et al. Hypertension in β-adducin deficient mice. *Hypertension* 2000; 36:449–453.
62. Casari G, Barlassina C, Cusi D, et al. Association of the alpha-adducin locus with essential hypertension. *Hypertension* 1995; 25:320–326.
63. Cusi D, Barlassina C, Azzani T, et al. Polymorphisms of alpha-adducin and salt sensitivity in patients with essential hypertension. *Lancet* 1997; 349:1353–1357.
64. Glorioso N, Filigheddu F, Cusi D, et al. Alpha-adducin 460Trp allele is associated with erythrocyte Na transport rate in North Sardinian primary hypertensives. *Hypertension* 2002; 39:357–362.
65. Bianchi G, Ferrari P, Staessen JA. Adducin polymorphism: detection and impact on hypertension and related disorders. *Hypertension* 2005; 45(3):331–340.
66. Blaustein MP. Sodium ions, calcium ions, and blood pressure regulation: a reassessment and hypothesis. *Am J Physiol* 1977; 232:C164–C173.
67. Ferrandi M, Minotti E, Salardi S, et al. Ouabain-like factor in the Milan hypertensive rats (MHS). *Am J Physiol* 1992; 263:739–748.
68. Manunta P, Ballabeni C, Ferandi M, et al. Modulation of endogenous ouabain response to salt challenge by alpha-adducin polymorphism in rats and humans. *Hypertension* 2002; 40:395.
69. Ferrari P, Torielli L, Ferrandi M, et al. PST2238: a new antihypertensive compound that antagonizes the long-term pressor effect of ouabain. *J Pharmacol Exp Ther* 1998; 285:83–94.
70. Wang JG, Staessen JA, Messaggio E, et al. Salt, endogenous ouabain and blood pressure interactions in the general population. *J Hypertens* 2003; 21:1475–1481.
71. Manunta P, Messaggio E, Ballabeni C, et al. Plasma ouabain-like factor during acute and chronic changes in sodium balance in essential hypertension. *Hypertension* 2001; 38:198–203.
72. Quadri L, Bianchi G, Cerri A, et al. 17 beta-(3-furyl)-5 beta-androstane-3 beta, 14 beta, 17 alpha-triol (PST 2238). A very potent antihypertensive agent with a novel mechanism of action. *J Med Chem* 1997; 40:1561–1564.
73. Ferrari P, Ferrandi M, Tripodi G, et al. PST 2238: A new antihypertensive compound that modulates Na,K-ATPase in genetic hypertension. *J Pharmacol Exp Ther* 1999; 288:1074–1083.
74. Ferrandi M, Barassi P, Minotti E, et al. PST 2238: a new antihypertensive compound that modulates renal Na-K pump function without diuretic activity in Milan hypertensive rats. *J Cardiovasc Pharmacol* 2002; 40:881–889.

10 | Attaching physiology to the genome

*Carol Moreno, Howard J. Jacob and
Allen W. Cowley Jr.*

INTRODUCTION

Blood pressure is a complex trait determined by several factors and regulated by many metabolic, hormonal and biochemical pathways that are controlled by different genes.[1–4] Common forms of hypertension are a result of gene–gene and gene–environmental interactions and it is necessary to link genes to all of the various determinants of blood pressure to understand the underlying causes of hypertension and related cardiovascular risk factors. In the search for the genes that determine blood pressure and hypertension, animal models have been proven very useful. For historic reasons, the rat has become the chosen model system to study hypertension and there are currently 11 hypertensive rat strains available for study (see: http://www.rgd.mcw.edu). Most of these rat strains have been extensively phenotyped and used to study the pathophysiology of hypertension. These data have proved to be of great utility in recent years in understanding the underlying basis of various forms of hypertension, related end-organ damage and in the hunt for genes for hypertension. The mouse, which is the generally preferred model system of geneticists and molecular biologists, has been less useful in this process because of the paucity of inbred mouse strains with hypertension.

USE OF INTERMEDIATE PHENOTYPES TO IDENTIFY MUTATIONS CONTRIBUTING TO COMMON FORMS OF HYPERTENSION

Identification of the genes contributing to the development of hypertension and the associated end-organ damage has been very difficult because of the polygenic nature of the disease,[5] the small effect of individual genes,[4] heterogeneity in onset of the disease[6] and the strong influence of the environment on the multiple pathways and genes controlling blood pressure.[7] Although a number of single gene mutations that influence the renal handling of sodium and blood pressure have been successfully identified,[1,8–10] efforts to identify common mutations in genes that contribute to hypertension and end-organ damage using whole genome scans have not been as successful.[11,12]

159

The failure to identify genes that contribute to variations in blood pressure has led to the view that there is a need to identify potential 'intermediate phenotypes' that might be better predictors of the onset and pathogenesis of hypertension than the level of pressure alone.[13–18] In principle, the intermediate phenotype mechanistically contributes to the blood pressure and is therefore closer to the causal gene(s). From a genetic perspective, intermediate phenotypes are expected to exhibit several basic characteristics. First, the phenotype is expected to map to the same region of the genome as blood pressure. Second, the phenotype must be correlated with blood pressure in the population studied. Third, the phenotype is expected to be linked closely to the primary action of genes that directly contribute to hypertension.[19]

The concept of 'intermediate phenotypes' arose from the widely recognized need to find traits that are relatively easy to measure and traits that are regulated by less redundant pathways than blood pressure itself. A number of phenotypes have been proposed to represent intermediate phenotypes and have been utilized in hypertension studies. These include measurements of free urinary cortisol in human hypertension,[20] kallikrein concentrations,[21] indices of sympathetic nervous system function[17] and plasma renin activity responses with changes in salt intake.[22] However, none of these putative intermediate phenotypes has yet been found to map to the same region of the genome as blood pressure, a prerequisite if the trait is to be used as a surrogate to map for blood pressure genes of hypertension.

In general, intermediate phenotypes are selected based on an assumed mechanistic relationship between a particular phenotype and hypertension, derived from some correlation between the phenotype and blood pressure. However, until they can be shown to map within the same genomic interval and to have a strong correlation with blood pressure, they must be considered to be 'potential intermediate phenotypes' or 'likely determinant phenotypes'. Others must be considered as 'secondary phenotypes', i.e. considered to be a consequence of high blood pressure that are significantly correlated with blood pressure but map to a region of the genome that does not contain a blood pressure quantitative trait locus (QTL). For example, if the severity of end-organ damage correlates with levels of blood pressure in an F2 population but does not map to a blood pressure QTL, it is likely to be a consequence of the hypertension not a cause of it.

FINDING GENES UNDERLYING BLOOD PRESSURE-RELATED TRAITS

There are several ways to link physiological data to the rat genome: QTL mapping, congenic and consomic strains, genetic manipulation, microarray expression and comparative mapping, to name a few. These tools not only facilitate gene identification and characterization but also contribute to the advance of systems biology at the whole organism level.

Genetic linkage of blood pressure and hypertension-related phenotypes

The main strategy used for the search of genes involved in the development of hypertension has been the identification of QTLs by genome-wide linkage analysis. According to the Rat Genome Database (see: http://www.rgd.mcw.edu), to date 589 hypertension-related traits have been mapped to the rat genome. These traits include blood pressure (systolic, diastolic and mean), blood pressure variability, end-organ damage indicators (aortic lesion, cardiac mass, kidney weight), lipid levels and levels of norepinephrine release after stress.

A QTL is defined as a chromosomal region that segregates with a quantitative phenotype in a cross between strains, at a defined statistical significance.[23,24] QTL mapping does not require prior knowledge of the causative genes for the disease. A large number of genomic resources are available for QTL mapping; currently, more than 10 000 microsatellite markers are available, of which 4200 have been used to screen 48 different strains of rats, some of them hypertensive, yielding a large number of potential crosses than can be used for genome-wide scans. QTL can be detected by linkage of a phenotype to genetic markers evenly spaced throughout the genome on a cosegregating population. The cosegregating population is constructed by crossing two strains that are distinct phenotypically (a hypertensive and a normotensive) and genetically (inbred) to produce a first filial (F1) generation. The F1 population is then either intercrossed to generate a second filial (F2) generation or backcrossed to one of the parental strains (N2 generation). Each rat in the second generation is unique in its genotype and is perhaps phenotypically unique, owing to recombination events during meiosis. Linkage analysis is then performed using computer software packages such as Mapmaker[23] or Map Manager,[25] which first construct a genetic linkage map and then detect the loci linked to the phenotype.

Genetic linkage analysis studies require large populations and a very accurate phenotyping measurement to achieve enough statistical power for QTL detection. Interaction of the genetic background with the environment, gene–gene interaction and incomplete penetrance (i.e. individuals who carry the gene but do not express the phenotype) can also have masking effects. Most of the genetic mapping studies to date have measured only blood pressure and end-organ damage. Only recently has there been an exhaustive study of the genetic determinants of blood pressure-related traits, intermediate, secondary and blood pressure-independent phenotypes.[3,4] Stoll et al[4] have developed a comprehensive genetic linkage map of 239 'likely determinant phenotypes' of blood pressure in the rat. This analysis was performed to build a model of the systems biology of the rat for renal, vascular and neurohumoral function, and to link it to the genome. To increase the power of QTL detection in this study, different types of stressor were utilized, such as salt loading, acute sodium and volume depletion, an electrical alerting stimulus, active versus resting blood pressures and stressors of vascular function such as angiotensin II, norepinephrine, acetylcholine, and the nitric oxide (NO) synthase inhibitor L-NAME. Among all the QTLs that mapped to the genome, Stoll et al found that many blood pressure-related traits mapped to the same genomic regions but that the phenotypes were, for the most part, independent, indicating that the trait clusters are likely to be the result of separate genes rather than gene pleiotropy. One particular aggregate of QTL on chromosome 18 was of particular interest to our research group.[4] This grouping of QTL could be divided into three functional groups: blood pressure salt sensitivity, plasma lipid concentrations, and renal function (Fig. 10.1). This collective profile of phenotypes on chromosome 18 is particularly interesting because it resembles syndrome X – the 'metabolic syndrome' in humans.[26] In addition, QTL related to blood pressure variability as determined by a time series analysis[27] and the change in blood pressure in response to an alerting stimulus were also found in

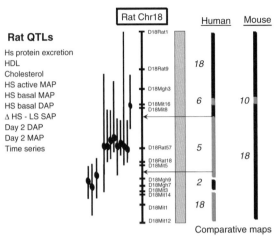

Fig. 10.1 Rat chromosome 18 contains aggregates of quantitative trait locus (QTL; the dot represents the peak of the LOD plot and the vertical line represents the 95% confidence limits of the QTL). Aggregates represent traits generally associated with the metabolic syndrome (syndrome X) in human populations. These include groups of QTL for hypertension, blood pressure salt sensitivity, early end-stage renal failure, and hyperlipidemia. Key: cholesterol, plasma cholesterol; day 2 DAP, average of second 3-h control day recording of basal diastolic arterial pressure; day 2 MAP, average of second 3-h control day recording of basal MAP; delta HS-LS SAP, reduction of basal systolic arterial pressure 36 h after salt depletion with Lasix and 0.4% salt diet; HDL, high-density plasma lipids; HS active MAP, mean arterial pressure after 3 weeks of 4% high-salt diet determined during the 3-h dark cycle recording with lights out; HS basal DAP, diastolic arterial pressure after 3 weeks of 4% high-salt diet determined during the 3-h light daytime cycle; HS basal MAP, MAP after 3 weeks of 4% high-salt diet determined during the 3-h light daytime cycle; HS protein excretion, 24-h protein excretion after 3 weeks of 4% high-salt diet; MAP, mean arterial pressure; time series, parameter representing blood pressure variability in time series analysis performed from data collected for 1 h at 1 Hz. Also shown are the homologous regions of this QTL of aggregated traits mapped to both human and mouse chromosomes by comparative mapping techniques. (Data from Stoll et al[4] with permission.)

the same region. Such functional cassettes have been observed in other areas of biomedical research, like autoimmune diseases.[28]

In a subsequent study, we performed a similar analysis in female rats in an attempt to assemble a genetic systems biology map of cardiovascular function in a female population.[3] The analysis was motivated by the lack of genetic information to explain the well-recognized sexual dimorphic pattern of hypertension and our initial observations that there were many sex differences in renal and cardiovascular function between rat strains. In general, very few genetic studies have focused exclusively on females, despite strong evidence of sexual dimorphism in the development of hypertension in human and animal studies.[29–31] Most of the blood pressure-related QTLs mapped to different regions of the genome with respect to the male population studied previously. This observation emphasizes the importance of separately analyzing linkage data based on sex. Aggregates of 8 to 11 QTLs were mapped to certain chromosomes and most of the traits that mapped within these QTL aggregates were not correlated with each other, similarly to what was observed in the male population. The finding of these functional cassettes of genetic regions that are important for the control of blood pressure and cardiovascular traits in male and female rats demonstrates the power of animal models in the dissection of multifactorial disorders, as well as the utility of this approach for studying complex diseases. The genomic regions harboring genes linked to many of the features of hypertension, and related metabolic and organ-damage phenotypes, delineate the locations in the genome where it will be especially interesting to search and test for candidate genes.

The detailed phenotyping of cardiovascular-related traits in linkage analysis studies also facilitates the identification of intermediate phenotypes, as any such leads might be useful in segregating hypertensive patient populations into more homogeneous subgroups, thereby reducing variance and facilitating the identification of genes that regulate blood pressure in humans. In our female study, kidney weight met the genetic definition of an intermediate phenotype, whereas the rest of the traits were classified as secondary phenotypes, potentially intermediate or blood pressure-unrelated phenotypes. Previous studies have indicated that the risk of hypertension and progressive renal disease is enhanced in subjects with reduced nephron numbers and greater kidney weight.[32,33] It has recently been reported that patients with hypertension had significantly fewer glomeruli per kidney than matched normotensive controls (702 379 versus 1 429 200 glomeruli).[33] Furthermore, kidney weight divided by body weight of the hypertensive subjects was 11% greater than in normotensive subjects.[33] Similar relationships have been described in the spontaneously hypertensive rats (SHR) compared with normotensive Wistar Kyoto (WKY) rats.[34] The observation indicates that kidney size or weight provides a useful subgroup to stratify in human populations.

These few examples illustrate that genetic linkage analysis is a powerful means to start the investigation of causes of hypertension, as well as providing a genomic map for cardiovascular function, and the identification of many chromosomal regions that segregate with traits that are important determinants of blood pressure and other aspects of cardiovascular function. These data can then be used to help find the genes, as well as to design physiological studies aimed at determining the mechanistic relationships between the clustered phenotypes.

Designer rats/mice in hypertension research

After linkage has been established, the next discovery phase requires a more detailed mechanistic, functional characterization of pathways to identify the specific genes and proteins responsible for the regulation of blood pressure. With linkage data, more discrete models can be built ('designer models'), which provide a reproducible source for phenotyping and increase the power of mapping traits. They also enable the measurement and replication of many phenotypes, because there is no limit in the number of animals that can be studied for each inbred genetic model. There are several different types of designer models that can be used for the search of genes that influence blood pressure.

Congenic/consomic strains
A congenic strain is developed by the integration of an individual piece of a chromosome containing a QTL, or a region with candidate genes of interest, into the genomic background of a recipient strain. Congenic strains are developed to confirm and narrow QTL regions of interest[5,35,36] and these model systems have proved very useful in the deconvolution of complex traits and the identification of candidate genes.[37–39] Several congenic lines have been developed for the

study of hypertension,[29,40–44] sometimes leading to the discovery of a causal gene.[36]

Congenic studies can be limited by losses or changes in a phenotype when a QTL is transferred to a different genetic background. As blood pressure is a complex trait, there might be epistatic interactions between or among QTLs.[45] This presumably occurs as a result of the loss of other loci in the original genetic background that contribute to or modify the phenotype.[46] Additional, more discrete phenotypes, or pharmacological agents (or other stressors) that can accelerate or exacerbate a trait, can also be used to overcome the problem of lost or altered phenotypes. Congenics can be generated in both directions, introgressing the susceptible QTL onto the resistant genome background, or the resistant QTL onto the susceptible background. However, development of congenic strains has been hindered by the time and expense involved in producing these strains. With the use of marker-assisted selection or 'speed' congenic breeding strategy[47] to identify the animals best suited for backcrossing in subsequent generations, the process of developing congenic strains requires generally 2 years and ~5 generations, rather than the traditional ten generations.

To overcome some of these limitations, a strategy for developing congenic lines from a consomic strain has been developed, that can accomplish this task in only two generations. In consomic strains, a whole chromosome is transferred to a different genomic background.[48–50] The use of reciprocal consomic strains has been described to study the role of chromosome Y in the development of hypertension on the SHR rat.[49,51,52] Further studies on this consomic strain revealed that the SHR Y chromosome has a locus that enhances SNS activity, which can raise systolic blood pressure and result in renal and cardiovascular tissue damage.[53] It also has an effect on lipid levels[54] and serum testosterone,[55] which are related to blood pressure. By using the SS (Dahl salt-sensitive) model of hypertension and the FHH (Fawn-Hooded Hypertensive) rats, our research group has developed a large panel of consomic rat strains, in which a single chromosome of the BN/Mcwi (Brown Norway) normotensive rat has been replaced, one at a time. This has allowed the assessment of the contribution of the genes on each chromosome, by extensive phenotyping, to several cardiovascular traits. These consomic rat panels consist of 22 inbred strains in which the chromosomes of the BN/Mcwi rats have been systematically transferred into the genomic background of the SS/Mcwi and 22 inbred stains in which BN/Mcwi chromosomes have been individually transferred into the background of the FHH/EurMcwi strain of rat. Environmental stressors used in the characterization of each consomic panel include chronic and acute hypoxia, acute hypercapnia, exercise and high-salt diets. These stressors were used to unmask deficiencies in the normal homeostatic mechanisms and idiopathic mechanisms that contribute to disease. The consomic panels have been characterized using more than 200 phenotypes specific to the heart, lung, kidney, vasculature and blood function (the results of this work are posted at http://www.pga.mcw.edu/). The measured phenotypes were selected to reveal alterations in a diverse set of underlying pathways that control these higher level functions. There are many applications for the use of consomic strains. They can be used for validation of QTLs, mapping of intermediate phenotypes to chromosomes, rapid development of congenic strains, and as control models for physiological studies. In complex traits like hypertension, the likelihood of having more than one trait-related gene is very high. These genes might interact in an additive or epistatic manner, complicating the search for the causative genes. One way to overcome this problem is to generate over-lapping congenic strains, derived from consomic, that cover the length of the chromosome, enabling one to localize and isolate the different QTLs within the chromosome.

Recombinant inbred strains

Production of recombinant inbred (RI) strains is accomplished by first inter-crossing two inbred strains. Then, the progeny is made inbred by 20 generations of brother × sister mating to generate a panel of inbred lines, each with a differ-ent combination of the progenitor genomes.[56] RI strains are therefore genetic mosaics of the two founding strains. This allows partitioning of individual com-plex traits into QTLs that, in some instances, have sufficient power to be studied as Mendelian loci. RI strains have been extensively used to study hypertension and its intermediate phenotypes.[56–60] Like consomic and congenic strains, it is possible to study the panel of RI strains at different conditions and ages, to reveal the gene–environment interactions.

Although there are several panels of rat and mouse RI strains,[61,62] only the rat HXB/BXH RI strain panels have been phenotypically characterized in sufficient detail to provide genetic determinants of hypertension and related traits.[59,63]

Other designer genetic models can be used in the study of complex diseases, and their phenotyping can aid in the discovery of the genetic determinants of hypertension. Recombinant congenics are a type of RI lines made by backcross-ing and randomly fixing parts of the genome by inbreeding so that each contains an average of 87.5% genes of a common background strain and 12.5% of a com-mon donor.[64] Advanced intercross lines are produced by crossing two parental strains. F1 rats are then intercrossed to produce F2s, and these are intercrossed through subsequent generations so that animals in an advanced intercross line accumulate new recombinants. Animals are maintained according to a pseudo-random breeding protocol to reduce loss of genetic variation in the population. An appropriate advanced intercross line could take at least 5 years to make but it can be used to map many loci. Advance intercross lines are being used to map blood pressure-related traits.[65]

Heterogeneous stocks

Genetically, heterogeneous stocks are derived from inbred strains through a series of progressive intercrosses. Existing heterogeneous stocks are derived from eight strains but any number can be used (an advanced intercross line is a heterogeneous stock derived from two strains). By subsequently maintaining the stock for many generations, using a pseudorandom breeding protocol, recombinants that allow high-resolution mapping are introduced. Traits are mapped by associating allelic variants with a phenotype, so that genotyping must be carried out for each experiment. Although mouse heterogeneous stocks have been used for mouse mapping experiments (the Boulder heterogeneous stock[66] and the Northport heterogeneous stock[67]), they have not yet been used for the study of hypertension.

Microarray

DNA microarray technology has introduced new opportunities in the field of integrative physiology by allowing the study of mRNA expression on a global scale, which then can be integrated with the physiological data, protein expression, and regulatory data to compose a 'biological atlas'[68] in which the genome is linked to the transcriptome, proteome and function. Microarray technology has been used in conjunction with other genetic strategies, such as QTL analysis,[29,69,70] congenic/consomic mapping,[71–74] or transgenic[75] and knock-out[76] techniques, to accelerate the search for genes underlying cardiovascular phenotypes. Genome-wide mRNA expression is particularly useful in the identification of genes with unknown function that could play a role in the development of hypertension.

Aitman et al[74] used rat congenic strains derived from the SHR and BN strains, in combination with microarray technology, to identify a strong positional and physiological candidate gene for insulin resistance, Cd36. McBride et al[71] utilized a similar strategy to identify candidate genes for blood pressure. The expression study was performed in congenic animals derived from the stroke-prone spontaneously hypertensive (SHRSP) and WKY and the two parental strains. Glutathione-S-transferase (Gstm1) was identified as a putative positional and physiological candidate as it participates in the defense against oxidative stress. Furthermore, differential expression of Gstm1 was confirmed by real-time quantitative polymerase chain reaction (RT-PCR).

The choice of tissue for gene expression profiling has been a matter of recent debate. The kidney is an ideal choice for 'gene hunting' experiments in hypertension, and several elegant transplantation experiments have shown that hypertension 'travels with the kidney'.[77,78] Liang et al[73] studied the temporal patterns of gene expression in the renal medulla of the SS rat when stimulated by a high-salt diet, and compared it with the consomic SS.BN13 rat, which exhibited reduced hypertension and renal damage. They identified a set of genes involved in different pathways known to be involved in the development of hypertension. The directional changes in the expression pattern of these genes were consistent with the reduced arterial pressure salt sensitivity and the absence of medullary interstitial fibrosis and reduced urinary protein excretion seen in the SS.BN13 consomic rat fed a high-salt diet. Only a handful of these differentially expressed genes mapped to chromosome 13. This indicates that extensive interchromosomal gene interactions occur that are probably secondarily related to the effects of high salt (e.g. changes in renin–angiotensin, sympathetic activity, vasopressin, volume changes). A physiologist would expect such responses because, as reflected by the complex physiological model diagram developed by Guyton et al[79] (Fig. 10.2),[80] initial changes in renal function alone in response to the high-salt diet would reverberate through the complex homeostatic system of cardiovascular controllers and result in the involvement of many other biological pathways.

Recent studies have combined the use of QTL mapping with microarray technology in the search for genetic loci that account for variation in the levels of gene expression, named expression quantitative loci (eQTL). This strategy combines expression profiling with linkage analysis in segregating populations, and further correlates them with phenotypes.[81] Transcript abundances serve as a surrogate for classical quantitative traits in that levels of expression are significantly correlated with the classical traits across members of a segregating population. Unlike traditionally defined quantitative traits, which often represent gross clinical measurements that can be far removed from the biological processes giving rise to them, the genetic linkages associated with transcript abundance afford a

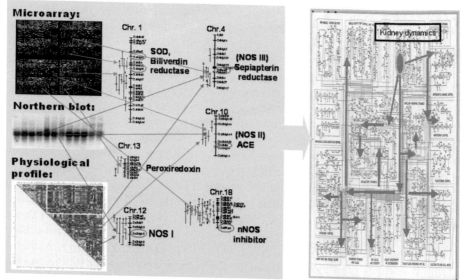

Fig. 10.2 How F2 linkage analysis, DNA microarrays and Northern blot analysis of renal medullary tissue, together with physiological profiling, converge to provide an initial understanding of the relationships between the expressions of genes and allelic variations that influence the complex regulatory pathways of the cardiovascular system. The Guyton model of cardiovascular regulation[79] (seen right) emphasizes that differences in gene expression with the renal medulla change kidney dynamics and thereby impact on many pathways of the system as influenced by changes in sodium and volume status, stimulation of autonomic pathways, a variety of endocrine responses, changes in blood flow to the brain and other regions of the circulation. Global responses to an initial stimulus such as salt intake therefore change the expression of genes throughout the genome. (From Cowley[80] with permission.)

closer look at cellular biochemical processes. Brem et al[82] were the first to demonstrate the utility of this strategy by completing the first dissection of transcriptional regulation in budding yeast. Schadt et al[69] further applied this strategy to study the molecular basis of fat pad mass in a murine cross and identified Mup1 as a candidate gene for obesity. In a similar study, Okuda et al[70] selected 11 genes differentially expressed between the SHR and WKY rats and subjected them to an F2 cosegregation analysis, together with blood pressure measurements. From the selected genes, it was found that the expression of two genes (monocarboxylate transporter 1 and glutathione-S-transferase Y(b) subunit) correlated with blood pressure in the F2 population, but they failed to associate the remaining genes with hypertension.

Linkage disequilibrium mapping

Linkage disequilibrium (LD) mapping offers yet another means by which to annotate genomic sequence with function and has been used by several investigators.[83-86] Genetic variation within species appears to be organized in discrete patterns or haplotype blocks, as a result of recombination over time. Although inbred strains should have no genetic variation among individuals, if comparisons are made between different strains, patterns of allelic similarities and differences among strains (strain-distribution patterns; SDPs) can be discerned for every variable locus.[86] This enables one to map mutations by correlating phenotype and genotype SDPs because a common phenotypic trait is most likely to be caused by a common ancestral polymorphism instead of independent newly acquired mutations in different strains.[86–88]

This strategy has been used to perform in-silico mapping of traits in mice.[86,88,89] For the rat, which has 11 different hypertensive inbred strains and several inbred models of cardiovascular disease, the construction of a high-density single nucleotide polymorphism (SNP) haplotype map is currently being developed. To complement the detailed phenotypic data available for numerous inbred strains, alleles of 48 common inbred strains have been determined for over 4328 simple sequence length polymorphisms (SSLPs) spanning the rat genome as part of the US Rat Genome Project. Furthermore, the National BioResource Project (NBRP) has determined 357 SSLP genotypes in 98 strains, including the 54 strains from their Rat Phenome Project. These data allow the construction of haplotypes across all major rat strains using publicly available tools such as the ACP Haplotyper (see: http://www.rgd.mcw.edu/ACPHAPLOTYPER/) to identify common haplotypes within models that have similar diseases. From these data, one can determine the 'evolutionary' relatedness of the various inbred strains of rats.[90] These allele data are now being greatly supplemented by the addition of over 45 000 SNPs identified across multiple rat strains (see: http://www.ncbi.nlm.nih.gov/SNP/snp_summary.cgi). These numbers will grow rapidly with two major SNP discovery projects underway in Europe (the Functional Genomics Group in the Netherlands and the Max-Delbruck Center for Molecular Medicine in Germany). Integration of the detailed phenotype information with haplotypes will provide a powerful tool for gene discovery.

Transgenic/knock-out/mutagenesis screens

Although QTL mapping is a powerful way to dissect the genetic components of complex disease, it is not the only way in which physiological data from the rat can be attached to the genome. Recently, with the advent of N-ethyl-N-nitrosourea (ENU) mutagenesis in the mouse,[91] there has been an increase in the screening of large numbers of phenotypes. Although this is a high-throughput approach, to evaluate single-gene function in model organisms the many animals that must be screened require global assessments of their phenotypes. Such general phenotypic screens do not always reflect the direct function of a gene. For example, an investigator who is studying the genetic basis of a complex trait, such as blood pressure or behavior, is evaluating a phenotype that is typically a clinical endpoint. This phenotype could be quite distant from the effects of the gene that is responsible for such mechanisms that might alter renal proximal tubule reabsorption or cause alterations in neuronal transmission.

The combination of QTL mapping and ENU mutagenesis offers considerable potential for accelerating the discovery of genes and gene function. So far, ENU has been predominantly used in the rat to cause neoplasia.[92] In the mouse, however, ENU mutagenesis is commonly used in phenotypic screens. ENU-induced modification of a quantitative trait could be useful to identify a gene that contributes to a QTL effect or that acts in the pathway that regulates the trait. ENU-induced mouse mutants that have similar phenotypes to quantitative traits being investigated in the rat can also inform rat studies, as investigators can use comparative mapping data to determine if the ENU mutation maps to a region that is in the conserved regions of the rat QTL being studied. In cases in which such mouse mutants exist, and the identity of the mutated gene is known, the orthologous rat gene can be further studied to see if it contributes to the effect of a QTL. Conversely, for investigators using the mouse, determining if mouse mutants map to a region of conservation in the rat genome that contains a QTL might provide additional phenotypes that could be used to facilitate gene identification. In this way, both species can be used as a source of additional alleles, which can then be used in the validation of candidate genes.

Mechanistic mapping

Two other approaches to generating physiological information can be mapped onto the genome: determination of a complex mechanistic response with mathematical modeling, and the use of physiological challenges to elicit specific responses. Most molecular genetic studies of complex diseases have focused on genes that are involved directly in generating the phenotype, rather than on physiological control or buffering systems, which can also affect a trait. Understanding the role of biological regulatory responses can be greatly enhanced through the development of mathematical modeling. Computer modeling can capture and characterize these complex events, as has recently been done to characterize the baroreceptor reflex in rats.[27] Evaluating this, and other similar reflexes, such as the chemoreceptor pathway for controlling respiration, requires the recording of several physiological responses at many time points. These reflexes are not easily captured as a single endpoint or trait because they often involve a series of steps, such as detecting a change in homeostasis, neuronally transmitting the recorded change, processing the message, transmitting a counter-response to effectors and the response of the effectors to restore homeostasis. Mathematical models allow such complex responses to be reduced to several parameters that correspond to quantitative measurements that can be mapped as discrete traits, thereby allowing the reflex to be attached to the genome. Such mapping data will inform investigators that a gene(s) in the region plays a role in a particular reflex.

Another approach to providing physiological information for mapping is the use of pharmacological agents that stimulate or inhibit various biological pathways. The observed responses enable one to assess the genetic basis of the pathway that is affected by an agent, and the counter regulatory pathways that compensate for its effects. This approach can be used in genetic crosses between disease and control strains, and in various inbred strains of rats, including congenics. For example, Vincent et al[93] have found an interaction between L-type calcium channel antagonists and a blood pressure locus on rat chromosome 2. Interestingly, this locus was not detected in a search for QTL that are linked to blood pressure. The drug created a stimulus that unmasked a genetic difference in a blood pressure response to this agent in the two rat strains studied. This allowed the investigators to dissect overall changes in blood pressure into a more specific phenotype: a change in blood pressure in response to an L-type calcium channel antagonist. The combined use of pharmacological challenges with QTL mapping allows various components of a complex phenotype to be mapped to the genome and can facilitate the discovery of the pathways that are involved in disease pathogenesis.

The power of comparative genomics

The ultimate reason for conducting research in an animal model is to provide key data to inform about how a process, gene or disease is likely to affect humans. Comparative genomics provides an effective, powerful method to facilitate this goal. For example, several years ago, a rat QTL linked to high blood pressure was mapped near to the rat angiotensin-converting enzyme (ACE) gene[94,95] and it was suggested then that another gene(s) near ACE might be the causative gene. After these publications, ACE was reported to be not linked to hypertension in humans;[96] however, genes in the vicinity of ACE could not be ruled out. Several years later, two publications reported a hypertension QTL in the region of ACE in humans,[95,97] indicating that the QTL identified in the rat might be indicative of where QTL for human hypertension might be found. Wilson et al further showed that the PRKWNK4 (protein kinase, lysine deficient 4) gene, which is located in the QTL that contains ACE, is responsible for the human hypertension disorder pseudohypoaldosteronism type II.[10] Nevertheless, the rat ortholog of PRKWNK4 appears not to play a role in some forms of hypertension in the rat.[98]

There are many QTL studies in humans and rats. As an example, we studied seven different rat crosses, which involve five hypertensive inbred rat strains, and identified 57 QTLs for 33 blood pressure traits. We determined which of these rat hypertension loci were conserved between rats, humans and mice and found that of the six QTLs for hypertension that had been reported in humans, five were in regions of conserved synteny with mapped hypertension QTL regions of the rat genome.[99] Because the different hypertensive rat strains show different etiologies of hypertension, integrating the results from all the crosses makes it possible to recapitulate the heterogeneous clinical picture of hypertension in humans and identify homologous human regions for further investigation. Sugiyama et al have also found significant concordance between mice, humans and rats for blood pressure QTLs[100] and a review of the literature of the growing numbers of QTLs for human hypertension shows that the predictions in 2000 are largely holding to be true.

Examples of QTLs that are conserved between species are not restricted to QTLs for hypertension. In both animal models and in humans, loci for obesity, autoimmune-related disorders and hypertension phenotypes have been identified and published, together with comparative map information.[28,99,101–103] Fig. 10.3 shows QTLs for specific disorders that map to equivalent regions in the rat, human and mouse genomes. It is striking that 11 obesity loci, four autoimmune loci and four hypertension loci lie in potentially evolutionarily conserved regions of the rat, human and mouse genomes. Furthermore, the number of QTLs that are in evolutionarily conserved segments, between at least two of the three species, is large: for 52 out of the 59 human chromosomal regions that are reported to contain genes that are involved in obesity-related phenotypes, a QTL for a similar phenotype has been mapped to a conserved region in another species.[56] Clearly, comparative mapping will continue to expand as more and more species are sequenced . These data when combined with physiological and pathophysiological data will lead to an increased understanding of the human.

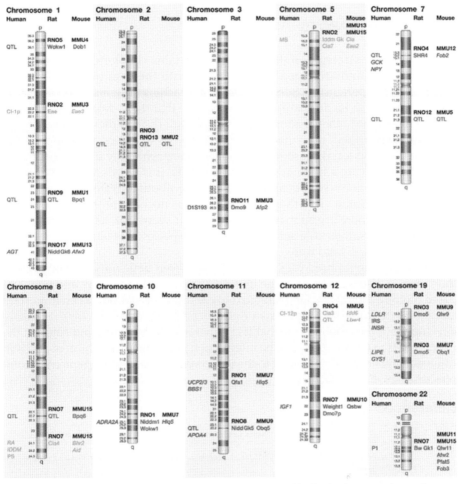

Fig. 10.3 Human ideograms annotated with loci associated with obesity, hypertension and autoimmune/inflammatory phenotypes in humans, rats and mice. Quantitative trait loci (QTLs) and comparative mapping information were obtained from the literature; map information relating to metabolic syndromes was obtained from the Human Obesity Gene Map: the 2000 update,[102] that for hypertension phenotypes from refs 104 and 105 and that for autoimmune/inflammatory disorders from refs 56 and 106. Each QTL shown has been mapped in one species and linked to a region of conserved synteny that contains a related locus in another species. Human loci (left of each ideogram) are shown by their locus name when available and by QTL when not. Homologous rat QTLs are shown to the right with their rat chromosomal (RNO) location and by locus name or QTL. Mouse homologous QTLs (far right) are shown with their likely chromosomal (MMU) location and locus name. Only QTLs that have been mapped in all three species are shown. As genetic intervals associated with QTLs are often not reported, chromosomal locations, rather than specific intervals, are shown. Key: ADRA2A, adrenergic, α-2A-receptor; Afp2, abdominal fat per cent 2; Afw3, abdominal fat weight QTL 3; AGT, angiotensinogen; Aid, activation-induced cytidine deaminase; APOA4, apolipoprotein A4; BBS1, Bardet-Biedl syndrome 1; Bhr2, bronchial hyperresponsiveness 2; Bpq, blood pressure QTL; Cia, collagen-induced arthritis; Dmo, diabetes mellitus OLETF; Dob1, dietary obesity 1; Eae3, susceptibility to experimental allergic encephalomyelitis 3; Fob2, F-line obesity QTL 2; GCK, glucokinase; GYS1, glycogen synthase 1; Hlq5, heat loss QTL 5; Idd6, insulin-dependent diabetes susceptibility 6; IDDM, insulin-dependent diabetes mellitus; IGF1, insulin-like growth factor 1; INSR, insulin receptor; IRS, insulin receptor substrate; Lbw4, lupus NZB NZW 4; LDLR; low-density lipoprotein receptor; LIPE, lipase; MS, multiple sclerosis; Nidd Gk, non-insulin-dependent diabetes glycerol kinase; Niddm1, non-insulin-dependent diabetes mellitus 1; NPY, neuropeptide Y; Obq5, obesity QTL 5; P1, P blood group; Pfat5, adiposity QTL; PS, psoriasis; Qfa1, weight QTL; Qlw, QTL late weight gain; Qsbw, Quackenbush-Swiss body weight QTL; RA, rheumatoid arthritis; SHR4, SHR (spontaneously hypertensive rat) body weight QTL; UCP2, uncoupling protein; Wokw, body weight QTL. (From Jacob & Kwitek.[19])

FUTURE PROSPECTS

Collectively, the strategies in the rat outlined in this chapter offer a means by which to start annotating genomic sequence with the determinants of blood pressure and hypertension. Some believe that attaching systems-level biology to the genome might be premature, but we believe that these data are essential to provide insight into the location of genes that underlie complex disease. If such genes are to be found, then many more phenotypes will need to be mapped to the genome to dissect disease mechanisms further, especially if functional gene clusters in QTLs are a hallmark of complex traits. It is worth noting that some investigators remain skeptical about inferring about physiology and QTLs across species. Some view these observations as nothing more than a chance occurrence, as there are so many QTLs. It is our view that, as more genes are found to play a similar role across the different species, it is likely that many of the predictions will hold true.

Given the many inbred rat strains that have been developed to model common human disease, and with the increasing power of sequence- and genome-based biology, the rat is well positioned to continue its tradition as an important animal model for studying human disease, particularly with respect to drug development. We would argue that it is imperative to look, test and conduct the experiments to truly determine the intersection between rat and human and that ultimately this research will lead to the understanding and management of complex diseases, like hypertension.

References

1. Lifton RP, Gharavi AG, Geller DS. Molecular mechanisms of human hypertension. *Cell* 2001; 104(4):545–556.
2. Garcia EA, Newhouse S, Caulfield MJ, et al. Genes and hypertension. *Curr Pharm Des* 2003; 9(21):1679–1689.
3. Moreno C, Dumas P, Kaldunski ML, et al. Genomic map of cardiovascular phenotypes of hypertension in female Dahl S rats. *Physiol Genomics* 2003; 15(3):243–257.
4. Stoll M, Cowley AW Jr, Tonellato PJ, et al. A genomic-systems biology map for cardiovascular function. *Science* 2001; 294(5547):1723–1726.
5. Rapp JP. Genetic analysis of inherited hypertension in the rat. *Physiol Rev* 2000; 80(1):135–172.
6. Samani NJ, Gauguier D, Vincent M, et al. Analysis of quantitative trait loci for blood pressure on rat chromosomes 2 and 13. Age-related differences in effect. *Hypertension* 1996; 28(6):1118–1122.
7. Hamet P, Pausova Z, Adarichev V, et al. Hypertension: genes and environment. *J Hypertens* 1998; 16(4):397–418.
8. Hansson JH, Nelson-Williams C, Suzuki H, et al. Hypertension caused by a truncated epithelial sodium channel gamma subunit: genetic heterogeneity of Liddle syndrome. *Nat Genet* 1995; 11(1):76–82.
9. Lifton RP, Dluhy RG, Powers M, et al. A chimaeric 11 beta-hydroxylase/aldosterone synthase gene causes glucocorticoid-remediable aldosteronism and human hypertension. *Nature* 1992; 355(6357):262–265.
10. Wilson FH, Disse-Nicodeme S, Choate KA, et al. Human hypertension caused by mutations in WNK kinases. *Science* 2001; 293(5532):1107–1112.
11. Kardia SL, Rozek LS, Krushkal J, et al. Genome-wide linkage analyses for hypertension genes in two ethnically and geographically diverse populations. *Am J Hypertens* 2003; 16(2):154–157.
12. Province MA, Kardia SL, Ranade K, et al. A meta-analysis of genome-wide linkage scans for hypertension:The National Heart, Lung and Blood Institute Family Blood Pressure Program. *Am J Hypertens* 2003; 16(2):144–147.
13. Gavras I, Manolis A, Gavras H. Genetic epidemiology of essential hypertension. *J Hum Hypertens* 1999; 13(4):225–229.
14. Kailasam MT, O'Connor DT, Parmer RJ. Hereditary intermediate phenotypes in African American hypertension. *Ethn Health* 1996; 1(2):117–128.

15. Kotchen TA, Kotchen JM, Grim CE, et al. Genetic determinants of hypertension: identification of candidate phenotypes. *Hypertension* 2000; 36(1):7–13.
16. Lucini D, Mela GS, Malliani A, et al. Impairment in cardiac autonomic regulation preceding arterial hypertension in humans: insights from spectral analysis of beat-by-beat cardiovascular variability. *Circulation* 2002; 106(21):2673–2679.
17. O'Connor DT, Insel PA, Ziegler MG, et al. Heredity and the autonomic nervous system in human hypertension. *Curr Hypertens Rep* 2000; 2(1):16–22.
18. Timberlake DS, O'Connor DT, Parmer RJ. Molecular genetics of essential hypertension: recent results and emerging strategies. *Curr Opin Nephrol Hypertens* 2001; 10(1):71–79.
19. Jacob HJ, Kwitek AE. Rat genetics: attaching physiology and pharmacology to the genome. *Nat Rev Genet* 2002; 3(1):33–42.
20. Litchfield WR, Hunt SC, Jeunemaitre X, et al. Increased urinary free cortisol: a potential intermediate phenotype of essential hypertension. *Hypertension* 1998; 31(2):569–574.
21. Kailasam MT, Martinez JA, Cervenka JH, et al. Racial differences in renal kallikrein excretion: effect of the ovulatory cycle. *Kidney Int* 1998; 54(5):1652–1658.
22. Williams GH, Dluhy RG, Lifton RP, et al. Non-modulation as an intermediate phenotype in essential hypertension. *Hypertension* 1992; 20(6):788–796.
23. Lander ES, Green P, Abrahamson J, et al. MAPMAKER: an interactive computer package for constructing primary genetic linkage maps of experimental and natural populations. *Genomics* 1987; 1(2):174–181.
24. Lander ES, Botstein D. Mapping Mendelian factors underlying quantitative traits using RFLP linkage maps. *Genetics* 1989; 121(1):185–199.
25. Manly KF, Cudmore RH, Jr., Meer JM. Map Manager QTX, cross-platform software for genetic mapping. *Mamm Genome* 2001; 12(12):930–932.
26. Ford ES, Giles WH, Dietz WH. Prevalence of the metabolic syndrome among US adults: findings from the third National Health and Nutrition Examination Survey. *JAMA* 2002; 287(3):356–359.
27. Kendziorski CM, Cowley AW, Jr., Greene AS, et al. Mapping baroreceptor function to genome: a mathematical modeling approach. *Genetics* 2002; 160(4):1687–1695.
28. Becker KG, Simon RM, Bailey-Wilson JE, et al. Clustering of non-major histocompatibility complex susceptibility candidate loci in human autoimmune diseases. *Proc Natl Acad Sci U S A* 1998; 95(17):9979–9984.
29. Yagil C, Sapojnikov M, Kreutz R, et al. Salt susceptibility maps to chromosomes 1 and 17 with sex specificity in the Sabra rat model of hypertension. *Hypertension* 1998; 31(1):119–124.
30. Clark JS, Jeffs B, Davidson AO, et al. Quantitative trait loci in genetically hypertensive rats. Possible sex specificity. *Hypertension* 1996; 28(5):898–906.
31. O'Donnell CJ, Lindpaintner K, Larson MG, et al. Evidence for association and genetic linkage of the angiotensin-converting enzyme locus with hypertension and blood pressure in men but not women in the Framingham Heart Study. *Circulation* 1998; 97(18):1766–1772.
32. Brenner BM, Garcia DL, Anderson S. Glomeruli and blood pressure. Less of one, more the other? *Am J Hypertens* 1988; 1(4 Pt 1):335–347.
33. Keller G, Zimmer G, Mall G, et al. Nephron number in patients with primary hypertension. *N Engl J Med* 2003; 348(2):101–108.
34. Skov K, Nyengaard JR, Korsgaard N, et al. Number and size of renal glomeruli in spontaneously hypertensive rats. *J Hypertens* 1994; 12(12):1373–1376.
35. Nabika T, Kobayashi Y, Yamori Y. Congenic rats for hypertension: how useful are they for the hunting of hypertension genes? *Clin Exp Pharmacol Physiol* 2000; 27(4):251–256.
36. Cicila GT, Garrett MR, Lee SJ, et al. High-resolution mapping of the blood pressure QTL on chromosome 7 using Dahl rat congenic strains. *Genomics* 2001; 72(1):51–60.
37. Yokoi N, Komeda K, Wang HY, et al. Cblb is a major susceptibility gene for rat type 1 diabetes mellitus. *Nat Genet* 2002; 31(4):391–394.
38. Ward CJ, Hogan MC, Rossetti S, et al. The gene mutated in autosomal recessive polycystic kidney disease encodes a large, receptor-like protein. *Nat Genet* 2002; 30(3):259–269.
39. MacMurray AJ, Moralejo DH, Kwitek AE, et al. Lymphopenia in the BB rat model of type 1 diabetes is due to a mutation in a novel immune-associated nucleotide (Ian)-related gene. *Genome Res* 2002; 12(7):1029–1039.
40. Eliopoulos V, Dutil J, Deng Y, et al. Severe hypertension caused by alleles from normotensive Lewis for a quantitative trait locus on chromosome 2. *Physiol Genomics* 2005; 22(1):70–75.
41. Bianchi G, Tripodi G, Casari G, et al. Two point mutations within the adducin genes are involved in blood pressure variation. *Proc Natl Acad Sci U S A* 1994; 91(9):3999–4003.
42. Ariyarajah A, Palijan A, Dutil J, et al. Dissecting quantitative trait loci into opposite blood pressure effects on Dahl rat chromosome 8 by congenic strains. *J Hypertens* 2004; 22(8):1495–1502.
43. Pravenec M, Landa V, Zidek V, et al. Transgenic expression of CD36 in the spontaneously hypertensive rat is associated with amelioration of metabolic disturbances but has no effect on hypertension. *Physiol Res* 2003; 52(6):681–688.

44. Sivo Z, Malo B, Dutil J, et al. Accelerated congenics for mapping two blood pressure quantitative trait loci on chromosome 10 of Dahl rats. *J Hypertens* 2002; 20(1):45–53.

45. Lander ES, Schork NJ. Genetic dissection of complex traits. *Science* 1994; 265(5181):2037–2048.

46. Nadeau JH, Frankel WN. The roads from phenotypic variation to gene discovery: mutagenesis versus QTLs. *Nat Genet* 2000; 25(4):381–384.

47. Lande R, Thompson R. Efficiency of marker-assisted selection in the improvement of quantitative traits. *Genetics* 1990; 124(3):743–756.

48. Nadeau JH, Singer JB, Matin A, et al. Analysing complex genetic traits with chromosome substitution strains. *Nat Genet* 2000; 24(3):221–225.

49. Negrin CD, McBride MW, Carswell HV, et al. Reciprocal consomic strains to evaluate y chromosome effects. *Hypertension* 2001; 37(2 Pt 2):391–397.

50. Cowley AW Jr, Liang M, Roman RJ, et al. Consomic rat model systems for physiological genomics. *Acta Physiol Scand* 2004; 181(4):585–592.

51. Ely DL, Daneshvar H, Turner ME, et al. The hypertensive Y chromosome elevates blood pressure in F11 normotensive rats. *Hypertension* 1993; 21(6 Pt 2):1071–1075.

52. Charchar FJ, Tomaszewski M, Strahorn P, et al. Y is there a risk to being male? *Trends Endocrinol Metab* 2003; 14(4):163–168.

53. Wiley DH, Dunphy G, Daneshvar H, et al. Neonatal sympathectomy reduces adult blood pressure and cardiovascular pathology in Y chromosome consomic rats. *Blood Press* 1999; 8(5–6):300–307.

54. Kren V, Qi N, Krenova D, et al. Y-chromosome transfer induces changes in blood pressure and blood lipids in SHR. *Hypertension* 2001; 37(4):1147–1152.

55. Toot J, Dunphy G, Turner M, et al. The SHR Y-chromosome increases testosterone and aggression, but decreases serotonin as compared to the WKY Y-chromosome in the rat model. *Behav Genet* 2004; 34(5):515–524.

56. Pravenec M, Klir P, Kren V, et al. An analysis of spontaneous hypertension in spontaneously hypertensive rats by means of new recombinant inbred strains. *J Hypertens* 1989; 7(3):217–221.

57. Hamet P, Sun YL, Malo D, et al. Genes of stress in experimental hypertension. *Clin Exp Pharmacol Physiol* 1994; 21(11):907–911.

58. Bottger A, van Lith HA, Kren V, et al. Quantitative trait loci influencing cholesterol and phospholipid phenotypes map to chromosomes that contain genes regulating blood pressure in the spontaneously hypertensive rat. *J Clin Invest* 1996; 98(3):856–862.

59. Pravenec M, Zidek V, Musilova A, et al. Genetic analysis of metabolic defects in the spontaneously hypertensive rat. *Mamm Genome* 2002; 13(5):253–258.

60. Pravenec M, Kren V. Genetic analysis of complex cardiovascular traits in the spontaneously hypertensive rat. *Exp Physiol* 2005; 90(3):273–276.

61. Shisa H, Lu L, Katoh H, et al. The LEXF: a new set of rat recombinant inbred strains between LE/Stm and F344. *Mamm Genome* 1997; 8(5):324–327.

62. Svenson KL, Cheah YC, Shultz KL, et al. Strain distribution pattern for SSLP markers in the SWXJ recombinant inbred strain set: chromosomes 1 to 6. *Mamm Genome* 1995; 6(12):867–872.

63. Pravenec M, Gauguier D, Schott JJ, et al. Mapping of quantitative trait loci for blood pressure and cardiac mass in the rat by genome scanning of recombinant inbred strains. *J Clin Invest* 1995; 96(4):1973–1978.

64. Moen CJ, van der Valk MA, Snoek M, et al. The recombinant congenic strains—a novel genetic tool applied to the study of colon tumor development in the mouse. *Mamm Genome* 1991; 1(4):217–227.

65. Wang X, Le Roy I, Nicodeme E, et al. Using advanced intercross lines for high-resolution mapping of HDL cholesterol quantitative trait loci. *Genome Res* 2003; 13(7):1654–1664.

66. McClearn GE, Wilson JR, Petersen DR, et al. Selective breeding in mice for severity of the ethanol withdrawal syndrome. *Subst Alcohol Actions Misuse* 1982; 3(3):135–143.

67. Demarest K, Koyner J, McCaughran J, Jr., et al. Further characterization and high-resolution mapping of quantitative trait loci for ethanol-induced locomotor activity. *Behav Genet* 2001; 31(1):79–91.

68. Vidal M. A biological atlas of functional maps. *Cell* 2001; 104(3):333–339.

69. Schadt EE, Monks SA, Drake TA, et al. Genetics of gene expression surveyed in maize, mouse and man. *Nature* 2003; 422(6929):297–302.

70. Okuda T, Sumiya T, Mizutani K, et al. Analyses of differential gene expression in genetic hypertensive rats by microarray. *Hypertens Res* 2002; 25(2):249–255.

71. McBride MW, Carr FJ, Graham D, et al. Microarray analysis of rat chromosome 2 congenic strains. *Hypertension* 2003; 41(3 Pt 2):847–853.

72. Liang M, Yuan B, Rute E, et al. Renal medullary genes in salt-sensitive hypertension: a chromosomal substitution and cDNA microarray study. *Physiol Genomics* 2002; 8(2):139–149.

73. Liang M, Yuan B, Rute E, et al. Insights into Dahl salt-sensitive hypertension revealed by temporal patterns of renal medullary gene expression. *Physiol Genomics* 2003; 12(3):229–237.

74. Aitman TJ, Glazier AM, Wallace CA, et al. Identification of Cd36 (Fat) as an insulin-resistance gene causing defective fatty acid and glucose metabolism in hypertensive rats. *Nat Genet* 1999; 21(1):76–83.

75. Kim S, Urs S, Massiera F, et al. Effects of high-fat diet, angiotensinogen (agt) gene inactivation, and targeted expression to adipose tissue on lipid metabolism and renal gene expression. *Horm Metab Res* 2002; 34(11–12):721–725.

76. Monti J, Gross V, Luft FC, et al. Expression analysis using oligonucleotide microarrays in mice lacking bradykinin type 2 receptors. *Hypertension* 2001; 38(1):E1–E3.

77. Liefeldt L, Schonfelder G, Bocker W, et al. Transgenic rats expressing the human ET-2 gene: a model for the study of endothelin actions in vivo. *J Mol Med* 1999; 77(7):565–574.

78. Churchill PC, Churchill MC, Bidani AK, et al. Genetic susceptibility to hypertension-induced renal damage in the rat. Evidence based on kidney-specific genome transfer. *J Clin Invest* 1997; 100(6):1373–1382.

79. Guyton AC, Coleman TG, Cowley AW Jr, et al. Systems analysis of arterial pressure regulation and hypertension. *Ann Biomed Eng* 1972; 1(2):254–281.

80. Cowley AW, Jr. Genomics and homeostasis. *Am J Physiol Regul Integr Comp Physiol* 2003; 284(3):R611–R627.

81. Abiola O, Angel JM, Avner P, et al. The nature and identification of quantitative trait loci: a community's view. *Nat Rev Genet* 2003; 4(11):911–916.

82. Brem RB, Yvert G, Clinton R, et al. Genetic dissection of transcriptional regulation in budding yeast. *Science* 2002; 296(5568):752–755.

83. Talbot CJ, Nicod A, Cherny SS, et al. High-resolution mapping of quantitative trait loci in outbred mice. *Nat Genet* 1999; 21(3):305–308.

84. Peissel B, Zaffaroni D, Zanesi N, et al. Linkage disequilibrium and haplotype mapping of a skin cancer susceptibility locus in outbred mice. *Mamm Genome* 2000; 11(11):979–981.

85. Kohn MH, Pelz HJ, Wayne RK. Natural selection mapping of the warfarin-resistance gene. *Proc Natl Acad Sci U S A* 2000; 97(14):7911–7915.

86. Grupe A, Germer S, Usuka J, et al. In silico mapping of complex disease-related traits in mice. *Science* 2001; 292(5523):1915–1918.

87. Wang X, Korstanje R, Higgins D, et al. Haplotype analysis in multiple crosses to identify a QTL gene. *Genome Res* 2004; 14(9):1767–1772.

88. Liao G, Wang J, Guo J, et al. In silico genetics: identification of a functional element regulating H2-alpha gene expression. *Science* 2004; 306(5696):690–695.

89. Pletcher MT, McClurg P, Batalov S, et al. Use of a dense single nucleotide polymorphism map for in silico mapping in the mouse. *PLoS Biol* 2004; 2(12):e393.

90. Thomas MA, Chen CF, Jensen-Seaman MI, et al. Phylogenetics of rat inbred strains. *Mamm Genome* 2003; 14(1):61–64.

91. Justice MJ. Capitalizing on large-scale mouse mutagenesis screens. *Nat Rev Genet* 2000; 1(2):109–115.

92. Previtali SC, Quattrini A, Pardini CL, et al. Laminin receptor alpha6beta4 integrin is highly expressed in ENU-induced glioma in rat. *Glia* 1999; 26(1):55–63.

93. Vincent M, Samani NJ, Gauguier D, et al. A pharmacogenetic approach to blood pressure in Lyon hypertensive rats. A chromosome 2 locus influences the response to a calcium antagonist. *J Clin Invest* 1997; 100(8):2000–2006.

94. Jacob HJ, Lindpaintner K, Lincoln SE, et al. Genetic mapping of a gene causing hypertension in the stroke-prone spontaneously hypertensive rat. *Cell* 1991; 67(1):213–224.

95. Hilbert P, Lindpaintner K, Beckmann JS, et al. Chromosomal mapping of two genetic loci associated with blood-pressure regulation in hereditary hypertensive rats. *Nature* 1991; 353(6344):521–529.

96. Staessen JA, Wang JG, Ginocchio G, et al. The deletion/insertion polymorphism of the angiotensin converting enzyme gene and cardiovascular-renal risk. *J Hypertens* 1997; 15(12 Pt 2):1579–1592.

97. Simon DB, Bindra RS, Mansfield TA, et al. Mutations in the chloride channel gene, CLCNKB, cause Bartter's syndrome type III. *Nat Genet* 1997; 17(2):171–178.

98. Monti J, Zimdahl H, Schulz H, et al. The role of Wnk4 in polygenic hypertension: a candidate gene analysis on rat chromosome 10. *Hypertension* 2003; 41(4):938–942.

99. Stoll M, Kwitek-Black AE, Cowley AW Jr, et al. New target regions for human hypertension via comparative genomics. *Genome Res* 2000; 10(4):473–482.

100. Sugiyama F, Churchill GA, Higgins DC, et al. Concordance of murine quantitative trait loci for salt-induced hypertension with rat and human loci. *Genomics* 2001; 71(1):70–77.

101. Griffiths MM, Encinas JA, Remmers EF, et al. Mapping autoimmunity genes. *Curr Opin Immunol* 1999; 11(6):689–700.

102. Perusse L, Chagnon YC, Weisnagel SJ, et al. The human obesity gene map: the 2000 update. *Obes Res* 2001; 9(2):135–169.

103. Tanase H, Suzuki Y, Ooshima A, et al. Genetic analysis of blood pressure in spontaneously hypertensive rats. *Jpn Circ J* 1970; 34(12):1197–1212.

104. Mansfield TA, Simon DB, Farfel Z, et al. Multilocus linkage of familial hyperkalaemia and hypertension, pseudohypoaldosteronism type II, to chromosomes 1q31-42 and 17p11-q21. *Nat Genet* 1997; 16(2):202–205.

105. Stoll M, Jacob HJ. Genetic rat models of hypertension: relationship to human hypertension. *Curr Hypertens Rep* 2001; 3(2):157–164.

106. Groot PC, Moen CJ, Dietrich W, et al. The recombinant congenic strains for analysis of multigenic traits: genetic composition. *Faseb J* 1992; 6(10):2826–2835.

11 | Genetic analysis of inherited hypertension in the rat

Bina Joe and Michael R. Garrett

SUMMARY

Blood pressure (BP) is a complex trait resulting from the concerted action of genetic and nongenetic factors. High BP (hypertension) is a leading risk factor of cardiovascular disease, including stroke, coronary heart disease, heart failure, peripheral vascular disease and renal failure. Because hypertension represents a major health problem that is also coupled with difficulties in identifying genetic determinants by human studies alone, researchers have selectively bred rats for high BP to provide animal models for the disease. Early work with these models was limited to studying the physiological control of BP. Subsequently, the development of genetic techniques and resources for the rat has enabled researchers to examine the underlying genetic causes of the disease. Typically, genetic linkage analyses and substitution mapping using congenic/consomic strains are performed to identify regions on the rat genome that harbor genes controlling BP. Genetic linkage analyses can only establish a statistical association of blood pressure with a particular chromosomal region. A congenic strain serves to confirm and help refine the chromosomal region containing the BP gene(s). Ultimately, the goal is to identify the allelic variants that are responsible for causing hypertension in the rat and to utilize this knowledge to improve clinical management strategies for the maintenance of normal physiological BP in humans. The purpose of this chapter is to address the current status of studies aimed at identifying BP causative genes using hypertensive rat models.

INTRODUCTION

Genetics, among many other factors, plays an important role in controlling blood pressure (BP) in humans. BP is a complex quantitative trait that results from the cumulative effects of many genetic loci (polygenic) and shows variation from low to high values (quantitative). It is hypothesized that elevated BP or hypertension, a leading risk factor for several cardiovascular diseases, is a result of abnormal functioning of genes that are primarily responsible for maintaining BP homeostasis. The identities of such genes are, however, largely unknown. It is for this reason that efforts, in the form of multiple genetic linkage analyses and association studies are currently used as techniques to identify the genes that cause high BP in humans.[1] Such efforts in humans are often thwarted by genetic heterogeneity, incomplete disease penetrance and other environmental factors. The effects of these factors that influence genetic analysis in humans are minimized in genetic studies conducted using inbred strains of hypertensive rats.[2,3]

Linkage analyses using rat models of hypertension have been very successful in identifying broad genomic regions that harbor causative genes for high blood pressure, also known as quantitative trait loci (QTL). Further, using these hypertensive rat models, several congenic strains were constructed and evaluated to corroborate the results obtained by genetic linkage analyses. In many instances these congenic strains confirmed the presence of the BP QTL. Such studies, however, lack the power to detect any single causative genetic factor within the large genomic segment containing the BP QTL. So, for the most part, the underlying genetic factors that influence the development of hypertension in these models remain elusive. However, by combining fine-mapping using congenic substrains, the available rat genomic sequence and emerging genomic techniques, the future looks good for discovering the genetic causes of hypertension in the rat. The expectation is, then, to utilize this information to better understand the disease in humans and develop better treatments.

GENETIC LINKAGE ANALYSES USING HYPERTENSIVE RAT STRAINS

Several inbred strains of hypertensive rats – each of which represents an individual genetic pool of naturally occurring alleles – exhibit an overall phenotype of high blood pressure. These include the Dahl salt-sensitive (S) rat, the spontaneously hypertensive rat (SHR), the stroke-prone SHR (SHRSP), the Milan hypertensive strain (MHS), the genetically hypertensive (GH) rat, the Sabra DOCA salt-sensitive (SBH) rat, the Lyon hypertensive (LH) rat, the fawn-hooded hypertensive (FHH) rat, the Prague hypertensive-hypertriglyceridemic (HTG) rat, the inherited stress-induced arterial hypertension (ISIAH) rat, the Prague hypertensive rat (PHR), albino surgery (AS) and the Munich Wistar Fromter (MWF) rat (these are reviewed in ref. 2 and additional information can be found at http://www.rgd.mcw.edu). The AS and MWF rats are not selectively bred strains but are genetically hypertensive rats. Determining the identity of alleles that are causative of high BP in these models is crucial to understanding the molecular basis of blood pressure control.

Genetic linkage analysis using the hypertensive rat models typically involves the generation of a segregating population using a hypertensive rat strain and an inbred strain with a contrasting phenotype, i.e. a normotensive rat (Table 11.1). On occasions, genetic linkage analyses for detecting BP QTL are also performed on populations derived from two hypertensive strains.[4,5] Using this approach, information on chromosomal location, the magnitude of the BP effect and the mode of inheritance of each causative locus, can be obtained. As can be seen from Table 11.1, the SHR is the most widely used hypertensive model for genetic linkage analysis, followed by the S rat and other hypertensive strains. Nevertheless, substantial data collected from all these linkage analyses indicate that there are a number of regions on the rat genome that contain BP QTL (Table 11.1).

Table 11.1 BP QTLs detected by genetic linkage analyses

RNO	Model	Linkage analysis	Sex	Diet	Approach	BP method	From marker	To marker	QTL location (Mb)	Reference
1	FHH/Eur	F1 (FHH x ACI) X FHH	M		GS	I	D1Mit17	D1Mit5	128–203	Brown DM et al. Nat Genet. 12: 44–51, 1996
	FHH/Eur	F2 (FHH x ACI)	M	LS	GS	I	D1Wox6	Mt1pa	132–186	Shiozawa M et al. J Am Soc Nephrol 11(11):2068–2078, 2000
	HTG	F2 (HTG x LEW)	C	LS	GS	D	D1Rat171	D1Mgh12	159–247[1]	Ueno T et al. J Mol Med. 81(1):51–60, 2003
	MHS/Gib	F2 (MHS x MNS)	C	LS	GS	B	D1Rat5	D1Mit9	11–44[2]	Zagato L et al. Hypertension. 36(5):734–739, 2000
	MWF/Fub	F1 (MWF x LEW) X MWF	M	LS	GS	I	D1Rat136		36	Schulz A et al. J Am Soc Nephrol. 13(11):2706–2714, 2002
	SBH/y	F2 (SBH x SBN)	C	IS	CS	I	D1Mgh2	D1Mit11	23–103	Yagil C et al. Hypertension 31: 119–124, 1998
	SBH/y	F2 (SBH x SBN)	C	IS	CS	I	D1Mit2	D1Mgh8	135–156	Yagil C et al. Hypertension 31: 119–124, 1998
	SHR	F2 (SHR x WKY)	M		CG	I	Sa		178	Iwai N et al. J Hypertension 10: 1155–1157, 1992
	SHR/NCrl	F2 (SHR x WKY)	M	LS	CG	B	Sa	Mt1pa	178	Samani NJ et al. J Clin Invest. 92: 1099–1103, 1993
	SHR	RI-SHR x BN		LS	CG	D	Kal		95	Pravenec M et al. Hypertension 17: 242–246, 1991
	SHR	F1 (SHR x F344) X SHR		LS	CS	I	D1Rat43	D1Mgh11	135–209	Ohno Y et al. Genetics.155(2): 785–792, 2000
	SHR/NHsd	F1 (S x SHR) X S	M	LS	GS	I	D1Rat189	D1Rat158	88–154	Garrett MR et al. J Am Soc Nephrol. 14(5):1175–1187, 2003
	SHR/Fub	F2 (S x SHR)	M	HS	GS	I	D1Rat1	D1Rat335	11–72	Siegel AK et al. Arterioscler Thromb Vasc Biol. 23(7):1211–1217, 2003
	SHR/Mol	F2 (SHR x BB)	C	LS	CS	I	Igf2	D1Mgh12	203–247	Kovacs P et al. Biochem Biophys Res Commun. 235: 343–348, 1997
	SHRSP/Heidelberg	F2 (W.S.10 x SHRSP)	C	IS	GS	D	Scnn1b		178	Kruetz R et al. Hypertension 29: 131–136, 1997
	SHRSP/Izm	F2 (SHRSP x WKY)	M	IS	GS	I	D1Wox29	Mt1pa	125–186	Mashimo T et al. Am J Hypertens. 12(11 Pt 1):1098–1104, 1999
	SHRSP/Izm	F2 (SHRSP x WKY)	C	IS	GS	I	D1Mgh5	Mt1pa	78–186	Kato N et al. J Hypertension. 21(2):295–303, 2003
	SHRSP/Izm	F1 (SHRSP x WKY) X SHRSP	M	LS	GS	I	D1Wox29	D1Wox10	125–221	Kato N et al. Hypertension. 42:1191–1197, 2003
	SS/Jr	F2 (S x LEW)	M	HS	GS	I	D1Wox1	Igf2	45–203	Garrett MR et al. Genome Res 8(7):711–723, 1998
	SS/Jr	F1 (S x SHR) X S	M	LS	GS	I	D1Rat189	D1Rat158	88–154	Garrett MR et al. J Am Soc Nephrol. 14(5):1175–1187, 2003

Continued

Table 11.1 BP QTLs detected by genetic linkage analyses

RNO	Model	Linkage analysis	Sex	Diet	Approach	BP method	From marker	To marker	QTL location (Mb)	Reference
1	SS/JrHSDMCwi	F2 (S x BN)	F	HS	GS	D	D1Rat265	D1Rat183	91–131	Moreno C et al. Genomics.15(3):243–257, 2003
	SS/JrHSDMCwi	F2 (S x BN)	F	HS	GS	D	D1Rat295	D1Rat301	214–235	Moreno C et al. Genomics.15(3):243–257, 2003
	SS/Fub	F2 (S x SHR)	M	HS	GS	I	D1Rat1	D1Rat335	11–72	Siegel AK et al. Arterioscler Thromb Vasc Biol. 23(7):1211–1217, 2003
2	AS	F2 (S x AS)	M	HS	GS	I	D2Uia17	D2Mco25	13–35	Garrett MR et al. J Hypertens. 20(12):2399–2406, 2002
	GH	F2 (GH x BN)	C	LS	CG	B	Gca		183[5]	Harris EL et al. J Hypertens. 13: 397–404, 1995
	LH	F2 (LH x LN)	M	LS	GS	D	D2Rat270		54	Bilusic M et al. Hypertension 44:1–7, 2004
	LH	F1 (LH x LN) X LH	M	LS	CS	D	D2Mit5	D2Wox20	67–181[1]	Vincent M et al. J Clin Invest 100: 2000–2006, 1997
	SHR/ NCrl	F2 (SHR x WKY)	M	LS	CS	B	D2Wox24	D2Mgh12	183–211	Samani NJ et al. Hypertension 28: 1118–1122, 1996
	SHR	F2 (SHR x BN)		IS	GS	D	Mt1pb	Gca	43–183	Schork NJ et al. Genome Res. 5: 164–172, 1995
	SHR/Ola	RI-SHR x BN, BN X SHR		LS	GS	D	D2N35		224	Pravenec M et al. J Clin Invest. 96: 1973–1978, 1995
	SHR/Mol	F1 (SHR x Wild) X SHR	C		GS	I	Fgg		175[5]	Kloting I et al. Biochem Biophys Res Commun. 284(5):1126–1133, 2001
	SHRSP/ Glasgow	F2 (SHRSP x WKY)	C	IS	GS	D	D2Mit5	Cpb	67–105	Clark JS et al. Hypertension 28: 898–906, 1996
	SHRSP/ Heidelberg	F2 (SHRSP x WKY)	C	IS	CG	D	Gca		183	Jacob HJ et al. Cell 67: 213–224, 1991
	SS/Hsd	F2 (S x R)	M	HS	CS	D	D2Mit10	D2Mit14	156–198	Herrera VL et al. J Clin Invest 102: 1102–1111, 1998
	SS/Jr	F2 (S x LEW)	M	HS	GS	I	D2Mit1	D2Mit6	3–78	Garrett MR et al. Genome Res. 1998; 8(7):711–723
	SS/Jr	F2 (S x MNS)	M	HS	CS	I	Fgg	Camk2d	175–224	Deng AY et al. J Clin Invest. 94: 431–436, 1994
	SS/Jr	F2 (S x WKY)	M	HS	CS	I	Fgg	Camk2d	175–224	Deng AY et al. J Clin Invest. 94: 431–436, 1994
	SS/Jr	F2 (S x AS)	M	HS	GS	I	D2Uia17	D2Mco25	13–35	Garrett MR et al. J Hypertens. 20(12):2399–2406, 2002

Chr	Strain	Cross					Marker 1	Marker 2	cM	Reference
3	hHTg	F2 (hHTg x BN)	M	LS	GS	D	D3Rat126	D3Rat17	121	Klimes I et al. Diabetologia 46(3):352–358, 2003
	HTG	F2 (HTG x LEW)	C	LS	GS	D	D3Wox3	D3Rat45	27–122	Ueno T et al. J Mol Med. 81(1):51–60, 2003
	SHR/NHsd	F2 (S x SHR)	M	HS	GS	—	D3Rat53	D3Rat45	0.3–39	Garrett MR et al. Physiol Genomics. 3(1):33–38, 2000
	SHR/Fub	F2 (S x SHR)	M	HS	GS	I	D3Mgh9	D3Rat75	4–51	Siegel AK et al. Arterioscler Thromb Vasc Biol. 23(7):1211–1217, 2003
	SHRSP/ Glasgow	F2 (SHRSP x WKY)	C	IS	GS	D	D3Mit10	D3Wox2	13–46	Clark JS et al. Hypertension 28: 898–906, 1996
	SHRSP/Izm	F2 (SHRSP x WKY)	M	IS	GS	—	D3Mgh16	D3Mgh8	6–14	Mashimo T et al. Am J Hypertens 12(11 Pt 1): 1098–1104, 1999
	SHRSP/Izm	F2 (SHRSP x WKY)	C	IS	GS	—	D3Mgh8	D3Wox10	14–48	Kato N et al. J Hypertension 21(2):295–303, 2003
	SHRSP/Izm	F1 (SHRSP x WKY) x SHRSP	M	LS	GS	—	D3Mit9		27	Kato N et al. Hypertension 42:1191–1197, 2003
	SS/Hsd	F2 (S x R)	M	HS	CS	—	D3Rat18	D3Rat6	120–148	Herrera VL et al. J Mol Med. 7(2):125–134, 2001
	SS/Jr	F2 (S x LEW)	M	HS	GS	—	D3Wox3	D3Mco21	27–68	Garrett MR et al. Genome Res. 8(7):711–723, 1998
	SS/Jr	F2 (S x BN)	M	HS	GS	—	D3Rat53	D3Rat45	0.3–39	Garrett MR et al. Physiol Genomics 3(1):33–38, 2000
	SS/Jr	F2 (S x BN)	M	HS	GS	—	D3Wox20	D3Wox1	124–168	Kato N et al. Mamm Genome 10: 259–265, 1999
	SS/Jr	F1 (S x R) X S	C	HS	CS	—	D3Mco16	D3Rat100	21–35	Cicila GT et al. Mamm Genome 10: 112–116, 1999
	SS/Jr	F1 (S x R) X S	C	HS	CS	—	D3Rat61	D3Rat59	148–163	Cicila GT et al. Mamm Genome 10: 112–116, 1999
	SS/Fub	F2 (S x SHR)	M	HS	GS	—	D3Mgh9	D3Rat75	4–51	Siegel AK et al. Arterioscler Thromb Vasc Biol. 23(7):1211–1217, 2003
4	AS	F2 (S x AS)	M	HS	GS	—	D4Uia1	D4Rat60	122–149	Garrett MR et al. J Hypertens. 20(12):2399–2406, 2002
	MHS	F2 (MHS x MNS)			CG	D	Add2		121[4]	Bianchi G et al. Proc Natl Acad Sci. USA 91: 3999–4003, 1994
	MWF/Fub	F1 (MWF x LEW) X MWF	M	LS	GS	—	D4Rat41	D4Rat41	97	Schulz A et al. J Am Soc Nephrol. 13(11):2706–2714, 2002
	SHR	F2 (SHR x WKY)	C	LS	CS	D	Npy	Npy	78	Katsuya T et al. Biochem Biophys Res Commun. 192: 261–267, 1993
	SHR	F2 (SHR x BN)		IS	GS	D	Npy	Npy	78	Schork NJ et al. Genome Res. 5: 164–172, 1995
	SHR/Ola	RI-SHR x BN, BN X SHR		LS	GS	D	Il6		0.5	Pravenec M et al. J Clin Invest. 96: 1973–1978, 1995
	SHR/Mol	F1 (SHR x BB) X BB		LS	CG	—	D4Mit2	D4Mit24	56–78	Kovacs P et al. Biophys Res Commun. 238: 586–589, 1997
	SHR/Sankyo	F2 (SHR x WKY)	C	LS	CS	D	Npy		78	Takami S et al. Hypertens Res. 19: 51–56, 1996

Continued

Table 11.1 BP QTLs detected by genetic linkage analyses

RNO	Model	Linkage analysis	Sex	Diet	Approach	BP method	From marker	To marker	QTL location (Mb)	Reference
4	SHRSP/Izm	F2 (SHRSP x WKY)	M	IS	GS	I	D4Mit2	Spr	56–120	Mashimo T et al. Am J Hypertens. 12(11 Pt 1):1098–1104, 1999
	SHRSP/Izm	F2 (SHRSP x WKY)	C	IS	GS	—	D4Mgh7	Try1	2–69	Kato N et al. J Hypertension 21(2):295–303, 2003
	SS/Jr	F2 (S x AS)	M	HS	GS	—	D4Rat160	D4Uia1	59–122	Garrett MR et al. J Hypertens. 20(12):2399–2406, 2002
5	hHTg	F2 (hHTg x BN)	M	LS	GS	D	D5Mgh9	D5Rat108	172	Klimes I et al. Diabetologia 46(3):352–358, 2003
	HTG	F2 (HTG x LEW)	C	LS	GS	D	D5Rat77		77–135	Ueno T et al. J Mol Med. 81(1):51–60, 2003
	MWF/Fub	F1 (MWF x LEW) X MWF	M	LS	GS	I	D5Rat41		155	Schulz A et al. J Am Soc Nephrol. 13(11):2706–2714, 2002
	SHR	F2 (SHR x WKY)	C		CG	D	D5Mgh14		150	Zhang L et al. Clin Exp Hypertens. 18: 1073–1087, 1996
	SHR	F2 (SHR x WKY)	C	LS	CS	D	D5Mgh5	D5Rat180	45–166	Ye P and West MJ. Clin Exp Pharmacol Physiol. 30(12):930–936, 2003
	SHR/Mol	F1 (SHR x Wild) X SHR	C		GS	I	Slc2a1	D5Mgh9	140–172[6]	Kloting I et al. Biochem Biophys Res Commun. 284(5):1126–1133, 2001
	SHR/NCrlBr	F2 (SHR x BN)	C	IS	CG	D	D5Rjr1		136	Stec DE et al. Hypertension 27: 1329–1336, 1996
	SHRSP/Izm	F2 (SHRSP x WKY)	C	IS	GS	—	D5Mgh2	D5Rat4	18–50	Kato N et al. J Hypertension 21(2):295–303, 2003
	SS/Jr	F2 (S x LEW)	M	HS	GS	I	D5Mit5	D5Mco2	109–149	Garrett MR et al. Genome Res 8(7):711–723, 1998
6	SHR/NIco	F2 (SHR x LEW)	C	LS	GS	I	D6Mit4	D6Rat84	60	Ramos A et al. Mol Psychiatry 4(5):453–462, 1999
	SHR	RI-SHR x BN, BN X SHR			GS	D	D6Rat46		13–36	Jaworski RL et al. Hypertension 39(2 Pt 2):348–352, 2002
	SHR/NHsd	F1 (S x SHR) X S	M	LS	GS	I	D6Rat180	D6Mit3	0.3–75	Garrett MR et al. J Am Soc Nephrol. 14(5):1175–1187, 2003
	SHR	F2 (S x SHR)	M	HS	GS	—	D6Rat80	D6Rat108	1–16	Siegel AK et al. Physiol Genomics 18(2):218–225, 2004
	SS/Jr	F1 (S x SHR) X S	M	LS	GS	—	D6Rat180	D6Mit3	0.3–75	Garrett MR et al. J Am Soc Nephrol. 14(5):1175–1187, 2003
	SS/Fub	F2 (S x SHR)	M	HS	GS	I	D6Rat80	D6Rat108	1–16	Siegel AK et al. Physiol Genomics 18(2):218–225, 2004

#	Strain	Cross					Marker 1	Marker 2	Range	Reference
7	SHR/Mol	F1 (SHR x Wild) X SHR	C		GS	I	Igf1		25[5]	Kloting I et al. Biochem Biophys Res Commun. 284(5):1126–1133, 2001
	SS/Jr	F1 (S x R) X S	C	HS	CG	I	Cyp11b1		113	Cicila GT et al. Nat Genet. 3: 346–353, 1993
8	AS	F2 (S x AS)	M	HS	GS		D8Mgh9	D8Mgh4	28–87	Garrett MR et al. J Hypertens. 20(12):2399–2406, 2002
	HTG	F2 (HTG x LEW)	C	LS	GS	D	D8Rat37	D8Rat117	54–122[1]	Ueno T et al. J Mol Med. 81(1):51–60, 2003
	SHR	F2 (SHR x BN)		IS	CG	D	D5Mit3	D5Mit5	85–109	Schork NJ et al. Genome Res. 5: 164–172, 1995
	SHR/Sankyo	F2 (SHR x WKY)	C	LS	CS	D	D8Mgh10		124	Takami S et al. Hypertens Res. 19: 51–56, 1996
	SHR	F2 (S x SHR)	M	HS	GS		D8Rat36	D8Rat133	57–95	Garrett MR et al. Physiol Genomics. 3(1):33–38, 2000
	SHR	RI-SHR x BN, BN X SHR			GS	D	D8Mit6	D8Rat40	10–49[7]	Jaworski RL et al. Hypertension 39(2 Pt 2):348–352, 2002
	SHRSP/Izm	F2 (SHRSP x WKY)	C	LS	GS		D8Mit1	Acaa	93–124	Kato N et al. J Hypertens 21(2):295–303, 2003
	SS/Iwai	F2 (S x WKY)	C	HS	CG		D8Mgh10		124	Takami S et al. Hypertens Res. 19: 51–56, 1996
	SS/Jr	F2 (S x LEW)	M	HS	GS		D8Mgh9	D8Wox2	28–61	Garrett MR et al. Genome Res. 8: 711–723, 1998
	SS/Jr	F2 (S x SHR)	M	HS	GS		D8Rat36	D8Rat133	57–98	Garrett MR et al. Physiol Genomics 3(1):33–38, 2000
	SS/Jr	F2 (S x AS)	M	HS	GS		D8Mgh9	D8Mgh4	28–87	Garrett MR et al. J Hypertens. 20(12):2399–2406, 2002
9	SHR/Sankyo	F2 (SHR x WKY)	C	LS	CS	D	D9Mit2		65	Takami S et al. Hypertens Res. 19: 51–56, 1996
	SHR/Fub	F2 (S x SHR)	M	HS	GS		D9Mit3	D9Rat5	56–85	Siegel AK et al. Arterioscler Thromb Vasc Biol. 23(7):1211–1217, 2003
	SHR/NHsd	F2 (S x SHR)	M	HS	GS		D9Uia10	D9Rat92	23–47	Garrett MR et al. Physiol Genomics 3(1):33–38, 2000
	SHRSP/Izm	F2 (SHRSP x WKY)	C	LS	CS		D9Wox18	D9Mit2	18–64	Kato N et al. J Hypertension 21(2):295–303, 2003
	SS/Jr	F2 (S x R)	C	HS	CS		D9Rat12	D9Rat4	65–91	Rapp JP et al. Genomics 51: 191–196, 1998
	SS/Jr	F2 (S x SHR)	M	HS	GS		D9Uia10	D9Rat92	23–47	Garrett MR et al. Physiol Genomics 3(1):33–38, 2000
	SS/Fub	F2 (S x SHR)	M	HS	GS		D9Mit3	D9Rat5	56–85	Siegel AK et al. Arterioscler Thromb Vasc Biol. 23(7):1211–1217, 2003
10	GH	F2 (GH x BN)	C	LS	CG	B	Ace		95[2,6]	Harris EL et al.J. Hypertens. 13: 397–404, 1995
	ISIAH	F2 (ISAH x WAG)			CG	D	D10Wox16		84[7]	Redina OE et al. Biochem Biophys. 380: 349–351, 2001
	MHS/Gib	F2 (MHS x MNS)	C		GS	B	D10Rat82	D10Rat73	33–46[3]	Zagato L et al. Hypertension 36(5):734–739, 2000
	SHR	F2 (SHR x WKY)	C	LS	CG	D	Ace		95	Zhang L et al. Clin Exp Hypertens. 18: 753–771, 1996
	SHR/NHsd	F1 (S x SHR) X S	M	LS	GS		D10Rat38	D10Mco66	32–82	Garrett MR et al. J Am Soc Nephrol. 14(5):1175–1187, 2003

Continued

Table 11.1 BP QTLs detected by genetic linkage analyses

RNO	Model	Linkage analysis	Sex	Diet	Approach	BP method	From marker	To marker	QTL location (Mb)	Reference
10	SHR/Mol	F2 (SHR x BB)	C	LS	CS	I	Abp	Ppy	56–91	Kovacs PB et al. Biochem Biophys Res Commun. 235: 343–348, 1997
	SHRSP/HD	F2 (SHRSP x WKY/HD-0)	C	LS	CS	D	Chrnb1		57	Kreutz R et al. Proc Natl Acad Sci USA 92: 8778–8782, 1995
	SHRSP/HD	F2 (SHRSP x WKY/HD-0)	C	LS	CS	D	Ace		95	Kreutz R et al. Proc Natl Acad Sci USA 92: 8778–8782, 1995
	SHRSP/ Heidelberg	F2 (SHRSP x WKY)	C	IS	CG	D	Ace		95	Jacob HJ et al. Cell 67: 213–224, 1991
	SHRSP/Izm	F2 (SHRSP x WKY)	M	IS	GS	I	Gh1	D10Mgh1	96–99	Mashimo T et al. Am J Hypertens. 12(11 Pt 1): 1098–1104, 1999
	SS/Jr	F2 (S x BN)	M	HS	GS	I	D10Mit4		37	Kato N et al. Mamm Genome 10: 259–265, 1999
	SS/Jr	F2 (S x WKY)	M	HS	GS	I	D10Mgh6		68	Kato N et al. Mamm Genome 10: 259–265, 1999
	SS/Jr	F2 (S x MNS)	M	HS	GS	I	D10Wox11	D10Wox6	54–82	Kato N et al. Mamm Genome 10: 259–265, 1999
	SS/Jr	F2 (S x LEW)	M	HS	GS	I	D10Mco30	D10Mco15	78–98	Garrett MR et al. Genome Res. 8(7):711–723, 1998
	SS/Jr	F1 (S x SHR) X S	M	LS	GS	I	D10Rat38	D10Mco66	32–82	Garrett MR et al. J Am Soc Nephrol. 14(5):1175–1187, 2003
11	SHR/Mol	F1 (SHR x Wild) X SHR	C		GS	I	D11Mgh4	D11Wox6	62–85[6]	Kloting I et al. Biochem Biophys Res Commun. 284(5):1126–1133, 2001
12	SHR/Nico	F2 (SHR x LEW)	C	LS	GS	I	D12Mit3	D12Wox8	24	Ramos A et al. Mol Psychiatry 4(5):453–462, 1999
	SS/Jr	F2 (S x WKY)	C	HS	GS	I	D12Wox16		28–39	Kato N et al. Mamm Genome 10: 259–265, 1999
	SS/JrHSDMCwi	F2 (S x BN)	F	HS	GS	D	D12Rat36	D12Rat22	35–46	Moreno C. et al. Genomics 15(3):243–257, 2003
13	LH	F2 (LH x LN)	M	LS	GS	D	D13Rat128	D13Mit3	67	Bilusic M et al. Hypertension 44:1–7, 2004
	SHR/NCrl	F2 (SHR x WKY)	M	LS	CS	B	D13Wox5		47–78	Samani NJ et al. Hypertension 28: 1118–1122, 1996
	SHR	F2 (SHR x WKY)	C	LS	CG	B	Ren		47	Sun L et al. Clin Exp Hypertens 15: 797–805, 1993
	SHR	F2 (SHR x WKY)	C		CG	B	Ren		47	Yu H et al. J Hypertension 16: 1141–1147, 1998

Chr	Strain	Cross					Marker	Marker	Range	Reference
	SHR/NCrlBr	F2 (SHR x LEW)	C	LS	CG	D	Ren		47	Kurtz TW et al. J Clin Invest. 85: 1328–1332, 1990
	SHR/Mol	F1 (SHR x BB) X BB		LS	CG	I	D13Uwm1		46	Kovacs P et al. Biophys Res Commun. 238: 586–589, 1997
	SHR/Ola	RI-SHR x BN	C	LS	CG	D	Ren		47	Pravenec ML et al. Genomics 9: 466–472, 1991
	SHRSP/Izm	F2 (SHRSP x WKY)	C	LS	GS	I	D13Mgh4	D13Mgh7	39–64	Kato N et al. J Hypertens. 21(2): 295–303, 2003
	SS/Jr	F2 (S x R)	C	HS	CS	I	D13Mgh3	D13Mit3	35–78	Zhang QY et al. Mamm Genome 8: 636–641, 1997
	SS/Jr	F2 (S x R) X S	C	HS	CG	I	Ren		47	Rapp JP et al. Am J Hypertens. 3: 391–396, 1990
	SS/JrHSDMCwi	F2 (S x BN)	F	HS	GS	D	D12Rat22		46	Moreno C et al. Physiol Genomics 15(3): 243–257, 2003
14	MHS/Gib	F2 (MHS x MNS)	C		GS	B	D14Rat90	D14Rat94	74–89[2]	Zagato L et al. Hypertension 36(5):734–739, 2000
	SS/JrHSDMCwi	F2 (S x BN)	F	LS	GS	D	D14Rat12		42	Moreno C et al. Physiol Genomics 15(3):243–257, 2003
15	SHRSP/Izm	F2 (SHRSP x WKY)	C	LS	GS	I	Ednrb	D15Mgh6	88–104	Kato N et al. J Hypertens. 21(2):295–303, 2003
	SS/JrHSDMCwi	F2 (S x BN)	F	HS	GS	D	D15Mgh9	D15Rat106	90–106	Moreno C et al. Physiol Genomics 15(3):243–257, 2003
16	SHR	F2 (SHR x BN)	M	IS	CG	D	D16Mit2	D16Mit5	1–13	Schork NJ et al. Genome Res. 5: 164–172, 1995
	SS/Jr	F2 (S x LEW)		HS	GS	I	D16Wox11	D16Mit3	18–47	Garrett MR et al. Genome Res. 8(7):711–723, 1998
17	FHH/Eur	F2 (FHH x ACI)	M	LS	GS	I	D17Rat54		26	Shiozawa M et al. J Am Soc Nephrol. 11(11):2068–2078, 2000
	LH	F2 (LH x LN)	M	LS	GS	D	D17Rat98	D17Mit4	64	Bilusic M et al. Hypertension 44:1–7, 2004
	SBH/y	F2 (SBH x SBN)	C	IS	CS	I	D17Mgh3		48–71	Yagil C et al. Hypertension 31: 119–124, 1998
	SS/Jr	F2 (S x LEW)	M	HS	GS	I	D17Mit2	D17Mco3	38–70	Garrett MR et al. Genome Res. 8(7):711–723, 1998
18	SHR/Mol	F2 (SHR x BB)	C	LS	CS	I	Ttr	D18Mit9	12–81	Kovacs PB et al. Biochem Biophys Res Commun. 235: 343–348, 1997
	SHRSP/Heidelberg	F2 (SHRSP x WKY)	C	IS	GS	D	D18Mit7		13	Jacob HJ et al. Cell 67: 213–224, 1991
	SS/Jr	F2 (S x LEW)	M	HS	GS	I	D18Mit1	D18Mco3	12–68	Garrett MR et al. Genome Res 8(7):711–723, 1998
	SS/JrHSDMCwi	F2 (S x BN)	M	HS	GS	D	D18Mit1	D18Mit8	12–62	Cowley AW Jr et al. Physiol Genomics 2(3):107–115, 2000

Continued

Table 11.1 BP QTLs detected by genetic linkage analyses

RNO	Model	Linkage analysis	Sex	Diet	Approach	BP method	From marker	To marker	QTL location (Mb)	Reference
19	SHR/Ola	RI-SHR x BN, BN x SHR	IS	GS		D	D19Mit7		45	Pravenec M et al. J Clin Invest 96: 1973–1978, 1995
20	GH	F2 (GH x BN)	M		CG	B	Tnf		4	Harris EI et al. Clin Exp Pharmacol Physiol. 25(3-4): 204–207.1998
	MHS	F2 (MHS x MNS)	C		GS	B	D20Rat44	D20Rat38	30–48	Zagato L et al. Hypertension 36(5):734–739, 2000
	SHR	RI-SHR x BN	C	LS	CG	D	D20Mgh4		8	Pravenec M et al. J Hypertension 7: 217–222, 1989
	SHRSP/Izm	F1 (SHRSP x WKY) x SHRSP	M	LS	GS	I	D20Mgh1		51	Kato N et al. Hypertension 42:1191–1197, 2003
X	SBH	F2 (SBH x SBN)	C	IS	CS	I	DXRat4	DXRat15	24–83	Yagil C et al. Hypertension 33 (part II): 261–265, 1999.
	SHRSP	F2 (SHRSP x WKY)	C	IS	GS	D	DXMgh5	DXMit4	40–80	Hilbert P et al. Nature 353: 521–529, 1991
Y	SHR	F2 (SHR x WKY)	C			I				Ely D et al. Hypertension 16: 277–281, 1990
	SHRSP	F2 (SHRSP x WKY)	C			B				Davidson AO et al. Hypertension 26: 452–459, 1995

BP QTLs that are reported in the literature are curated in this table by their location on the rat genome and organized by chromosome. The full names of hypertensive rat models are provided earlier in the article under the sub-heading 'Genetic linkage analyses using hypertensive rat strains'. For details on all other inbred strains, please refer to the rat genome database (*www.rgd.mcw.edu*). Sex-F, female; M, male; C, combined population of males and females. Diet-LS, Low salt (<1% NaCl); IS, Intermediate salt diet (1 to <4% NaCl); HS= High salt (≥ 4% NaCl). Approach-CG, Candidate gene; CS, Chromosome scan; GS, Genome scan. BP method-I, Indirect by tail-cuff method; D, Direct; B, Both by tail-cuff and direct methods. 'From marker' indicates the marker that defines the p terminal end of the BP QTL region. 'To marker' indicates the marker that defines the q terminal end of the BP QTL region. The physical location in Mb of each BP QTL was obtained by BLAST searching the rat genome (v 3.1) using the 'From marker' and the 'To marker' at the website: *http://rgd.mcw.edu/* and the 'To marker' at the website: *http://www.ensembl.org/Rattus_norvegicus/* in Nov 2004. Whenever the markers were not listed at this website, alternate markers at the closest position on the radiation hybrid map were obtained from *http://rgd.mcw.edu/* and used instead for the BLAST search. ¹QTL detected in response to drug; ²QTL by direct BP method only; ³QTL by indirect BP method only; ⁴QTL detected as interaction with RNO14; ⁵QTL detected in males only; ⁶QTL detected in females only; ⁷QTL detected in response to stress. In some cases, data are listed twice because the linkage analysis was performed using two hypertensive strains (e.g. F2 (S x AS), both S and AS are hypertensive strains). Blank spaces in all columns represent data that are insufficient or not provided in the original publications.

The major findings from these multiple linkage analyses are as follows:

- Every rat chromosome harbors at least one BP QTL, confirming that the overall genetic control of BP is complex and facilitated by a large number of genetic elements.
- Some BP QTL, such as the ones on rat chromosome (RNO)1, RNO2 and RNO10 are repeatedly detected in multiple genetic linkage analyses of several different hypertensive strains, demonstrating that these QTL might play a more important role in BP regulation than those on other chromosomes.
- The type of segregating population (i.e. the genetic background) studied has an important effect on whether a given QTL will be detected. For example, a BP QTL was detected on RNO7 in a backcross population involving the Dahl S, but not detected in an F2 population.
- Environmental changes, such as diet (salt-feeding) and stress can influence the power of detection of a QTL.
- BP QTL can be sex dependent, i.e. detected in males and not in females, or vice versa.
- Some BP QTL might be developmental specific genetic factors, i.e. they are detected only at specific ages.

The significance of these observations in the context of BP regulation in rats remains unclear until the genetic elements/genes underlying each of the detected BP QTL are identified.

Linkage analysis is a valuable tool that allows for the identification of genomic regions that contain genes linked to BP. However, there are two recognizable problems associated with linkage analysis: (1) detection of QTL by linkage analysis relies heavily on predictions based on statistical criteria; and (2) linkage analysis results in the identification of broad genomic regions in the range of 10 to 50 cM as being confidence intervals for the presence of a BP QTL.[6,7] A genetic interval of this size typically corresponds in humans and rodents to 10 to 50 Mb of DNA, or ~100 to 500 genes.[6,7] Considering the size of the rat genome (2.75 Gb), the localization of a BP QTL to be at least one out of 100 to 500 genes can be considered remarkable, but this resolution of localization is too low to be able to identify the actual BP controlling gene.

SUBSTITUTION MAPPING USING CONGENIC STRAINS

Linkage analysis is only a first step and requires additional corroborative genetic experiments to confirm and refine the QTL. To this end, consomic or congenic strains of rats are constructed and studied. Developing congenic strains involves substituting a segment of chromosome, or in the case of a consomic,[8] the entire chromosome, from one inbred strain (the donor strain) into another inbred strain (the recipient strain). This process is termed substitution mapping. The standard procedure has been to first develop a congenic strain that contains a large genomic interval to confirm the QTL. Subsequently, smaller congenic strains are developed to refine the location of the BP QTL to a small genomic interval. This step is usually an iterative process and continues until the interval contains a small set of genes. To date, many BP QTL have only been confirmed using large congenic strains and very few have been localized to small genomic intervals. Congenic strains are indicated by the following notation: 'Recipient strain. Donor strain', wherein, 'recipient strain' is the strain to whose genome a known genomic region from the 'donor strain' is introgressed. For example, SHR.BN refers to the introgression of a segment of Brown Norway (BN) rats into the SHR genetic background. The following section is a compilation of the results obtained from the analysis of congenic strains specifically constructed to validate the BP QTL detected by genetic linkage analysis. For clarity of presentation these results are sorted by chromosome.

RNO1

Evidence from the large number of linkage analyses that identified BP QTL on RNO1 (see Table 11.1) led to follow-up studies by substitution mapping using congenic strains. In the recent past, congenic strains with relatively small regions of RNO1 were developed and tested. These congenic strains include the transfer of Sabra hypertension-prone rat (SBH/y) into Sabra hypertension-resistant rat (SBN/y) and vice versa,[9] BN into SHR,[10] LEW (Lewis) into S,[11-14] SHRSP (SHR stroke-prone) into Wistar Kyoto (WKY),[15] SHR into WKY,[16,17] WKY into SHR,[17] WKY/Izm into SHRSP/Izm,[18] SHR into BB/OK (Biobreeding/Ottawa Kloting)[19] and SHRSP/Izm to WKY/Izm.[20,21] Fig. 11.1 shows the physical location of all BP QTL on the rat genome confirmed by these substitution mapping studies. It is evident from the figure that these studies vary widely in terms of the resolution to which the locations of BP QTL have been determined. For example, in Fig. 11.1, RNO1 a–d are localized within small regions from 2 to 20 Mb, whereas the majority of the other BP QTL represented are within large genomic regions of > 125 Mb. Interestingly, many of the BP QTL, with the exception of a and f, are clustered in the region ~100–225 Mb on RNO1. The present localization of BP QTL on RNO1 from multiple animal models is not sufficient to determine if allelic forms of the same gene(s) underlie the BP QTL found in each of the hypertensive models.

RNO2

As shown in Table 11.1, genetic studies using multiple F2 populations with the Dahl S rat as one of the parentals revealed BP QTL on RNO2. A few of these are corroborated by substitution mapping. Congenic strains introgressing the low BP QTL alleles from WKY or MNS (Milan normotensive strain) into the S rat proved the existence of a major BP QTL on RNO2.[22] The congenic strain with the WKY donor was further dissected by substitution mapping and found to comprise two BP QTL, QTL1 and QTL2.[23] These QTL are represented in Fig. 11.1, RNO2 a and b. A third BP QTL, called QTL3, was also suggested to be in the region represented by RNO2, c.[23] However, experimental evidence for this QTL was weak.[23] A congenic strain with the MNS donor on the S background localized a BP QTL to a 15 cM region.[24] This BP QTL region, shown in the figure at RNO2, d, was further localized to a 5.7 cM region on RNO2.[25]

BP QTL have also been localized on RNO2 using SHR as one of the parental strains (see Table 11.1). Recently, reciprocal congenic strains using SHR and

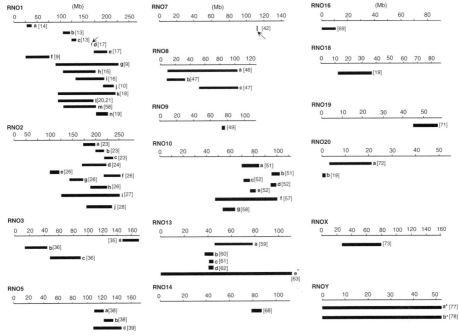

Fig. 11.1 Physical locations of blood pressure quantitative trait loci (BP QTL) on the rat genome that are defined by substitution mapping. The data presented are organized by rat chromosome (RNO) numbers, i.e. each panel represents the BP QTL defined on one rat chromosome. The x-axis for each panel represents the length of the corresponding rat chromosome in megabases (Mb). The length of the rat Y chromosome was not available and it was therefore calculated based on the relative length of the human Y chromosome to the human X chromosome. Bars represent the locations of BP QTL that are defined by flanking markers. These markers were manually curated from the respective original research articles and locations of each of these markers on the physical map of the rat genome (v. 3.1) were determined by BLAST searching the Ensembl website (http://www.ensembl.org/Rattus_norvegicus/) in November 2004. Whenever the markers were not listed at this website, alternate markers at the closest position on the radiation hybrid map were obtained from http://www.rgd.mcw.edu/ and used instead for the BLAST search. Alphabets alongside of each bar represent the QTL discussed under the appropriate chromosome number in the text. The numbers in square brackets next to each letter represent the number of the cited reference. Arrows represent BP QTLs that have been localized to relatively small genomic intervals of < 2 Mb and 177 kb respectively. * Indicates a study wherein a consomic strain is reported; microsatellite markers used to derive this consomic strain are not mentioned, therefore bars are drawn to represent the entire chromosomes.

WKY rats were studied.[26] This study resulted in the identification of at least four independent BP QTL.[26] The locations of these BP QTL are shown in Fig. 11.1 at RNO2, e–h. SHR alleles at three of the BP QTL shown in the figure at RNO2, e–g, increase BP, whereas SHR alleles at the BP QTL shown at RNO2, h, decrease BP. BN alleles from RNO2 introgressed into SHR rats to derive SHR.BN congenics are also reported to lower BP in SHR rats.[27] As seen at RNO2, i, the BP QTL detected in this study using SHR.BN congenic strain is large and overlaps with most of the BP QTL localized by other substitution mapping studies. Taken together, all these results indicate that, as on RNO1, RNO2 is also abundant in BP regulatory genes.

McBride et al[28] used microarray gene expression analysis as a complementary technique to detect superior candidate genes from among all the candidate genes within the BP QTL region (see Fig. 11.1, RNO2, j). The objective was to identify the gene(s) underlying the BP QTL on RNO2 that was previously defined by substitution mapping using SHRSP.WKY congenic strains.[29,30] Differentially expressed genes were sought among the parental SHRSP, WKY and SHRSP.WKY congenic rats by genome-wide gene expression analysis. A significant reduction in expression of glutathione-S-transferase type 1 (*Gstm1*) was observed.[28] This gene also mapped within the BP QTL region on RNO2. *Gstm1* is involved in the defense against oxidative stress.[28] In the SHRSP rat, endothelial dysfunction has been attributed to increased generation of superoxide anions, which in turn leads to vascular oxidative stress.[31-33] Induction of chronic oxidative stress by glutathione depletion can cause severe hypertension in normotensive rats.[34] These data suggest that *Gstm1* is both a positional and physiological candidate gene for the BP QTL on RNO2.[28]

RNO3

Linkage analysis has detected BP QTL on RNO3 using several models of hypertension, including the Dahl S, SHR, SHRSP, and HTG (Prague hypertriglyceridemic) strains (see Table 11.1). There appear to be two distinct BP QTLs, one located at the proximal and another at the distal region of RNO3. In 1999, a BP QTL located towards the distal end of RNO3 was confirmed by Cicila et al[35] (see Fig. 11.1, RNO3, a). Palijan et al[36] constructed and studied multiple S.LEW congenic strains spanning the proximal region of RNO3 and confirmed that the region contained a BP QTL (Fig. 11.1, RNO3, b) wherein alleles from the LEW rat lowered BP.[36] In addition to these two BP QTL, a third BP QTL located towards the middle region of RNO3 (Fig. 11.1, RNO3, c) was also identified.[36] LEW alleles at this QTL enhanced BP in S.LEW congenic rats. This study demonstrates the utility of congenic strains to dissect and detect closely linked alleles with opposing effects on BP.

RNO4

As shown in Table 11.1, linkage analyses using many hypertensive rat models have identified BP QTL on RNO4. A congenic strain containing a 12 cM region from the SHR rat introgressed into the BB/OK rat is also reported on chromosome 4.[37] Although these congenics provided strong evidence for the presence of genes on RNO4 involved in obesity and related phenotypes, the mean and diastolic BP of this congenic strain were not different from that in the parental BB/OK rat. Therefore, the existence of a BP QTL on RNO4 could not be confirmed using the BB.SHR congenic strain.

RNO5

Segregating populations derived from Dahl S, SHR, SHRSP, MWF and HTG strains show linkage to BP on RNO5. Substitution mapping using S.LEW congenic rats indicates that there are two closely linked interactive BP QTL on RNO5 (Fig. 11.1, RNO5 a and b).[38] The QTL was found to be interactive because strains with congenic segments that contained either one of the genomic regions depicted as a or b in Fig. 11.1, RNO5, did not show a BP effect, but strains with congenic segments that contained both a and b did show a significant BP effect. A BP QTL on RNO5 has also been localized using SHR.BN rats (Fig. 11.1, RNO5, c).[39] This BP QTL spans a large genomic interval that overlaps with both the QTL identified using S.LEW congenic strains.[38] Further substitution mapping is required to determine whether the BP QTL colocalized to this region using SHR.BN rats (Fig. 11.1, RNO5, c) also comprises multiple BP QTL that might interact.

RNO6

Although several linkage analyses have detected BP QTL on RNO6, to date no congenic strains have been developed to confirm the BP QTL reported on this chromosome.

RNO7

Only linkage analysis from populations derived from either the Dahl S or SHR have detected BP QTL on RNO7 (see Table 11.1). Unlike the other BP QTLs that remain unidentified to date, the BP causative gene on RNO7 in the Dahl S rat was suggested as early as the 1970s to be the steroid biosynthetic enzyme 11-β hydroxylase.[40] Substitution mapping using S.R congenic strains also pointed to the same gene.[41, 42] The interesting features of this study are: (1) that it is the only study that has been completed from QTL to gene in the field of hypertension research using rat models; and (2) that the introgressed region (177 kb) used to define the BP QTL on RNO7 represents one of the best 'minimal' regions isolated among rat congenic strains constructed to date (Fig. 11.1, RNO7).[42] This study demonstrates that substitution mapping can indeed achieve the limit of resolution required to identify a candidate BP causative gene to be one among a handful of genes. Due to compelling evidence supported by coding sequence mutations[41,43] and by functional studies on 11-β hydroxylase,[40,44,45] it was concluded that the gene responsible for the observed BP QTL on RNO7 in S rats is 11-β hydroxylase.

RNO8

Of the several independent genetic linkage studies that provide evidence for BP QTL on RNO8 (see Table 11.1), two were conducted using experimental crosses involving two hypertensive strains: F2 (S × SHR) and F2 (S × AS) populations.[4,5] Substitution mapping for corroborating these observations has not been done. An SHR.Lx (Lx = BN.Lx/Cub) congenic strain has successfully 'trapped' a BP QTL in the region (Fig. 11.1, RNO8, a).[46] Recently, using S.LEW congenic strains, two BP QTL with opposite effects of S alleles were identified.[47] S alleles of the QTL shown in Fig. 11.1, RNO8, b, significantly increase BP, whereas the S alleles of the QTL shown in Fig. 11.1, RNO8, c, decrease BP.[47]

RNO9

Even though genetic linkage analyses using F2 populations derived from (SHR × WKY), (S × R) and (S × SHR) rats independently detected BP QTL on RNO9 (see

Table 11.1), only the study involving the S and R has confirmed the BP QTL using congenic strains.[48] A recent study[49] has further localized this BP QTL to be within a relatively smaller genomic region of ~2.4cM on rat RNO9 (Fig. 11.1, RNO9).

RNO10

Multiple linkage analyses with several hypertensive strains including the Dahl S, SHR, SHRSP, GH (Genetically Hypertensive), MHS and ISIAH rats have detected BP QTL on RNO10 (see Table 11.1). BP QTL on RNO10 detected in F2 (S × MNS) and F2 (S × LEW) populations were confirmed using initial congenic strains containing introgressed regions from either MNS[50] or LEW[11] as the donors of large regions of RNO10 to the S genome. Subsequently, multiple congenic substrains have been constructed and characterized for fine-mapping of these BP QTL.[51,52] These studies localized two RNO10 BP QTLs, QTL1 and QTL2, to intervals of < 2.6 cM and < 3.2 cM, respectively.[51] Interestingly, QTL1 (Fig. 11.1, RNO10, a) from the MNS congenic series and the QTL defined with the LEW congenic series colocalize to the same region of RNO10, implying that both LEW and MNS carry alleles that are functionally the same but are contrasting to those in the S rat for BP QTL1. In contrast to QTL1, QTL2 (Fig. 11.1, RNO10, b) was only identified in the congenic substrains derived from MNS. Additional studies using S.LEW congenic substrains to localize BP QTL on RNO10 by telemetry were reported recently.[52,53] These studies by telemetry have corroborated the findings earlier reported by the tail-cuff method[51] and resulted in further fine-mapping the QTL1 and QTL2 regions to ~ 5.79 Mb and ~ 4.75 Mb on RNO10 (Fig. 11.1, RNO10, c, d). Also, this study[52] detected another BP QTL called QTL3 (Fig. 11.1, RNO10, e), which is within the QTL1 region reported by Garrett et al.[51]

Additionally, linkage analyses of an F2(S × MNS) population found statistical evidence of an interaction between BP QTL on RNO2 and RNO10. This interaction was tested by constructing a double congenic strain that contained introgressed regions from the WKY on RNO2 and from the MNS on RNO10.[54] The introgressed region on RNO2 was a large genomic segment derived from WKY that contained the BP QTL represented in Fig. 11.1, RNO2, a, b and c. The introgressed region on RNO10 was also a large genomic segment derived from the MNS that contained the BP QTL represented in Fig. 11.1, RNO10, a and b. The double congenic strain had a much greater reduction in BP than either of the single congenic strains alone or their combined effects, proving that there is a highly significant interaction between BP QTL on RNO2 and RNO10.

Wnk4 is causally linked to human pseudohypoaldosteronism type II, which is a rare Mendelian form of arterial hypertension in humans.[55,56] WKY.SHRSP congenic strains constructed around the *Wnk4* locus were used to evaluate the candidacy of *Wnk4* for BP control in rats.[57] This congenic strain contained a BP QTL (represented in Fig. 11.1, RNO10, f). However, there were no mutations detected in the coding sequence of *Wnk4* in SHRSP and WKY rats. Also, *Wnk4* was not differentially expressed between SHRSP and WKY rats. Therefore, *Wnk4* was reasonably ruled out as a candidate gene for this QTL.[57] Using WKY.SHRSP congenic strains, a genetic interaction for the regulation of systolic BP is reported between the BP QTL on RNO10 (shown in Fig. 11.1, RNO10, g)[58] and the BP QTL on RNO1 (shown in Fig. 11.1, RNO1, m). However, there are some inconsistencies with the congenic strain named as WKY-1.SHRSP-Mt1pa/D1Rat200,[15] which represents the RNO1 BP QTL. In one study, this congenic strain is reported to have no significant changes in systolic BP compared to that in the parental WKY rats,[58] but in a previous study, this same congenic strain was reported to have a significant systolic BP effect independent of RNO10.[15] Therefore, the reported genetic interaction is inconclusive and needs further clarification.

RNO11 and RNO12

Evidence of BP QTL using linkage analysis was found on RNO11 (involving SHR) and on RNO12 (involving either Dahl S or SHR). No substitution mapping has been reported on these chromosomes.

RNO13

Linkage of BP to RNO13 was detected using the renin locus (*Ren*) as a candidate gene in an F2(S × R) population (see Table 11.1). Since then, using other hypertensive rat models, BP QTL on RNO13 have been reported around the *Ren* locus (see Table 11.1). However, by using S.R congenic strains, the *Ren* locus was ruled out as the BP QTL.[59] The BP QTL was instead localized to a segment shown in Fig. 11.1, RNO13, a, which excludes the *Ren* locus.[59] Two other congenic strains using S and R rats have been studied (Fig. 11.1, RNO13, b,[60] and Fig. 11.1, RNO13, c[61]). These congenic strains do not include the QTL region defined by Zhang et al,[59] but include the *Ren* locus. Surprisingly, higher BP was associated with the R alleles, which is the opposite of what would be expected based on the linkage analysis of S and R rats.[59] A reasonable explanation for all these observations is perhaps that the QTL detected by genetic linkage analysis is composed of at least two different BP causative genes with opposing effects. While Zhang et al[59] 'captured' the BP lowering alleles of the S rat, Jiang et al[60] and St Lezin et al[61] isolated the closely linked BP enhancing alleles of the S rat.

A congenic strain introgressing the *Ren* locus of BN into SHR also detected similar but minor BP differences in the direction opposite of that expected based on the linkage analysis (Fig. 11.1, RNO13, d).[62] In this case, the authors concluded that the RNO13 BP QTL must be outside the introgressed region (*Ren* to D13N1). The only conclusive evidence by substitution mapping comes from a consomic strain constructed by replacing the entire RNO13 of the S rat with that from the BN rat. This strain was reported to have markedly low BP compared to the S rat (Fig. 11.1, RNO13, e).[63]

RNO14

Two linkage analyses have detected BP QTL on RNO14 (involving either Dahl S or MHS). Evidence from physiological, biochemical and genetic studies has demonstrated the involvement of adducin in BP regulation in MHS and in a subset of patients with essential hypertension.[64–67] The alpha subunit of adducin (*Add1*) is a locus on RNO14. Therefore, the role of this subunit in BP regulation was studied by constructing reciprocal congenic strains of MHS and MNS,[68] both encompassing the *Add1* locus (Fig. 11.1, RNO14; *Note*: identical QTL region studied in both reciprocal congenic strains). Systolic BP of MNS.MHS-*Add1* was significantly higher than that of MNS, whereas systolic BP of MHS.MNS-*Add1* was significantly lower than that of MHS.[68] Therefore, the BP QTL on RNO14 around the *Add1* locus stands confirmed.

RNO15

Linkage analyses using Dahl S or SHRSP as the hypertensive parental strains have detected BP QTL on RNO15 (see Table 11.1). However, no congenic strains for studying BP QTL have been reported on this chromosome.

RNO16

There is only suggestive evidence for linkage of BP to RNO16 in F2 (SHR × BN) and F2 (S × LEW) populations (see Table 11.1). The BP QTL on RNO16 is localized to ~10 Mb using S.LEW congenic strains (Fig. 11.1, RNO16).[69]

RNO17

Conclusive experimental evidence for or against the existence of BP QTL on RNO17 is lacking. This is because two independent genetic linkage analyses using F2 (S × LEW)[11] and F2 (SBH × SBN)[70] rats detected BP QTL on RNO17. However, an S.LEW congenic strain did not corroborate the identification of the BP QTL found using the F2 (S × LEW) population.[11] The reason for this remains unknown, although it was suggested that the BP QTL detected by linkage could have been missed by the introgressed region on the congenic strain.[2] There are no additional studies for detecting or confirming BP QTL on RNO17 by substitution mapping.

RNO18

Several independent genetic linkage studies provide evidence for BP QTL on RNO18 (see Table 11.1). By constructing a BB.SHR (RNO18) congenic strain, Kloting et al[19] observed an increase in BP compared to the parental BB rats, thus confirming the presence of BP QTL on RNO18 (Fig. 11.1, RNO18).

RNO19

Based on linkage studies using the SHR, which suggested a BP QTL on RNO19 in the vicinity of the angiotensinogen gene,[71] an SHR.BN congenic strain was constructed (Fig. 11.1, RNO19).[71] This congenic strain had BN alleles at the angiotensinogen locus and successfully 'captured' a BP QTL. There were no major changes in plasma angiotensinogen or renin activities between this congenic strain and the parental SHR strain. Therefore, the BP QTL 'trapped' in this congenic strain is not linked to differences in either plasma angiotensinogen levels or angiotensinogen expression.

RNO20

In the past, the region around the major histocompatibility complex RT1 on RNO20 has retained much of the attention from substitution mapping studies.[2] The effect of high-fat diet on BP was studied recently[72] using SHR and SHR.1N (1N = BN.*Lx*/*Cub*) congenic rats. Replacing BN alleles at an ~30 cM region resulted in higher BP in these congenic rats (Fig. 11.1, RNO20, a). In this study, the authors were interested in examining the role of the tumor necrosis factor-α (TNFα) locus, which was included in the introgressed region. A number of sequence differences between SHR and SHR.1N rats in the regulatory regions of the TNFα gene were identified. However, because no significant gene–diet interactions in its mRNA expression were observed,[72] TNFα was excluded as a candidate gene for the QTL on RNO20 that controls high-fat-diet-induced changes in BP. Another congenic strain was constructed by transferring SHR alleles from the RT1 region to the BB rat (Fig. 11.1, RNO20, b).[19] Elevated BP was observed in this congenic strain, thereby confirming the BP QTL on RNO20.

RNOX

Evidence from two genetic linkage analyses using F2 (SHRSP × WKY)[73] and F2 (SBH × SBN) populations[74] indicated the presence of BP QTL on RNOX (see Table 11.1). A congenic strain constructed by introgressing SHR alleles into the BB rat genome[19] corroborated the QTL reported by Hilbert et al (Fig. 11.1, RNOX).[73]

RNOY

Hypertension in the SHR is linked to the Y chromosome.[75,76] Transferring RNOY from BN (= BN.*Lx/Cub*) to the SHR decreased systolic and diastolic blood pressures in the SHR.BN-Y consomic strain (Fig. 11.1, RNOY, a).[77] Reciprocal consomic strains were used to study the effect of RNOY in SHRSP and WKY.[78] Replacing RNOY of SHRSP rat with RNOY from WKY rat significantly reduced systolic BP compared with the BP of parental SHRSP (Fig. 11.1, RNOY, b).[78] Systolic BP was increased in the reciprocal WKY.SHRSP consomic strain compared to the WKY parental strain.[78] Neither the origin of the Y chromosome nor the sex of the parental strain had any influence on the blood pressure response to salt loading in the SBH model of hypertension.[9]

SUBSTITUTION MAPPING STUDIES-WHAT DO WE KNOW SO FAR?

As can be seen from Fig. 11.1, several laboratories have invested substantial amounts of time and effort to construct and characterize primary congenic strains with large introgressed segments (> 50–80 cM). With the exception of the BP QTL on RNO4, RNO6, RNO15 and RNO17, most of the BP QTL identified by linkage analysis were corroborated by the construction and characterization of congenic strains.

In the past, the area of study involving congenic rat strains was rather slow. The major rate-limiting factor in the construction of congenic substrains (used to fine-map the QTL) was that the development of microsatellite markers in a given target region was difficult due to the non-availability of rat genome sequence information. The availability of mouse, [79–81] and subsequently, rat genome sequences[82] has facilitated the identification of microsatellite markers in any targeted region of the rat genome, which are easily tested for polymorphisms and used to expedite the characterization of congenic strains. Single nucleotide polymorphisms (SNPs) within expressed sequences of the rat genome are also becoming available.[83] These are also useful in expediting the construction of congenic strains.

One of the major outcomes of such genetic dissections is the understanding that, unlike the BP QTL on RNO7,[42] a majority of the BP QTL detected by linkage analyses comprises multiple underlying causative genes. This phenomenon of each BP QTL being composed of multiple BP QTLs poses problems for identifying all the causative genes for high BP. For example, the single BP QTL on RNO1 detected by genetic linkage analysis of S and LEW rats[11,12] was later shown to comprise at least three independent BP QTLs.[13] Further dissection of each of these BP QTLs is possible only as long as the phenotypic effects of these BP QTL are detectable, i.e. the magnitude of genetic variation has to be greater than the effect of nongenic or environmental fluctuations. This is often a problem when the BP effects being monitored between congenic strains and parental control strains are small (i.e. < 10 mmHg). Thus, even though the construction of additional congenic substrains is not an insurmountable problem any more because of the availability of genetic markers, the ability to detect BP differences accounted by the BP QTL becomes a major rate-limiting factor. Researchers tend to believe that the telemetry method of BP measurement is more accurate, sensitive and therefore reliable compared to the tail-cuff method.[84,85] However, there are no conclusively supportive data to support this observation. On the contrary, in one of the recent studies on RNO1, BP measurements in congenic and S rats were reported to be concordant between the telemetry and tail-cuff methods.[14]

Nevertheless, the results obtained by genetic analysis using substitution mapping in rats can be summarized as follows:

- Substitution mapping has revealed that BP QTL detected by genetic linkage analyses are often composed of multiple underlying BP causative genes. Therefore, the actual number of genetic factors controlling BP in any given hypertensive rat model is greater than would be estimated by the number of BP QTL identified by genetic linkage analyses.
- The BP QTL 'trapped' within a congenic strain exert their effect independent of the other BP QTL detected in a genetic linkage analysis.
- These primary congenic strains serve as tools and are available as starting material to fine-map and identify BP QTL.

Most of the studies have used congenic substrains to localize BP QTL within several megabases (see Fig. 11.1). So far, only one report provides a reasonable 'proof-of-principle' for substitution mapping using congenic strains as a means for advancing from QTL localization to BP causative gene identification.[42] This study utilized several iterations of congenic substrains to fine-localize the BP QTL on RNO7 to a region < 177 kb on the rat genome. Progress in identification of the other BP QTL in rat models is eagerly awaited.

APPLICABILITY OF COMPLEMENTARY TECHNIQUES

The results reviewed in this article indicate that the path for genetic dissection from QTL to gene identification is an intense endeavor in terms of time, effort and resources. With a view to expedite this process, complementary approaches are sought or are being contemplated. Most of these are tailored to detect additional properties of causative elements within a QTL region. Microarray gene expression analysis is one such approach wherein gene expressions of positional candidates are used to prioritize the search for the causative QTL. Aitman et al[86] successfully identified CD36 as a molecule responsible for insulin resistance in the SHR by performing a comparative global gene expression analysis between a congenic strain with a relatively large introgressed region and one of the parental strains. The success of this study is encouraging for using global gene expression analysis as a complementary technique to expedite BP-causative gene identification using congenic strains. In the field of substitution mapping for finding hypertension causative genes, a study by McBride et al[28] has used gene expression analysis in combination with substitution mapping and identified glutathione-S-transferase (*Gstm1*) as a BP-causative candidate gene. Such experiments, however, require additional compelling evidence to progress from the identification of '*a* BP-causative candidate gene' to validation of it being '*the* BP-causative gene'. For example, transgenic rescue experiments were used by Pravenec et al[87] to establish unequivocally that CD36 is an insulin resistance QTL in the SHR. As there are not many reports documenting success, using microarray analysis in conjuction with substitution mapping may remain unpredictable for outcomes.[88]

It also remains to be seen whether some of the other emerging techniques that are used in mouse models of disease such as proteomics,[89] silencer RNA molecules (SIRNA)[90] or bioinformatics approaches such as haplotype analysis[91] can be applied as complementary approaches to expedite identifying causative BP QTL in rats.

PERSPECTIVES

Despite all the above-documented difficulties associated with substitution mapping, data from genetic studies using animal models of hypertension indicate that it is possible to utilize substitution mapping to not only confirm that genomic regions harbor BP QTL but also define, with improved resolution, the physical limits of the genomic regions surrounding each of these BP QTL. Further improving the resolution of localization by additional substitution mapping is a required exercise for advancing from BP QTL detection and confirmation to BP QTL identification in rats.

References

1. Lifton RP, Gharavi AG, Geller DS. Molecular mechanisms of human hypertension. *Cell* 2001; 104:545–556.
2. Rapp JP. Genetic analysis of inherited hypertension in the rat. *Physiol Rev* 2000; 80:135–172.
3. Stoll M, Kwitek-Black AE, Cowley AW Jr, et al. New target regions for human hypertension via comparative genomics. *Genome Res* 2000; 10:473–482.
4. Garrett MR, Saad Y, Dene H, et al. Blood pressure QTL that differentiate Dahl salt-sensitive and spontaneously hypertensive rats. *Physiol Genomics* 2000; 3:33–38.
5. Garrett MR, Joe B, Dene H, et al. Identification of blood pressure quantitative trait loci that differentiate two hypertensive strains. *J Hypertens* 2002; 20:2399–2406.
6. Glazier, AM, Nadeau JH, Aitman TJ. Finding genes that underlie complex traits. *Science* 2002; 298:2345–2349.
7. Darvasi A, Pisante-Shalom A. Complexities in the genetic dissection of quantitative trait loci. *Trends Genet* 2002; 18:489–491.
8. Cowley AW Jr, Liang M, Roman RJ, et al. Consomic rat model systems for physiological genomics. *Acta Physiol Scand* 2004; 181:585–592.
9. Yagil C, Hubner N, Kreutz R, et al. Congenic strains confirm the presence of salt-sensitivity QTLs on chromosome 1 in the Sabra rat model of hypertension. *Physiol Genomics* 2003; 12:85–95.
10. St Lezin E, Liu W, Wang JM, et al. Genetic analysis of rat chromosome 1 and the Sa gene in spontaneous hypertension. *Hypertension* 2000; 35:225–230.

11. Garrett MR, Dene H, Walder R, et al. Genome scan and congenic strains for blood pressure QTL using Dahl salt-sensitive rats. *Genome Res* 1998; 8:711–723.

12. Saad Y, Garrett MR, Lee SJ, et al. Localization of a blood pressure QTL on rat chromosome 1 using Dahl rat congenic strains. *Physiol Genomics* 1999; 1:119–125.

13. Saad Y, Garrett MR, Rapp JP. Multiple blood pressure QTL on rat chromosome 1 defined by Dahl rat congenic strains. *Physiol Genomics* 2001; 4:201–214.

14. Joe B, Garrett MR, Dene H, et al. Substitution mapping of a blood pressure quantitative trait locus to a 2.73 Mb region on rat chromosome 1. *J Hypertens* 2003; 21:2077–2084.

15. Hubner N, Lee YA, Lindpaintner K, et al. Congenic substitution mapping excludes Sa as a candidate gene locus for a blood pressure quantitative trait locus on rat chromosome 1. *Hypertension* 1999; 34:643–648.

16. Iwai N, Tsujita Y, Kinoshita M. Isolation of a chromosome 1 region that contributes to high blood pressure and salt sensitivity. *Hypertension* 1998; 32:636–638.

17. Frantz S, Clemitson JR, Bihoreau MT, et al. Genetic dissection of region around the Sa gene on rat chromosome 1:evidence for multiple loci affecting blood pressure. *Hypertension* 2001; 38:216–221.

18. Kato N, Nabika T, Liang Y-Q, et al. Isolation of a chromosome region affecting blood pressure and vascular disease traits in the stroke-prone rat mode. *Hypertension* 2003; 42:1191–1197.

19. Kloting I, Voigt B, Kovacs P. Metabolic features of newly established congenic diabetes-prone BB.SHR rat strains. *Life Sci* 1998; 62:973–979.

20. Cui ZH, Ikeda K, Kawakami K, et al. Exaggerated response to restraint stress in rats congenic for the chromosome 1 blood pressure quantitative trait locus. *Clin Exper Pharmacol Physiol* 2003; 30:464–469.

21. Cui ZH, Ikeda K, Kawakami K, et al. Exaggerated response to cold stress in a congenic strain for the quantitative trait locus for blood pressure. *J Hypertens* 2004; 22:2103–2109.

22. Deng AY, Dene H, Rapp JP. Congenic strains for the blood pressure quantitative trait locus on rat chromosome 2. *Hypertension* 1997; 30:199–202.

23. Garrett MR, Rapp JP. Multiple blood pressure QTL on rat chromosome 2 defined by congenic Dahl rats. *Mamm Genome* 2002; 13:41–44.

24. Dutil J, Deng AY. Further chromosomal mapping of a blood pressure QTL in Dahl rats on chromosome 2 using congenic strains. *Physiol Genomics* 2001; 6:3–9.

25. Dutil J, Deng AY. Mapping a blood pressure quantitative trait locus to a 5.7-cM region in Dahl salt-sensitive rats. *Mamm Genome* 2001; 12:362–365.

26. Alemayehu A, Breen L, Krenova D, et al. Reciprocal rat chromosome 2 congenic strains reveal contrasting blood pressure and heart rate QTL. *Physiol Genomics* 2002; 10:199–210.

27. Pravenec M, Zidek V, Musilova A, et al. Genetic isolation of a blood pressure quantitative trait locus on chromosome 2 in the spontaneously hypertensive rat. *J Hypertens* 2001; 19:1061–1064.

28. McBride MW, Carr FJ, Graham D, et al. Microarray analysis of rat chromosome 2 congenic strains. *Hypertension* 2003; 41:847–853.

29. Jeffs B, Negrin CD, Graham D, et al. Applicability of a 'speed' congenic strategy to dissect blood pressure quantitative trait loci on rat chromosome 2. *Hypertension* 2000; 35:179–187.

30. Carr FJ, Negrin CD, Clark JS, et al. Chromosome 2 reciprocal congenic strains to evaluate the effect of the genetic background on blood pressure. *Scott Med J* 2002; 47:7–9.

31. Grunfeld S, Hamilton CA, Mesaros S, et al. Role of superoxide in the depressed nitric oxide production by the endothelium of genetically hypertensive rats. *Hypertension* 1995; 26:854–857.

32. Kerr S, Brosnan MJ, McIntyre M, et al. Superoxide anion production is increased in a model of genetic hypertension: role of the endothelium. *Hypertension* 1999; 33:1353–1358.

33. Hamilton CA, Brosnan MJ, McIntyre M, et al. Superoxide excess in hypertension and aging: a common cause of endothelial dysfunction. *Hypertension* 2001; 37:529–534.

34. Vaziri ND, Wang XQ, Oveisi F, et al. Induction of oxidative stress by glutathione depletion causes severe hypertension in normal rats. *Hypertension* 2000; 36:142–146.

35. Cicila GT, Choi CR, Dene H, et al. Two blood pressure/cardiac mass quantitative trait loci on chromosome 3 in Dahl rats. *Mamm Genome* 1999; 10:112–116.

36. Palijan A, Dutil J, Deng AY. Quantitative trait loci with opposing blood pressure effects demonstrating epistasis on Dahl rat chromosome 3. *Physiol Genomics* 2003; 15:1–8.

37. Kloting I, Kovacs P, van den Brandt J. Congenic BB.SHR (D4Mit6-Npy-Spr) rats: a new aid to dissect the genetics of obesity. *Obes Res* 2002; 10:1074–1077.

38. Garrett MR Rapp JP. Two closely linked interactive blood pressure QTL on rat chromosome 5 defined using congenic Dahl rats. *Physiol Genomics* 2002; 8:81–86.

39. Pravenec M, Kren V, Krenova D, et al. Genetic isolation of quantitative trait loci for blood pressure development and renal mass on chromosome 5 in the spontaneously hypertensive rat. *Physiol Res* 2003; 52:285–289.

40. Rapp JP, Dahl LK. Mendelian inheritance of 18- and 11beta-steroid hydroxylase activities in the adrenals of rats genetically susceptible or resistant to hypertension. *Endocrinology* 1972; 90:1435–1446.

41. Cicila GT, Garrett MR, Lee SJ, et al. High-resolution mapping of the blood pressure QTL on chromosome 7 using Dahl rat congenic strains. *Genomics* 2001; 72:51–60.
42. Garrett MR, Rapp JP. Defining the blood pressure QTL on chromosome 7 in Dahl rats by a 177kb congenic segment containing Cyp11b1. *Mamm Genome* 2003; 14:268–273.
43. Cicila GT, Rapp JP, Wang J-M, et al. Linkage of 11b-hydroxylase mutations with altered steroid biosynthesis and blood pressure in the Dahl rat. *Nat Genet* 1993; 3:346–353.
44. Rapp JP, Dahl LK. Mutant forms of cytochrome P-450 controlling both 18- and 11b-steroid hydroxylation in the rat. *Biochemistry* 1976; 15:1235–1242.
45. Nonaka Y, Fujii T, Kagawa N, et al. Structure/function relationship of CYP11B1 associated with Dahl's salt-resistant rats. Expression of rat CYP11B1 and CYP11B2 in *Escherichia coli*. *Eur J Biochem* 1998; 258:869–878.
46. Kren V, Pravenec M, Lu S, et al. Genetic isolation of a region of chromosome 8 that exerts major effects on blood pressure and cardiac mass in the spontaneously hypertensive rat. *J Clin Invest* 1997; 99:577–581.
47. Ariyarajah A, Palijan A, Dutil J, et al. Dissecting quantitative trait loci into opposite blood pressure effects on Dahl rat chromosome 8 by congenic strains. *J Hypertens* 2004; 22:1495–1502.
48. Rapp JP, Garrett MR, Dene H, et al. Linkage analysis and construction of a congenic strain for a blood pressure QTL on rat chromosome 9. *Genomics* 1998; 51:191–196.
49. Meng H, Garrett MR, Dene H, et al. Localization of a blood pressure QTL to a 2.4-cM interval on rat chromosome 9 using congenic strains. *Genomics* 2003; 81:210–220.
50. Dukhanina OI, Dene H, Deng AY, et al. Linkage map and congenic strains to localize blood pressure QTL on rat chromosome 10. *Mamm Genome* 1997; 8:229–235.
51. Garrett MR, Zhang X, Dukhanina OI, et al. Two linked blood pressure quantitative trait loci on chromosome 10 defined by Dahl rat congenic strains. *Hypertension* 2001; 38:779–785.
52. Palijan A, Lambert R, Dutil J, et al. Comprehensive congenic coverage revealing multiple blood pressure quantitative trait loci on Dahl rat chromosome 10. *Hypertension* 2003; 42:515–522.
53. Sivo Z, Malo B, Dutil J, et al. Accelerated congenics for mapping two blood pressure quantitative trait loci on chromosome 10 of Dahl rats. *J Hypertens* 2002; 20:45–53.
54. Rapp JP, Garrett MR, Deng AY. Construction of a double congenic strain to prove an epistatic interaction on blood pressure between rat chromosomes 2 and 10. *J Clin Invest* 1998; 101:1591–1595.
55. Wilson FH, Disse-Nicodeme S, Choate KA, et al. Human hypertension caused by mutations in WNK kinases. *Science* 2001; 293:1107–1112.
56. Kahle KT, Wilson FH, Leng Q, et al. WNK4 regulates the balance between renal NaCl reabsorption and K+ secretion. *Nat Genet* 2003; 35:372–376.
57. Monti J, Zimdahl H, Schulz H, et al. The role of Wnk4 in polygenic hypertension:a candidate gene analysis on rat chromosome 10. *Hypertension* 2003; 41:938–942.
58. Monti J, Plehm R, Schulz H, et al. Interaction between blood pressure quantitative trait loci in rats in which trait variation at chromosome 1 is conditional upon a specific allele at chromosome 10. *Hum Mol Genet* 2003; 12:435–439.
59. Zhang Q-Y, Dene H, Deng AY, et al. Interval mapping and congenic strains for a blood pressure QTL on rat chromosome 13. *Mamm Genome* 1997; 8:636–641.
60. Jiang J, Stec DE, Drummond H, et al. Transfer of a salt-resistant renin allele raises blood pressure in Dahl salt-sensitive rats. *Hypertension* 1997; 29:619–627.
61. St Lezin EM, Pravenec M, Wong AL, et al. Effects of renin gene transfer on blood pressure and renin gene expression in a congenic strain of Dahl salt-resistant rats. *J Clin Invest* 1996; 97:522–527.
62. St Lezin E, Liu W, Wang N, et al. Effect of renin gene transfer on blood pressure in the spontaneously hypertensive rat. *Hypertension* 1998; 31:373–377.
63. Cowley AW Jr, Roman RJ, Kaldunski ML, et al. Brown Norway chromosome 13 confers protection from high salt to consomic Dahl S rat. *Hypertension* 2001; 37:456–461.
64. Bianchi G, Tripodi G, Casari G, et al. Two point mutations within the adducin genes are involved in blood pressure variation. *Proc Natl Acad Sci U S A* 1994; 91:3999–4003.
65. Tripodi G, Szpirer C, Reina C, et al. Polymorphism of gamma-adducin gene in genetic hypertension and mapping of the gene to rat chromosome 1q55. *Biochem Biophys Res Commun* 1997; 237:685–689.
66. Efendiev R, Krmar RT, Ogimoto G, et al. Hypertension-linked mutation in the adducin alpha-subunit leads to higher AP2-mu2 phosphorylation and impaired Na+,K+-ATPase trafficking in response to GPCR signals and intracellular sodium. *Circ Res* 2004; 95:1100–1108.
67. Bianchi G, Manunta P. Adducin, renal intermediate phenotypes, and hypertension. *Hypertension* 2004; 44:394–395.
68. Tripodi G, Florio M, Ferrandi M, et al. Effect of Add1 gene transfer on blood pressure in reciprocal congenic strains of Milan rats. *Biochem Biophys Res Commun* 2004; 324:562–568.
69. Moujahidine M, Dutil J, Hamet P, et al. Congenic mapping of a blood pressure QTL on chromosome 16 of Dahl rats. *Mamm Genome* 2002; 13:153–156.

70. Yagil C, Sapojnikov M, Kreutz R, et al. Salt susceptibility maps to chromosomes 1 and 17 with sex specificity in the Sabra rat model of hypertension. *Hypertension* 1998; 31:119–124.

71. St Lezin E, Zhang L, Yang Y, et al. Effect of chromosome 19 transfer on blood pressure in the spontaneously hypertensive rat. *Hypertension* 1999; 33:256–260.

72. Pausova Z, Sedova L, Berube J, et al. Segment of rat chromosome 20 regulates diet-induced augmentations in adiposity, glucose intolerance, and blood pressure. *Hypertension* 2003; 41:1047–1055.

73. Hilbert P, Lindpaintner K, Beckmann JS, et al. Chromosomal mapping of two genetic loci associated with blood–pressure regulation in hereditary hypertensive rats. *Nature* 1991; 353:521–529.

74. Yagil C, Sapojnikov M, Kreutz R, et al. Role of chromosome X in the Sabra rat model of salt-sensitive hypertension. *Hypertension* 1999; 33:261–265.

75. Ely DL, Turner ME. Hypertension in the spontaneously hypertensive rat is linked to the Y chromosome. *Hypertension* 1990; 16:277–281.

76. Ely D, Turner M, Milsted A. Review of the Y chromosome and hypertension. *Braz J Med Biol Res* 2000; 33:679–691.

77. Kren V, Qi N, Krenova D, et al. Y-chromosome transfer induces changes in blood pressure and blood lipids in SHR. *Hypertension* 2001; 37:1147–1152.

78. Negrin CD, McBride MW, Carswell HV, et al. Reciprocal consomic strains to evaluate y chromosome effects. *Hypertension* 2001; 37:391–397.

79. Waterston RH, Lindblad-Toh K, Birney E, et al. Initial sequencing and comparative analysis of the mouse genome. *Nature* 2002; 420:520–562.

80. Guigo R, Dermitzakis ET, Agarwal P, et al. Comparison of mouse and human genomes followed by experimental verification yields an estimated 1,019 additional genes. *Proc Natl Acad Sci U S A* 2003; 100:1140–1145.

81. Pennacchio LA. Insights from human/mouse genome comparisons. *Mamm Genome* 2003; 14:429–436.

82. Gibbs RA, Weinstock GM, Metzker ML, et al. Genome sequence of the Brown Norway rat yields insights into mammalian evolution. *Nature* 2004; 428:493–521.

83. Zimdahl H, Nyakatura G, Brandt P, et al. A SNP map of the rat genome generated from cDNA sequences. *Science* 2004; 303:807.

84. Whitesall SE, Hoff JB, Vollmer AP, et al. Comparison of simultaneous measurement of mouse systolic arterial blood pressure by radiotelemetry and tail-cuff methods. *Am J Physiol Heart Circ Physiol* 2004; 286:H2408–2415.

85. Bunag R, Butterfield J. Tail-cuff blood pressure measurement without external preheating in awake rats. *Hypertension* 1982; 4:898–903.

86. Aitman TJ, Glazier AM, Wallace CA, et al. Identification of Cd36 (Fat) as an insulin-resistance gene causing defective fatty acid and glucose metabolism in hypertensive rats. *Nat Genet* 1999; 21:76–83.

87. Pravenec M, Landa V, Zidek V, et al. Transgenic rescue of defective CD36 ameliorates insulin resistance in spontaneously hypertensive rats. *Nat Genet* 2001; 27:156–158.

88. Pravenec M, Wallace C, Aitman TJ, et al. Gene expression profiling in hypertension research: a critical perspective. *Hypertension* 2003; 41:3–8.

89. Kovarova H, Halada P, Man P, et al. Proteome study of Francisella tularensis live vaccine strain-containing phagosome in Bcg/Nramp1 congenic macrophages: resistant allele contributes to permissive environment and susceptibility to infection. *Proteomics* 2002; 2:85–93.

90. Buckingham SD, Esmaeili B, Wood M, et al. RNA interference:from model organisms towards therapy for neural and neuromuscular disorders. *Hum Mol Genet* 2004; 13 Spec No 2:R275–288.

91. Yalcin B, Fullerton J, Miller S, et al. Unexpected complexity in the haplotypes of commonly used inbred strains of laboratory mice. *Proc Natl Acad Sci U S A* 2004; 101:9734–9739.

12 | Transgenic rats and hypertension

Tara Collidge and John J. Mullins

INTRODUCTION

Hypertension is a complex disease influenced by the interaction of multiple genetic and environmental factors. Various experimental approaches have been used to increase our understanding of the pathophysiology of hypertension over the years, with transgenic models becoming increasingly important since the early 1990s. A transgenic animal is created by inserting exogenous genetic material coding for a gene (or genes) of interest from the same or different species, into a fertilized embryo by pronuclear microinjection to produce live, transgenic offspring harboring that gene. Transgenic technologies complement existing experimental techniques for investigating hypertension by potentially providing a causal link between phenotype and candidate genes. Additionally, some transgenic models emulate human disease closely and as such, form good experimental models in their own right.

Despite the lack of embryonic stem cell lines in the rat, which allow the development of 'knockout' strains and gene-titration experiments in mice, several hypertensive transgenic models have been developed in the rat. This species is attractive due to: its tendency to develop experimental hypertension; larger size, that allows a wide range of physiological and surgical interventions; and because many good models of hypertension already exist in this species.

In the rat, hypertension can readily be selected by breeding and phenotypic screening, which has resulted in a variety of strains being generated including the spontaneously hypertensive rat (SHR) strains, Dahl salt-sensitive rats and Lyon hypertensive rats. These phenotype-driven models of hypertension can mimic the polygenetic nature of human hypertension (e.g. SHR) and have demonstrated the importance of strain, i.e. genetic background, on complex traits such as hypertension, where the interaction of multiple gene effects produces the phenotype, making subtle strain differences important.[1,2]

The advantage of transgenic, gene-driven models over traditional phenotype-selected strains is that they have a clearly defined (mono)genetic cause for their hypertension, permitting the study of a specific candidate gene as well as more conventional pathophysiological investigation. Their disadvantage is that transgene integration is random and can result in multiple copies of the gene and/or expression in numerous tissues, resulting in gross and often ectopic gene expression. However, concordant results in more than one transgenic line favor the candidate gene being responsible for the phenotype rather than the integration site. Due to their relative genetic simplicity, transgenic animals on an inbred background form a powerful tool with which to investigate the role of candidate genes in hypertension (and other conditions) and to answer specific questions posed by the experimenter. An increasing number of transgenic rat models have been developed (Tables 12.1 and 12.2) and for the purpose of this review we have grouped them according to whether they directly involve the renin–angiotensin system (RAS).

TRANSGENIC MODELS OVEREXPRESSING COMPONENTS OF THE RENIN–ANGIOTENSIN SYSTEM

TGR(mRen2)27

The TGR(mRen2)27 was the first transgenic hypertensive rat described.[3] The mouse *Ren2* gene encoding renin, together with large 5′ and 3′ flanking sequences including the endogenous promoter and other control elements, was inserted into single-cell rat embryos and one of the resulting founders, named TGR(mRen2)27, was used to establish a lineage of hypertensive rats. This model was originally developed to investigate mouse *Ren2* gene expression and function under the control of its own promoter in the rat, which unlike the mouse and in common with man, possesses a single renin gene. Although not designed to emulate human hypertension, it has provided an excellent model of hypertension, exhibiting many phenotypic similarities with the human disease. It remains one of the widest used experimental models of hypertension and has been extensively reviewed.[4,5]

Animals have severe, chronic hypertension with systolic blood pressures reaching 240 mmHg in heterozygous males and 290 mmHg in homozygotes by 8–10 weeks of age. Death from hypertensive crisis due to malignant transformation occurs in some homozygotes but is unpredictable. Chronic treatment with angiotensin-converting enzyme (ACE) inhibitors is required to prevent death and to maintain a breeding line. Reaction kinetics for angiotensin II generation in the rat and man suggest that renin is rate limiting. Hence, insertion of extra copies of the renin gene is a powerful way of driving the RAS in this species. Mouse prorenin is highly expressed in the adrenal gland, which is a major source of circulating renin activity in the TGR(mRen2)27 model,[6] but expression occurs at many sites including the kidney, heart, resistance vasculature and brain.[3,7] Expression is absent from the rat submandibular gland in contrast to the DBA/2 mouse where Ren2 is expressed at high levels in this tissue, suggesting that other unidentified factors capable of activating Ren2 exist within the mouse submandibular gland that are absent in the rat.[3,8]

Females exhibit less severe hypertension and lower mortality than males, with female homozygotes equivalent to heterozygote males in terms of blood pressure. Such sexual dimorphism has been observed in other hypertensive rat strains including SHRs and the deoxycorticosterone acetate (DOCA) salt model.[9,10] Large human epidemiological studies also suggest that being female

Table 12.1 Summary of transgenic rat models with altered blood pressure

Name	TGR (mREN2)27	Inducible hypertensive rat	TGR(hAT-mRen2)	TGR(hAT-rpR)	TGR (hAOGEN/hRen)
Transgene	Mouse Ren2 complete gene plus 3′ and 5′ flanking sequences	Cyp1a1 promoter fused to mouse Ren2 cDNA (integrated onto Y chromosome)	Human α1AT promoter fused to mouse Ren2 cDNA	Human α1AT promoter fused to rat Renin cDNA	Human angiotensinogen and renin genes
Back-ground	Hanover Sprague–Dawley	Fisher F334	Fisher F334	Fisher F334	Sprague–Dawley
Phenotype	SBP 200 mmHg at 9 weeks (heterozygote) > 250 mmHg (homozygote)	Normal prior to induction. SBP 220 mmHg after 7 days	SBP 190 mmHg at 7 weeks	Not hypertens-ive at 10 weeks	SBP 200 mmHg at 7 weeks
Sex influence	Male > female	All male	Not determined	Males >> females	Not reported
Drug correction	ACE inhibitors AT antagonism Not spironolactone	Salt sensitivity attenuated by superoxide dismutase mimetic	ACE inhibitors		ACE inhibition Human renin inhibitor Bosentan Cyclosporin NFκB inhibitor
Expression site	Widespread Mostly adrenal cortex	Mostly liver	Liver	Liver	Widespread for both transgenes but hRenin great-est in kidney and hAngio-tensinogen in the liver
End-organ injury	Vascular remodeling, cardiac hypertrophy and fibrosis, nephrosclerosis and stroke Variable malignant hypertension	Fibrinoid necrosis of mesentery, coronary and renal circulations. Cardiac hypertrophy	Vascular remodeling Cardiac hypertrophy and fibrosis Nephrosclerosis Transformation to malignant hypertension	Cardiac fibrosis and nephrosclero-sis	Cardiac hypertrophy, nephrosclerosis and malignant hypertension.
Plasma levels	10–20 × mouse prorenin levels Dispute over other RAS components but not greatly elevated	10^5 × mouse prorenin levels Elevated angiotensin II and aldosterone	10^3 × mouse prorenin levels Other RAS components normal	400 × rat prorenin levels Renin, angiotensin II normal	Human prorenin and angiotensinogen elevated. Plasma angiotensin II elevated

ACE, angiotensin-converting enzyme; AT, angiotensin; RAS, renin–angiotensin system.

is cardioprotective.[11] Androgens are capable of modulating *Ren2* expression in the mouse and administration of androgens to female mice results in higher levels of submandibular *Ren2* transcription.[12] Additionally, levels of circulating RAS components appear to be higher in male rats compared to females.[13] Hence,

Table 12.2 Further summary of transgenic rat models with altered blood pressure

Name	DAHL SS TGR(α1NK-ATPase)	1. TGR(ASRAOGEN) 2. TGR(ASHAOGEN – mREN2)	NPY-TgR	TGR(DbH-ETB:ETBsl:sl)	TGR(hKLK1)
Transgene	Rat wild-type α1Na-K-ATP-ase cDNA and promoter	200-bp reverse orientation construct producing anti-sense oligonucleotide to rat angiotensino-gen. Driven by GFAP	Rat NPY gene and promoter	DbH-ETB rescue of spotting lethal	Human tissue kallikrein under the mouse metallothionein promoter
Background Phenotype	Dahl-salt sensitive Improves hypertension and glomeru-losclerosis	1. Sprague–Dawley 2. TGR(mRen2)27 Hypotension and polyuria. Reduced hypertension in TGR(mRen2)27 cross	Sprague–Dawley Stress-induced hypertension Increased vascular resistance and pressor response Reduced hypotension	Spotting lethal Salt sensitive hypertension	Sprague–Dawley Hypotension Reduced hypertrophy and fibrosis to pressor agents Altered circadian rhythm
Drug correction				Amiloride	B$_2$ antagonist
Expression site	Heart, brain, kidney, aorta	Brain	Heart, vessels, spleen	Adrenergic tissue	Heart
Plasma levels		Normal plasma angiotensinogen. 90% reduction in brain level Reduced AVP	Normal at rest NPY elevated post-hemorrhage	ET-1 increased	

AVP, arginine-vasopressin; DbH-ETB, rat endothelin B cDNA under control of human dopamine hydroxylase promoter; ET-1, endothelin-1; GFAP, glial fibrillary acidic protein; NPY, neuropeptide Y.

in the TGR(mRen2)27 model, enhanced expression of the transgene mediated by androgens could account for the increased severity of the male phenotype rather than a pre-existing, sexual predisposition.

Vascular remodeling in TGR(mRen2)27 occurs in resistance as well as in large blood vessels and nephrosclerosis with proteinuria is seen as early as 8 weeks.[14–18] In common with other hypertensive models, vascular remodeling of resistance vessels is associated with medial hyperplasia while medial hypertrophy and polyploidy are associated with larger vessels such as the aorta.[19] In malignant hypertensive disease, this progresses to the two features of malignant vascular injury; fibrinoid necrosis and endarteritis proliferans. Young animals show changes of left ventricular hypertrophy progressing to failure by 30 weeks. The hypertrophic response has molecular features, such as reduced response to the inotropic effects of isoprenaline and phenylephrine, in common with human left ventricular hypertrophy and other animal models.[15,17] The similarity between this model and human hypertensive pathology is striking and the underlying mechanisms in TGR(mRen2)27 rats are likely to have relevance in the human setting.

The development of end-organ pathology appears to be angiotensin II dependent. Antihypertensive agents will lower blood pressure but are not as effective in attenuating end-organ damage as drugs specifically targeting the RAS.[20,21] In TGR(mRen2)27 transgenic rats, transgene-derived prorenin is elevated whereas endogenous rat renin is appropriately suppressed. Angiotensin I and II are both decreased in the plasma. The levels of transgene-derived prorenin and angiotensin II at the tissue level, however, are likely to be more relevant than circulating levels in predicting end-organ injury in this and other animal models. Administration of low-dose lisinopril (0.5 mg/kg/day) to TGR(mRen2)27 rats resulted in partial attenuation of blood pressure, lower cardiac to body mass ratio and reduced renal injury in association with decreased renal angiotensin II levels. Dihydralazine-treated animals, despite correction of blood pressure to control levels, displayed no improvement in target-organ injury or alteration in renal angiotensin II levels.[21] Low doses of the angiotensin II receptor blocker telmisartan reduced renal and cardiac injury in TGR(mRen2)27 animals with only modest effect on hypertension[20] and low-dose ramipril treatment (5 mg/kg/day) resulted in increased survival and failure to transform from benign to malignant hypertension, without lowering blood pressure. Tissue, but not plasma, ACE activity was decreased, suggesting that the paracrine RAS is important for transformation to malignant hypertension and lethality in this model, independent of blood pressure.[22] Although the tail-cuff plethysmography used by Montgomery et al failed to detect subtle or intermittent changes in blood pressure, their treatment group had comparable medial hypertrophy to control animals, suggesting a similar level of hypertension.[22] However, identical subdepressor ramipril treatment of TGR(mRen2)27 rats could not prevent left ventricular hypertrophy and fibrosis developing or perivascular fibrosis within the right ventricle, implicating pressure, rather than the RAS, as the dominant effector for hypertrophic cardiac remodeling in this model.[23] Minute falls or fluctuations in blood pressure with so-called 'subdepressor doses' of agents antagonizing the RAS are difficult to exclude as no studies of this type have used continuous arterial monitoring via telemetry. As such, pressure effects may partially contribute to the outcome of tissue RAS inhibition discussed above.

Increasingly, there is evidence that individual tissues can regulate their own RAS and all components of the RAS are present in some vessels.[24] Cardiomyocytes release angiotensin II on mechanical stretch[25] and the brain has an isolated RAS with important roles in systemic blood pressure regulation in addition to nonhemodynamic effects.[26,27] The demonstration that mouse *Ren2* expression in the TGR(mRen2)27 rat occurs in all tissues exhibiting injury, suggests strongly, but does not prove, that local angiotensin II formation is enhanced and could mediate organ injury. Evidence suggesting upregulation of the paracrine RAS and the powerful effect of agents that block this system (even administered at doses that have little or no effect on blood pressure) strongly links angiotensin II with target-organ injury in a variety of hypertensive states. Direct and indirect pressure effects are also important and might be the dominant effector in certain types of target-organ response.

Constitutive tissue-specific renin-expressing transgenics

To address the role of (pro)renin in the development of cardiovascular pathology, and to bypass target organ expression, a constitutive prorenin expressing model – TGR(hAT-mRen2) – has been developed using the human α1 antitrypsin (hAT) promoter to drive ectopic mouse *Ren2* cDNA expression in the liver. Elevated plasma mouse prorenin levels and hypertension (190 mmHg systolic by 7 weeks of age) were observed in transgenic animals. Circulating prorenin levels were elevated 1×10^3-fold in this model, compared with only a 10- to 20-fold elevation in TGR(mRen2)27; in both models, angiotensin II and aldosterone were not elevated. Initial studies suggested that left ventricular hypertrophy occurred prior to the onset of significant hypertension, which suggests that transgene expression, rather than hypertension *per se*, was important in the pathogenesis of end-organ injury in this model.[28] It is likely that this model will provide additional information on the role of prorenin in the development of hypertensive pathology.

A closely related strain, the TGR(hAT-rpR), which expresses rat instead of mouse prorenin, was not hypertensive (determined by tail plethysmography) but did develop end-organ damage in the form of cardiac fibrosis, hypertrophy, glomerulosclerosis and large vessel remodeling. Rat prorenin levels were 400-fold elevated in the plasma of male animals but other components of the RAS were similar to nontransgenic controls.[29] Sexual dimorphism is also observed in TGR(hAT-rpR) rats, with males having a 60-fold greater plasma prorenin level than female animals, and only male animals displaying target-organ pathology.[29] Again, in the absence of hypertension in young adults, it is tempting to speculate that pathology in this model is mediated by elevated, circulating prorenin.

The double 'human' transgenic rat

Double transgenic rats carrying the human renin and angiotensinogen genes have been established. Species specificity within the RAS means that rats expressing either human renin or angiotensinogen are normotensive. Intercrossing rats from these strains generated a double transgenic on a Sprague–Dawley background, heterozygous for each transgenic site and capable of angiotensin II formation. Both transgenes used genomic sequences driven by their endogenous promoters and as such expression was observed from many sites including target organs.[30] These double transgenic animals exhibited severe hypertension (200 mmHg by 7 weeks) and developed malignant hypertension with typical end-organ injury.[30]

The resulting double transgenic strain allows the development of targeted treatment in humans. In addition to the human renin antagonist Ro42-5892, which corrected hypertension and pathology, blood pressure could also be reduced and end-organ damage ameliorated by the nuclear factor kappa B (NFκB) inhibitor pyrrolidine dithiocarbamate.[31] NFκB is a pro-inflammatory transcription factor upregulated in this model along with activator protein 1 (AP-1). Ciclosporin, an immunosuppressant acting via calcineurin inhibition to block interleukin-2 (IL-2) dependent T-cell responses, was also able to significantly attenuate vascular proliferation and monocyte infiltration in the presence of only a small reduction in systolic blood pressure.[32] Treatment of double transgenic rats with dexamethasone resulted in amelioration of renal injury and inflammatory cell infiltration independent of blood pressure. Similar results were seen with the more specific immunosuppressant agents Mycophenolate Mofetil and soluble tumor necrosis factor receptor, entanercept.[33]

As with other forms of vascular injury, especially angiotensin-II-mediated injury, perivascular monocyte accumulation and cell adhesion molecule upregulation is described in association with vascular injury.[34–36] It is significant that, in this setting, anti-inflammatory treatment attenuated both inflammatory cell accumulation and target organ injury. However, to date more specific proinflammatory mediators have not been mechanistically implicated in the pathogenesis of malignant hypertension in this model.

Brain-specific angiotensinogen depletion

Systemic blood pressure can be regulated via central mechanisms and agents such as methyldopa owe their mode of action to as yet poorly understood central mechanisms. The extent to which neurological mechanisms contribute to human hypertension, or experimental animal models, is unclear. In health, the blood–brain barrier excludes circulating angiotensin II from the brain, which has an independent RAS capable of angiotensin II generation with roles in regulating salt–water balance and vascular tone via arginine–vasopressin, adrenocorticotropic hormone, mineralocorticoids and sympathetic outflow. Additionally, intracerebroventricular injections of renin or angiotensin II into the brains of rats will result in marked salt–water thirst and increased drinking behavior.[37] Some strains of SHR and the TGR(mRen2)27 line have elevated protein levels of angiotensinogen or angiotensins within the brain and central administration of RAS antagonists can attenuate hypertension.[38]

With the purpose of dissecting out the relative importance of neurological influences, a transgenic rat was developed to express a reverse orientation sequence encoding the 5′ end, exon 1 and partial exon 2 of the rat angiotensinogen gene. The construct was driven by a glial fibrillary acid protein promoter localizing expression to the central nervous system and put onto a Hanover Sprague–Dawley background. This new strain TGR(ASRAOGEN) exhibited a 90% reduction in brain angiotensinogen protein while plasma levels remained unchanged. The animals were mildly hypotensive (systolic pressure 5 mmHg lower than controls) and passed larger quantities of dilute urine and this corresponded to reduced plasma arginine–vasopressin. In response to intracerebroventricular renin injection they exhibited an attenuated drinking response and the degree of hypertension and left ventricular hypertrophy induced during systemic subcutaneous angiotensin II infusion was reduced.[39]

An additional cross was performed onto the TGR(mRen2)27 background.[40] This cross exhibited less hypertension (systolic pressures of 200 mmHg compared with 220 mmHg), suggesting that in the TGR(mRen2)27, as with other hypertensive models, the central nervous system contributes to the etiology of hypertension and target-organ injury.

The inducible hypertensive rat

As already mentioned, transgenic approaches can result in high and ectopic levels of gene expression not typical of human hypertension. However, it is now possible to insert genes in a highly regulated way and control both the level and site of transgene expression. Both forms of control have been used in the Inducible Hypertensive Rat (IHR).[48] In the IHR, mouse *Ren2* cDNA is regulated by the *Cyp1a1* promoter and expressed only in the presence of specific inducing agents (Fig. 12.1). There are three important differences from the earlier TGR(mRen2)27 strain. First, mouse prorenin is expressed from an extrarenal site and not from organs affected by hypertensive injury. Second, expression is

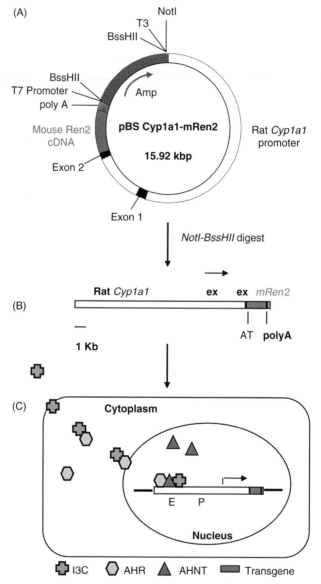

Fig. 12.1 Transgene structure and regulation. (A) pBluescript Cyp1a1-mRen2 structure. The Cyp1a1-mRen2 transgene comprised the rat *Cyp1a1* promoter, including exon1 and partial exon 2, fused to 1.2 kb mRen2 cDNA with SV40 polyadenylation site (polyA). (B) The transgene was excised by *NotI-BssHII* digest. (C) Transgene regulation following integration. E, *Cyp1a1* enhancer; P, *Cyp1a1* promoter; I3C, indole-3-carbinol; AHR, aryl hydrocarbon receptor; AHNT, aryl hydrocarbon nuclear translocator.

inducible and reversible so that hypertension can be generated reproducibly and at will. Third, because constitutive transcription is absent, hypertension is generated *de novo* and does not influence cardiovascular development. It is appreciated that manipulation of the RAS early in life can alter vascular development, renal morphology and blood pressure in adult animals, including humans, and this phenomenon might complicate the adult phenotype of constitutive transgenics: 50% of the fetuses from women taking angiotensin II receptor antagonists during early pregnancy developed renal abnormalities and oligohydramnios.[42] Components of the RAS are expressed in characteristic patterns throughout nephrogenesis and inhibition of this system during late (neonatal) nephrogenesis in the rat results in vascular, tubular and papillary abnormalities. Additionally, gene deletion studies of ACE, angiotensinogen and $AT1_{A/B}$ show similar renal malformations.[43,44] Such abnormalities result in reduced nephron number, which is postulated to contribute to adult hypertension.[45]

As part of the hepatic cytochrome p450 system, *Cyp1a1* expression is directly regulated by lipophilic xenobiotics such as indole-3 carbinol (I3C) acting via the aryl hydrocarbon receptor. *Cyp1a1* is not constitutively expressed and induction occurs when I3C binds the aryl hydrocarbon receptor (AHR) in the cytoplasm. This complex translocates to the nucleus and binds the aryl hydrocarbon nuclear translocator (ARNT). Both AHR and ARNT are basic helix-loop-helix transcription factors that bind aromatic hydrocarbon responsive elements within the enhancer region resulting in structural changes within the promoter which favor transcription.[46,47] Inclusion of dietary I3C results in rapid expression and secretion of mouse prorenin from the liver (see Fig. 12.1). Very low levels of expression are also found in the skin and small intestine but these tissues do not suffer hypertensive injury in this model.[48]

The transgene was introduced onto an inbred Fisher F334 background with good breeding characteristics, to yield a pure inbred strain with a highly reproducible phenotype. Only male animals carry the transgene due to integration into the Y chromosome. Within 24 hours of addition of I3C to standard feed, blood pressure rises and peaks at 7 days, remaining stable at a level of 220 mmHg systolic. Due to the potentially beneficial effects of I3C on human breast cancer, there is a history of human exposure to this compound without adverse effects.[49,50] Animals develop malignant hypertension over 14 days and display clinical signs consistent with accelerated hypertension such as polyuria, weight loss, hemolysis and reduced appetite. Fibrinoid necrosis and proliferative endarteritis are seen in the mesenteric and cardiac circulations by day seven and renal bed by day 14 (Fig. 12.2).

The cerebral circulation is spared. The reason for this hierarchy of vascular bed susceptibility is unknown, but may relate to the differential autoregulatory capacity within these organs. All components of the RAS are significantly elevated in the plasma. Transgene derived prorenin is 5×10^4 times greater, active renin 1×10^2 times greater and circulating angiotensin II double compared to Fisher F334 controls by day seven. Prorenin elevation occurs rapidly together with an elevation in blood pressure, which precedes the rise in circulating active renin and angiotensin II. This suggests that processing of the transgene at a local, tissue level is responsible in part for the phenotype. For example, it has been suggested that one percent of prorenin can exist in an active form without cleavage via conformational shift alone.[51] If this occurs in the IHR model it would result in significant levels of circulating 'active' renin. Endogenous rat renin

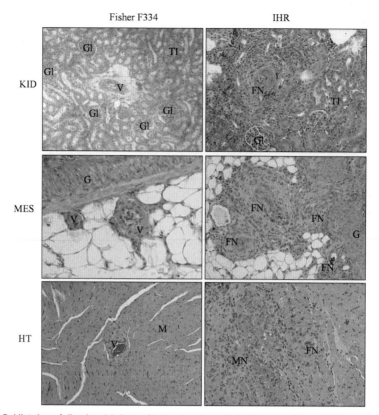

Fig. 12.2 Histology following 14 days of induction in the IHR. Fisher F334 and IHRs were induced for 14 days with 0.3% w/w I3C. Fibrinoid necrosis (FN) is seen in the kidney (KID), mesentery (MES) and heart (HT). MN, myocardial necrosis; G, gut wall; Gl, glomerulus; TI, tubulointerstitium; V, normal vessel; M, myocardium.

within the kidney is undetectable by immunostaining during the early development of hypertension, suggesting appropriate suppression.

Recently, the IHR model has been shown to display salt sensitivity if transient induction and hypertension are allowed to develop. Blood pressure levels returned to normal when induction was stopped, but increased if the animals were fed a diet containing 8% sodium chloride. If a superoxide dismutase (SOD) mimetic was coadministered, salt sensitivity was attenuated suggesting that, in the IHR, superoxide production plays a role in this mechanism.[52]

This novel model is extremely versatile and the experimenter is able to switch transgene expression on and off at will. Notably, blood pressure can return to normal after 14 days of induction,[52] therefore offering the opportunity to study repair mechanisms without excessive mechanical or pharmacological manipulation. Patients with malignant hypertension also have activation of the RAS and frequently present with established renal and cardiac impairment. As such, this model provides an excellent opportunity to observe the development of this condition, without surgical or pharmacological manipulation, for the first time.

The abrupt onset of transgene expression in the IHR might account for the severity of the hypertensive phenotype compared to the TGR(mRen2)27 strain. Adaptive changes within the vasculature of TGR(mRen2)27 animals due to constitutive expression and continuous prorenin exposure may favor the development of a chronic, rather than malignant, hypertension in this model. Another factor influencing the severity of the phenotype seen in the IHR model appears to be the genetic background, which differs from TGR(mRen2)27. Indeed, when the transgene in the TGR(mRen2)27 strain was moved onto Fisher F334 and Lewis backgrounds, differences in lethality were observed between the two transgenic strains.[53] Linkage analysis suggested that this trait was influenced by two loci spanning the *ACE* and *AT1* genes.[41] Plasma ACE activity is significantly higher in Fisher F334 rats compared to Lewis rats, suggesting involvement of the RAS in modulating this phenotype.

As there is no transgene expression in target organs or in the kidney, and endogenous renin is downregulated, this model provides us with an opportunity to dissect the role of the paracrine RAS. Initial studies looking at cardiomyocytes *in vitro* and *in vivo* suggested that transgene-derived prorenin was elevated. This raises the possibility of uptake and activation of prorenin within cardiac and perhaps other tissues.[54] This has been alluded to in other studies where prorenin binding and uptake by vessels and cardiomyocytes via a renin receptor has been suggested.[55–58]

Given that agents blocking the RAS are highly efficacious in treating these and other animal models of hypertension and that direct infusion of angiotensin II results in vascular remodeling and hypertensive end-organ injury, much attention has focused on the role of angiotensin II and the molecular mechanisms involved. In addition to regulating vascular tone and salt–water balance, angiotensin II behaves as a cytokine influencing a variety of cellular processes including oxidative stress via nicotinamide adenine dinucleotide phosphate (NADPH) oxidase,[59,60] growth and inflammation.[61,62] Within vessels, angiotensin II has been shown to affect tone, inflammation, matrix remodeling and thrombosis via actions on endothelial cells, vascular smooth muscle cells and fibroblasts. The resulting angiotensin-II-induced endothelial dysfunction has been suggested as critical in mediating vascular remodeling in hypertensive states as well as other conditions where vascular remodeling is central, such as atherosclerosis.[63] Although the list of molecular effectors of angiotensin II is still incomplete, evidence suggests that alteration in the redox state of cells is an important and early event in the molecular cascade leading to aberrant vascular function. Angiotensin II can stimulate the formation of reactive oxygen species (ROS) *in vitro* via a membrane-bound NAD(P)H oxidase.[59] ROS, in turn, avidly inactivates nitric oxide (NO) necessary for normal endothelial function.[64] The consequence of NO inactivation, in addition to vasoconstriction, is NFκB activation through loss of inhibitory factor kappa B (IκB) stabilization triggering expression of proinflammatory cytokines, leukocyte adhesion and vascular smooth muscle cell proliferation and migration.[65–67] Evidence also exists for increased levels of ROS in certain hypertensive conditions. Infusion of angiotensin II into rats increased the levels of NAD(P)H-derived ROS. Both hypertension and NAD(P)H expression were decreased by pretreatment with SOD.[68] Heparin-binding SOD, targeted to the endothelium, was capable of reducing blood pressure in a SHR model known to have high levels of vascular ROS.[69]

Angiotensin II is also capable of inducing leukocyte recruitment and activation by ROS-dependent pathways. Vascular cell adhesion molecule-1 (VCAM-1) binds circulating leukocytes initiating adhesion of inflammatory cells. Endothelial VCAM-1 expression is induced by angiotensin II via NFκB and inhibited by an antioxidant.[70] Angiotensin II has also been found to increase VCAM-1 expression in rat vascular smooth muscle cells.[71]

The role of macrophages and other inflammatory cells is increasingly a target for investigation, not only in malignant vascular injury but also in vasculopathy related to atheroma, diabetes, postangioplasty restenosis and benign hypertension. Whereas the association of inflammatory cells with such lesions is not in dispute, their significance is still unclear, although it would seem that they are not necessarily a response to tissue injury. Factors that initiate the recruitment of these cells are also receiving attention. Macrophage chemoattractant protein 1 (MCP-1), a member of the C-C chemokine family, is a macrophage chemoattractant that acts via the CCR2 receptor and is upregulated in the arteries of animals rendered hypertensive by angiotensin II infusion.[72]

NON-RENIN–ANGIOTENSIN SYSTEM TRANSGENIC MODELS INFLUENCING BLOOD PRESSURE

Transgenic rescue of defective Cd36 in spontaneously hypertensive rats

Hypertension, dyslipidemia, obesity and insulin resistance coexist in humans in a metabolic disorder called syndrome X. SHRs exhibit a similar disorder and linkage analysis has identified regions likely to harbor genes that influence this complex phenotype.[73] Cd36 encodes a fatty acid receptor involved in transport of long-chain fatty acids in muscle and adipose. Its location on chromosome 4 was identified by differential expression studies using DNA microarrays of congenic strains (SHR NIH strain X Brown-Norway) and coincides with a region of peak linkage to metabolic defects in the SHR.[74] Additionally, Aitman et al identified multiple sequence variants in the coding sequence and undetectable levels of Cd36 protein, suggesting that Cd36 deficiency contributes to the defects in fatty acid and glucose metabolism linked to chromosome 4 in the SHR.[74] The SHR congenic for the Brown-Norway chromosome 4 segment containing Cd36 (approximately 35cM), exhibited improvements in carbohydrate and lipid metabolism as well as systolic hypertension.[75] Transgenic expression of wild-type Cd36 in the SHR was able to ameliorate insulin resistance but not improve hypertension.[76,77] Candidate genes such as leptin, neuropeptide Y and endothelial nitric oxide, linked to Cd36 within the differential chromosome segment of the congenic SHR, might influence hypertension in this model.

In man, Cd36 deficiency is associated with altered myocardial fatty-acid metabolism, inherited hypertrophic cardiomyopathy and ischemic heart disease.[78,79]

The interaction between hypertension and metabolic parameters such as insulin resistance and fatty-acid metabolism is complex and is likely to be influenced by multiple gene effects.

Neuropeptide Y transgenic

Neuropeptide Y (NPY) is a ubiquitous neuropeptide, which co-localizes with norepinephrine in the secretory vesicles of central and peripheral neurons. Exogenous administration results in persisting pressor and vasoconstrictor responses and in some instances might potentiate the effects of other vasoactive substances such as angiotensin II or norepinephrine.[80,81] SHRs have higher NPY levels within the myocardium and an enhanced pressor response to NPY administration and the NPY locus has been shown to segregate with blood pressure.[82,83]

Little is known regarding human hypertension but links to exercise induced blood pressure elevation have been made.[84] To examine the role of overexpression of this peptide during rest and stress, transgenic animals were created expressing the rat NPY gene under control of its own promoter on a Sprague–Dawley genetic background.[85] Animals had increased levels of NPY protein in many organs, mirroring the distribution of the endogenous peptide. In a resting state, transgenic animals displayed a greater total peripheral resistance than nontransgenic controls. Interestingly, blood pressure determined by direct arterial measurement was normal but found to be elevated when estimated using tail-cuff plethesmography. The authors confirmed an enhanced stress response by illustrating greater pressor responses to noradrenaline infusion and a reduced fall in blood pressure and heart rate induced by hemorrhage. They suggest that in this setting NPY acts by modulating α-adrenoreceptor sensitivity, shedding light on an important aspect of blood pressure regulation. Rats harboring the NPY transgene demonstrated a reduced pressor response to nitric oxide inhibition with N-(omega)-nitro-L-arginine methyl ester. This effect was centrally mediated and could be mimicked by intracerebroventricular infusion of NPY and inhibited by an NPY antagonist.[86] As both NPY and nitric oxide act as inhibitory neurotransmitters, sometimes within the same neural circuits, it is plausible that one can compensate for deficiency of the other.

Human kallikrein transgenic

The kallikrein kinin system is widespread and can exert powerful vasodilatory, antioxidant, antiproliferative and antithrombotic effects. This system is also interconnected with the RAS and the contribution of kinins to the efficacious effects of ACE inhibitors has long been debated (Fig. 12.3). The effects of kinins

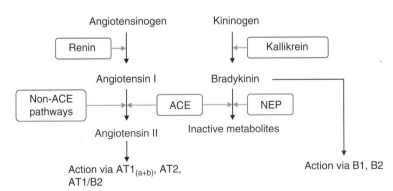

Fig. 12.3 The renin–angiotensin system and kallikrein kinin system. ACE, angiotensin-converting enzyme – identical to kininase II and active principally within the pulmonary circulation; AT, angiotensin II receptor; AT1 subdivisions AT1$_{a+b}$, exist only in rodents; B1/2, bradykinin receptor type 1/2; NEP, neural endopeptidase; nonACE pathways, include cathepsin G, chymostatin-sensitive angiotensin II generating enzyme (CAGE), chymase, tonin and tissue plasminogen activator (tPA) and are important in nonpulmonary tissues and might account for 40% of angiotensin II generation in humans.

are mediated mostly via its receptor B2, which is constitutively and widely expressed.[87] B2 expression on the renal collecting duct may mediate natriuresis via prostaglandin E_2 generation.[88,89] Kinins can also inhibit the actions of vasopressin (ADH), contributing to their diuretic effect.[90]

Human essential hypertension is associated with low urinary kininogen excretion.[91] This defect is more common within the salt-sensitive subpopulation and it has been suggested that kinins mediate excretion of excess salt and counter the effects of the sympathetic system and RAS activation.[92,93] Reduced kallikrein expression was found in three rodent models displaying salt sensitivity: the nitric oxide inhibition model, the four-fifths nephrectomy model and the protein overload model.[94] Administration of kallikrein to humans and rats was able to lower blood pressure but only in salt-sensitive individuals[95,96] and B2 null mice develop salt-sensitive hypertension at a young age.[97]

A transgenic rat that overexpresses human kallikrein under the mouse metallothionein promoter was generated and the cardiovascular effects assessed.[98] High levels of expression were observed in the hearts of these animals and expression was also seen in the kidney, lung and brain. Transgenic animals were hypotensive (5 mmHg lower) and had a reduced response in terms of left ventricular hypertrophy, atrial natriuretic peptide expression and fibrosis to isoproterenol infusion. Hypotension was improved – but not corrected – by a B2 antagonist, suggesting that increased kinin generation is at least partially responsible. An additional finding was that the circadian rhythm in these animals was altered such that the amplitude of the dominant 24-hour period was reduced, suggesting that the kallikrein kinin system might have a role in regulating blood pressure at the level of circadian rhythm.

Rescuing spotting-lethal

Endothelins (ETs) 1–3 with their potent vasoconstrictor and mitogenic actions have been implicated in the development of accelerated hypertension.[99,100] The effects of ETs are mediated in mammals through two functionally distinct classes of receptor: ETA and ETB. ETB displays a dual role, able to induce vasoconstriction when situated on vascular smooth muscle cells, as well as nitric-oxide-mediated vasodilatation on endothelial cells. Angiotensin II can induce ET expression, suggesting the possibility of crosstalk between the renin– angiotensin and ET systems. In animals, ET(s) infusion results in increases in blood pressure and vascular resistance.[101,102] Induction of ET expression within vascular endothelial cells occurs in response to low levels of shear stress, and in response to mediators such as thrombin, and angiotensin II,[100] which could be involved in the pathogenesis of malignant hypertension. Pressure alone, without inducing shear stress, caused an increase in ET-1 release *in vitro* via a mechanism involving protein kinase C and phospholipase C.[103] As mentioned above, elevated ET-1 levels have been reported in 'low-renin' as well as some 'high-renin' models of hypertension, including the DOCA–salt model and chronic administration of caffeine to Goldblatt rats.[104,105] Renal ET-1 mRNA levels were also increased in the TGR(mRen2)27 Edinburgh Sprague–Dawley cross HanRen2/Edin-with malignant hypertension, but administration of bosentan, a combined ETA/ETB antagonist, failed to attenuate hypertension or affect outcome.[106]

A natural deletion of the ETB gene exists called spotting-lethal. Animals with this condition die neonatally from aganglionic megacolon, the rodent equivalent of Hirschsprung's disease (where ETB mutations compose 5%). Genetic rescue of these animals by targeting the rat ETB cDNA under the direction of the human dopamine hydroxylase promoter replaces ETB at adrenergic sites including the enteric nervous system [termed TGR(DBH-ETB:ETBsl/sl)].[107] As mentioned above, ETB can induce vasoconstriction or vasodilatation depending on location and promotes natriuresis when situated on renal tubular epithelium. The rescued phenotype lacked ETB receptor expression within the kidney and appeared healthy and normotensive on a low-salt diet. However, they exhibited a hypertensive response to high (8%) dietary sodium chloride that corrected with amiloride, implicating abnormal epithelial sodium channel (ENaC) activity, known to be important in sodium handling within the distal nephron. Under salt stress, the renin–angiotensin system in these animals is appropriately suppressed, consistent with ETB providing tonic inhibition of endothelial sodium channel during the normal maintenance of blood pressure. A gain of function mutation of the ENaC gene results in one of the few monogenetic causes of human hypertension, Liddle syndrome.[108,109]

Although ETA antagonists are beneficial in DOCA-salt treated rats, ETB antagonism can sometimes be detrimental. To address this, TGR(DBH-ETB:ETBsl/sl) rats were treated with unilateral nephrectomy and DOCA-salt. The result was worsening of hypertension and end-organ injury in the form of left ventricular hypertrophy and renal dysfunction, again suggesting a protective role for ETs acting via ETB.[110] The authors mention that an increase of ETA-mediated activity rather than reduced ETB activation cannot be excluded.

Endothelins have also been implicated in renal injury through their actions on mesangial cell proliferation[111] and are associated with human renal injury such as cyclosporin nephropathy and lupus nephritis.[112,113] TGR(hET-2)37 is a transgenic rat line generated by insertion of the human ET-2 gene under the control of its own promoter. ET-2 is highly expressed within the glomerulus of transgenic rats but absent from normal rat kidney. TGR(hET-2)37 rats were normotensive but developed glomerulosclerosis with proteinuria by 12 months of age, suggesting a role for ET-2 in the development of fibrotic injury within the kidney independent of blood pressure. The maintenance of normotension in these animals, despite a 2-fold elevation in circulating ET-2, is unclear but might be partially accounted for by activation of the nitric oxide system, since inhibition of this system resulted in greater than expected hypertension. However, this line also exhibited developmental abnormalities within the kidneys and heart, which might also contribute to overall blood pressure.[114,115]

Rescuing Dahl salt-sensitive rats

Renal salt handling has been proposed as central to the etiology of hypertension in human disease and animal models. Clear examples exist where altered sodium handling results directly in hypertension such as Liddle syndrome. Here, dominantly inherited mutations of the sodium channel on the collecting tubule lead to sustained activation with sodium retention and associated hypertension. A transgenic strategy was employed to investigate the role of the sodium potassium ATP-ase (Na-K-ATPase) in hypertension and salt handling in the kidney. Dahl salt-sensitive (D S-S) rats have a mutation in the α1 Na-K-ATPase that segregates with hypertension.[116] The authors went on to express the wild-type α1 Na-K-ATPase under the control of its own promoter on a D S-S background to obtain a reduction in blood pressure and glomerulosclerosis, suggesting that α1 Na-K-ATPase acts as a susceptibility factor in salt sensitive hypertension in this model. However, the existence of the α1 Na-K-ATPase mutation is debatable: the transversion proposed by Herrera et al to result in a single amino acid substitution and altered protein function could not be confirmed and might have resulted from a reverse transcriptase error in cDNA synthesis.[117] Transgenic expression of 'wild-type' protein might have resulted in relative hypotension due to overexpression of α1 Na-K-ATPase.[1] In response, Herrera suggested the mutation was missed as a consequence of a nonrandom error in Taq polymerase.[118]

CURRENT DEVELOPMENT AND FUTURE PROSPECTS

Constitutive transgenics are disadvantaged by transgene expression during cardiovascular development, which might permit 'adaptation' and alter phenotype, the inability to switch transgene expression on at will and expression in multiple tissues including those subject to injury. Techniques have evolved to overcome these problems and allow the generation of conditional and tissue-specific transgenics. When placed on an inbred background these animals show small interanimal variation in pathology and comprise a stronger experimental model. As such, the IHR offers a unique opportunity to investigate hypertensive vascular remodeling without these constraints.

More recently, a P1 artificial chromosome transgenic rat for the 150kb *Ian5* gene has been developed that demonstrated transgenic rescue of T cell lymphopenia in the biobreeding diabetic rat strain.[119] This illustrates that bacterial artificial chromosome-based clones, carrying large transgenes, can be used to test the function of novel genes and narrow quantitative trait loci regions.

A far greater and more sophisticated degree of genetic manipulation could be achieved through gene targeting and, as a wealth of knowledge has accumulated from the many rat models of hypertension, it would be ideal to apply such knockout technology to the rat. The vast majority of gene knock-out experiments have been achieved in the mouse, where embryonic stem (ES) cells suitable for homologous targeting of endogenous genes, are readily obtainable. To date, the production of germline-competent rat ES cells for gene-targeting has proved elusive. Two groups have reported the culture of rat ES-like cells for many generations,[120,121] making them available for transfection with targeting constructs. Recently, nuclear cloning has been achieved using two-cell stage embryos as donor and recipient cells.[122] It might be possible, in the future, to use targeted ES-like cells as a source of nucleus for nuclear transfer, thus circumventing the need for germline-competence.[123]

One alternative strategy for the production of knockout rats is the use of ethyl-nitroso-urea (ENU) mutagenesis,[124] which randomly introduces point mutations into the genome through intercalation of ENU into the DNA. An appropriate screening protocol is necessary to look for mutations in genes of interest.[124]

Chemically synthesized small interfering RNAs (siRNAs) and short hairpin RNAs (shRNAs) have recently been shown to transiently or stably knockdown gene expression in transgenic mice and, significantly, in rats.[125–128] This technology also promises to widen the application of transgenic technology to the rat and other species.

A new possibility for germline modification follows from the identification of exogenous growth factors and serum-free culture conditions, which allow continuous culture of mouse spermatogonial stem cells (SSCs) for periods in excess of 6 months.[129] The stem cells, generated from neonate, pup and adult testes, can be transplanted into recipient seminiferous tubules, after extensive culture, and can reconstitute long-term spermatogenesis, or even restore fertility to infertile recipients. In-vitro proliferation of SSCs should make genetic manipulation, such as targeted modification, possible and such strategies could prove invaluable for species such as the rat.

The increasing array of transgenic tools available to modify the rat genome has been recently reviewed.[130] These techniques, together with our knowledge of the rat genome,[131,132] should increase the diversity of transgenic rat models available to investigate human disease and gene function.

CONCLUSIONS

Transgenic technology has resulted in the development of constitutive transgenics that can directly test the role of candidate genes. This has expanded research into the regulation of blood pressure and the pathological effects of hypertension. The role of renal salt handling and vasoactive systems, especially the RAS, has been shown to be important not only for the development of hypertension, but in the development of end-organ injury independent of blood pressure.

Transgenic lines like the TGR(mRen2)27 and the IHR provide good experimental models of hypertensive end-organ injury and share many characteristics with human hypertensive disease.

It is hoped that advances in our understanding of the molecular mechanisms underlying hypertension in this model will have relevance beyond this species. Additionally, the insertion of a wild-type gene can be used to test the contribution of an existing mutation to the overall phenotype. With the rapid advances in transgenic technology, one can anticipate the introduction of increasingly sophisticated and subtle genomic alterations in order to understand the genetic basis of hypertension. Equally exciting is the potential for applying knockout technology to alter genes in classical animal models, such as SHR, in an attempt to rescue the hypertensive phenotype. At present caution must be used before extrapolating the findings from transgenic rats to the human setting but these animals will undoubtedly form an increasingly important tool in the experimental armory of hypertension research.

References

1. Rapp JP. Genetic analysis of inherited hypertension in the rat. *Physiol Rev* 2000; 80:135–172.
2. Rapp JP, Wang SM, Dene H. Effect of genetic background on cosegregation of renin alleles and blood pressure in Dahl rats. *Am J Hypertens* 1990; 3:391–396.
3. Mullins JJ, Peters J, Ganten D. Fulminant hypertension in transgenic rats harbouring the mouse Ren-2 gene. *Nature* 1990; 344:541–544.
4. Engler S, Paul M, Pinto YM. The TGR(mRen2)27 transgenic rat model of hypertension. *Regul Pept* 1998; 77:3–8.
5. Lee MA, Bohm M, Pau M, et al. Physiological characterization of the hypertensive transgenic rat TGR(mREN2)27. *Am J Physiol* 1996; 270:E919–E929.
6. Tokita Y, Franco-Saenz R, Mulrow PJ, Ganten D. Effects of nephrectomy and adrenalectomy on the renin-angiotensin system of transgenic rats TGR(mRen2)27. *Endocrinology* 1994; 134:253–257.

7. Hilgers KF, Peters J, Veelken R, et al. Increased vascular angiotensin formation in female rats harboring the mouse Ren-2 gene. *Hypertension* 1992; 19:687–691.

8. Zhao Y, Bader M, Kreutz R, et al. Ontogenetic regulation of mouse Ren-2d renin gene in transgenic hypertensive rats, TGR(mREN2)27. *Am J Physiol* 1993; 265:E699–E707.

9. Crofton JT, Share L, Brooks DP. Gonadectomy abolishes the sexual dimorphism in DOC-salt hypertension in the rat. *Clin Exp Hypertens* 1989; A11:1249–1261.

10. Ganten U, Schroder G, Witt M, et al. Sexual dimorphism of blood pressure in spontaneously hypertensive rats: effects of anti-androgen treatment. *J Hypertens* 1989; 7:721–726.

11. Kannel WB, Dawber TR, McGee DL. Perspectives on systolic hypertension. The Framingham study. *Circulation* 1980; 61:1179–1182.

12. Wagner D, Metzger R, Paul M, et al. Androgen dependence and tissue specificity of renin messenger RNA expression in mice. *J Hypertens* 1990; 8:45–52.

13. Chen YF, Naftilan AJ, Oparil S. Androgen-dependent angiotensinogen and renin messenger RNA expression in hypertensive rats. *Hypertension* 1992; 19:456–463.

14. Bachmann S, Peters J, Engler E, et al. Transgenic rats carrying the mouse renin gene – morphological characterization of a low-renin hypertension model. *Kidney Int* 1992; 41:24–36.

15. Bohm M, Moll M, Schmid B, et al. Beta-adrenergic neuroeffector mechanisms in cardiac hypertrophy of renin transgenic rats. *Hypertension* 1994; 24:653–662.

16. Springate JE, Feld LG, Ganten D. Renal function in hypertensive rats transgenic for mouse renin gene. *Am J Physiol* 1994; 266:F731–F737.

17. Tawfik-Schlieper H, Moll M, Schmid B, et al. Alterations of cardiac alpha- and beta-adreno-ceptors and inotropic responsiveness in hypertensive transgenic rats harbouring the mouse renin gene (TGR(mREN2)27). *Clin Exp Hypertens* 1995; 17:631–648.

18. Thybo NK, Korsgaard N, Mulvany MJ. Morphology and function of mesenteric resistance arteries in transgenic rats with low-renin hypertension. *J Hypertens* 1992; 10:1191–1196.

19. Brosnan MJ, Devlin AM, Clark JS, et al. Different effects of antihypertensive agents on cardiac and vascular hypertrophy in the transgenic rat line TGR(mRen2)27. *Am J Hypertens* 1999; 12:724–731.

20. Bohm M, Lee M, Kreutz R, et al. Angiotensin II receptor blockade in TGR(mREN2)27: effects of renin-angiotensin-system gene expression and cardiovascular functions. *J Hypertens* 1995; 13:891–899.

21. Lee MA, Bohm M, Kim S, et al. Differential gene expression of renin and angiotensinogen in the TGR(mREN-2)27 transgenic rat. *Hypertension* 1995; 25:570–580.

22. Montgomery HE, Kiernan LA, Whitworth CE, et al. Inhibition of tissue angiotensin converting enzyme activity prevents malignant hypertension in TGR(mREN2)27. *J Hypertens* 1998; 16:635–643.

23. Bishop JE, Kiernan LA, Montgomery HE, et al. Raised blood pressure, not renin-angiotensin systems, causes cardiac fibrosis in TGR m(Ren2)27 rats. *Cardiovasc Res* 2000;47:57–67.

24. Gibbons GH. The pathophysiology of hypertension: the importance of angiotensin II in cardiovascular remodeling. *Am J Hypertens* 1998; 11:177S–181S.

25. Sadoshima J, Xu Y, Slayter HS, Izumo S. Autocrine release of angiotensin II mediates stretch-induced hypertrophy of cardiac myocytes in vitro. *Cell* 1993; 75:977–984.

26. Culman J, Blume A, Gohlke P, Unger T. The renin–angiotensin system in the brain: possible therapeutic implications for (AT1 receptor) blockers. *J Hum Hypertens* 2002; 16(suppl 3):S64–S70.

27. Veerasingham SJ, Raizada MK. Brain renin-angiotensin system dysfunction in hypertension: recent advances and perspectives. *Br J Pharmacol* 2003; 139:191–202.

28. Ogg D. Characterisation of rat lines transgenic for the mouse Ren-2(d) cDNA. Thesis. Edinburgh University; 1997.

29. Veniant M, Menard J, Bruneval P, et al. Vascular damage without hypertension in transgenic rats expressing prorenin exclusively in the liver. *J Clin Invest* 1996; 98:1966–1970.

30. Bohlender J, Fukamizu A, Lippoldt A, et al. High human renin hypertension in transgenic rats. *Hypertension* 1997; 29:428–434.

31. Muller DN, Dechend R, Mervaala EM, et al. NF-kappaB inhibition ameliorates angiotensin II-induced inflammatory damage in rats. *Hypertension* 2000; 35:193–201.

32. Mervaala E, Muller DN, Park J-K, et al. Cyclosporin A protects against angiotensin II-induced end-organ damage in double transgenic rats harboring human renin and angiotensinogen genes. *Hypertension* 2000; 35:360–366.

33. Muller DN, Shagdarsuren E, Park JK, et al. Immunosuppressive treatment protects against angiotensin II-induced renal damage. *Am J Pathol* 2002; 161:1679–1693.

34. Grafe M, Auch-Schwelk W, Zakrzewicz A, et al. Angiotensin II-induced leukocyte adhesion on human coronary endothelial cells is mediated by E-selectin. *Circ Res* 1997; 81:804–811.

35. Mervaala EMA, Muller DN, Park J-K, et al. Monocyte infiltration and adhesion molecules in a rat model of high human renin hypertension. *Hypertension* 1999; 33:389–395.

36. Muller DN, Mervaala EMA, Schmidt F, et al. Effect of bosentan on NF-{kappa}B, inflammation, and tissue factor in angiotensin II-induced end-organ damage. *Hypertension* 2000; 36:282–290.

37. Fitzsimons JT. Angiotensin, thirst, and sodium appetite. *Physiol Rev* 1998; 78:583–686.
38. DiNicolantonio R, Hutchinson JS, Mendelsohn FA. Exaggerated salt appetite of spontaneously hypertensive rats is decreased by central angiotensin-converting enzyme blockade. *Nature* 1982; 298:846–848.
39. Baltatu O, Silva JA Jr, Ganten D, Bader M. The brain renin-angiotensin system modulates angiotensin II-induced hypertension and cardiac hypertrophy. *Hypertension* 2000; 35:409–412.
40. Schinke M, Baltatu O, Bohm M, et al. Blood pressure reduction and diabetes insipidus in transgenic rats deficient in brain angiotensinogen. *Proc Natl Acad Sci U S A* 1999; 96:3975–3980.
41. Kantachuvesiri S, Haley CS, Fleming S, et al. Genetic mapping of modifier loci affecting malignant hypertension in TGRmRen2 rats. *Kidney Int* 1999; 56:414–420.
42. Serreau R, Luton D, Macher MA, et al. Developmental toxicity of the angiotensin II type 1 receptor antagonists during human pregnancy: a report of 10 cases. *Br J Obstet Gynaecol* 2005; 112:710–712.
43. Sequeira Lopez ML, Gomez RA. The role of angiotensin II in kidney embryogenesis and kidney abnormalities. *Curr Opin Nephrol Hypertens* 2004; 13:117–122.
44. Wu J, Edwards D, Berecek K. Changes in renal angiotensin II receptors in spontaneously hypertensive rats by early treatment with the angiotensin-converting enzyme inhibitor captopril. *Hypertension* 1994; 23:819–822.
45. Woods LL, Rasch R. Perinatal ANG II programs adult blood pressure, glomerular number, and renal function in rats. *Am J Physiol* 1998; 275:R1593–R1599.
46. Elferink CJ, Whitlock JP Jr. 2,3,7,8-Tetrachlorodibenzo-*p*-dioxin-inducible, Ah receptor-mediated bending of enhancer DNA. *J Biol Chem* 1990; 265:5718–5721.
47. Okino ST, Whitlock JP Jr. Dioxin induces localized, graded changes in chromatin structure: implications for Cyp1A1 gene transcription. *Mol Cell Biol* 1995; 15:3714–3721.
48. Kantachuvesiri S, Fleming S, Peters J, et al. Controlled hypertension, a transgenic toggle switch reveals differential mechanisms underlying vascular disease. *J Biol Chem* 2001; 276:36727–36733.
49. Bradlow HL, Michnovicz JJ, Halper M, et al. Long-term responses of women to indole-3-carbinol or a high fiber diet. *Cancer Epidemiol Biomarkers Prev* 1994; 3:591–595.
50. Wong GY, Bradlow L, Sepkovic D, et al. 1997 Dose-ranging study of indole-3-carbinol for breast cancer prevention. *J Cell Biochem* 1997; Suppl 28–29, 111–116.
51. Yamauchi T, Nagahama M, Watanabe T, et al. Site-directed mutagenesis of human prorenin. Substitution of three arginine residues in the propeptide with glutamine residues yields active prorenin. *J Biochem (Tokyo)* 1990; 107:27–31.
52. Howard LL, Patterson ME, Mullins JJ, Mitchell KD. Salt-sensitive hypertension develops after transient induction of ANG II-dependent hypertension in Cyp1a1-Ren2 transgenic rats. *Am J Physiol Renal Physiol* 2005; 288:F810–F815.
53. Whitworth CE, Fleming S, Kotelevtsev Y, et al. A genetic model of malignant phase hypertension in rats. *Kidney Int* 1995; 47:529–535.
54. Peters J, Farrenkopf R, Clausmeyer S, et al. Functional significance of prorenin internalization in the rat heart. *Circ Res* 2002; 90:1135–1141.
55. Danser AH, van Kats JP, Admiraal PJ, et al. Cardiac renin and angiotensins. Uptake from plasma versus in situ synthesis. *Hypertension* 1994; 24:37–48.
56. Prescott G, Silversides DW, Chiu SM, Reudelhuber TL. Contribution of circulating renin to local synthesis of angiotensin peptides in the heart. *Physiol Genomics* 2000; 4:67–73.
57. Saris JJ, Derkx FH, De Bruin RJ, et al. High-affinity prorenin binding to cardiac man-6-P/IGF-II receptors precedes proteolytic activation to renin. *Am J Physiol Heart Circ Physiol* 2001; 280:H1706–H1715.
58. van Kesteren CA, Danser AH, Derkx FH, et al. Mannose 6-phosphate receptor-mediated internalization and activation of prorenin by cardiac cells. *Hypertension* 1997; 30:1389–1396.
59. Griendling KK, Minieri CA, Ollerenshaw JD, Alexander RW. Angiotensin II stimulates NADH and NADPH oxidase activity in cultured vascular smooth muscle cells. *Circ Res* 1994; 74:1141–1148.
60. Ushio-Fukai M, Zafari AM, Fukui T, et al. p22phox is a critical component of the superoxide-generating NADH/NADPH oxidase system and regulates angiotensin II-induced hypertrophy in vascular smooth muscle cells. *J Biol Chem* 1996; 271:23317–23321.
61. Brasier AR, Recinos A 3rd, Eledrisi MS. Vascular inflammation and the renin-angiotensin system. *Arterioscler Thromb Vasc Biol* 2002; 22:1257–1266.
62. Ruiz-Ortega M, Lorenzo O, Suzuki Y, et al. Proinflammatory actions of angiotensins. *Curr Opin Nephrol Hypertens* 2001; 10:321–329.
63. Dzau VJ. 2001 Theodore Cooper Lecture: tissue angiotensin and pathobiology of vascular disease: a unifying hypothesis. *Hypertension* 2001; 37:1047–1052.
64. Harrison DG. Cellular and molecular mechanisms of endothelial cell dysfunction. *J Clin Invest* 1997; 100:2153–2157.

65. De Caterina R, Libby P, Peng HB, et al. Nitric oxide decreases cytokine-induced endothelial activation. Nitric oxide selectively reduces endothelial expression of adhesion molecules and proinflammatory cytokines. *J Clin Invest* 1995; 96:60–68.

66. Dubey RK, Jackson EK, Luscher TF. Nitric oxide inhibits angiotensin II-induced migration of rat aortic smooth muscle cell. Role of cyclic-nucleotides and angiotensin1 receptors. *J Clin Invest* 1995; 96:141–149.

67. Peng HB, Libby P, Liao JK. Induction and stabilization of I kappa B alpha by nitric oxide mediates inhibition of NF-kappa B. *J Biol Chem* 1995; 270:14214–14219.

68. Laursen JB, Rajagopalan S, Galis Z, et al. Role of superoxide in angiotensin II-induced but not catecholamine-induced hypertension. *Circulation* 1997; 95:588–593.

69. Nakazono K, Watanabe N, Matsuno K, et al. Does superoxide underlie the pathogenesis of hypertension? *Proc Natl Acad Sci U S A* 1991; 88:10045–10048.

70. Pueyo ME, Gonzalez W, Nicoletti A, et al. Angiotensin II stimulates endothelial vascular cell adhesion molecule-1 via nuclear factor-kappaB activation induced by intracellular oxidative stress. *Arterioscler Thromb Vasc Biol* 2000; 20:645–651.

71. Tummala PE, Chen XL, Sundell CL, et al. Angiotensin II induces vascular cell adhesion molecule-1 expression in rat vasculature: A potential link between the renin-angiotensin system and atherosclerosis. *Circulation* 1999; 100:1223–1229.

72. Bush E, Maeda N, Kuziel WA, et al. CC chemokine receptor 2 is required for macrophage infiltration and vascular hypertrophy in angiotensin II-induced hypertension. *Hypertension* 2000; 36:360–363.

73. Aitman TJ, Gotoda T, Evans AL, et al. Quantitative trait loci for cellular defects in glucose and fatty acid metabolism in hypertensive rats. *Nat Genet* 1997; 16:197–201.

74. Aitman TJ, Glazier AM, Wallace CA, et al. Identification of Cd36 (Fat) as an insulin-resistance gene causing defective fatty acid and glucose metabolism in hypertensive rats. *Nat Genet* 1999; 21:76–83.

75. Pravenec M, Zidek V, Simakova M, et al. Genetics of Cd36 and the clustering of multiple cardiovascular risk factors in spontaneous hypertension. *J Clin Invest* 1999; 103:1651–1657.

76. Pravenec M, Landa V, Zidek V, et al. Transgenic expression of CD36 in the spontaneously hypertensive rat is associated with amelioration of metabolic disturbances but has no effect on hypertension. *Physiol Res* 2003; 52:681–688.

77. Pravenec M, Landa V, Zidek V, et al. Transgenic rescue of defective Cd36 ameliorates insulin resistance in spontaneously hypertensive rats. *Nat Genet* 2001; 27:156–158.

78. Tanaka T, Sohmiya K, Kawamura K. Is CD36 deficiency an etiology of hereditary hypertrophic cardiomyopathy? *J Mol Cell Cardiol* 1997; 29:121–127.

79. Watanabe K, Toba K, Ogawa Y, et al. [Different patterns of 123I-BMIPP myocardial accumulation in patients with type I and II CD36 deficiency]. *Kaku Igaku* 1997; 34:1125–1130.

80. Dahlof C, Dahlof P, Lundberg JM. Neuropeptide Y (NPY): enhancement of blood pressure increase upon alpha-adrenoceptor activation and direct pressor effects in pithed rats. *Eur J Pharmacol* 1985; 109:289–292.

81. Wahlestedt C, Hakanson R, Vaz CA, Zukowska-Grojec Z. Norepinephrine and neuropeptide Y: vasoconstrictor cooperation in vivo and in vitro. *Am J Physiol* 1990; 258:R736–R742.

82. Katsuya T, Higaki J, Zhao Y, et al. A neuropeptide Y locus on chromosome 4 cosegregates with blood pressure in the spontaneously hypertensive rat. *Biochem Biophys Res Commun* 1993; 192:261–267.

83. Westfall TC, Han SP, Knuepfer M, et al. Neuropeptides in hypertension: role of neuropeptide Y and calcitonin gene related peptide. *Br J Clin Pharmacol* 1990; 30 (suppl 1):75S–82S.

84. Solt VB, Brown MR, Kennedy B, et al. Elevated insulin, norepinephrine, and neuropeptide Y in hypertension. *Am J Hypertens* 1990; 3:823–828.

85. Michalkiewicz M, Michalkiewicz T, Kreulen DL, McDougall SJ. Increased blood pressure responses in neuropeptide Y transgenic rats. *Am J Physiol Regul Integr Comp Physiol* 2001; 281:R417–R426.

86. Michalkiewicz M, Zhao G, Jia Z, et al. Central neuropeptide Y signaling ameliorates N(omega)-nitro-L-arginine methyl ester hypertension in the rat through a Y1 receptor mechanism. *Hypertension* 2005; 45:780–785.

87. Bhoola KD, Figueroa CD, Worthy K. Bioregulation of kinins: kallikreins, kininogens, and kininases. *Pharmacol Rev* 1992; 44:1–80.

88. Garcia-Perez A, Smith WL. Apical-basolateral membrane asymmetry in canine cortical collecting tubule cells. Bradykinin, arginine vasopressin, prostaglandin E2 interrelationships. *J Clin Invest* 1984; 74:63–74.

89. Stokes JB, Kokko JP. Inhibition of sodium transport by prostaglandin E2 across the isolated, perfused rabbit collecting tubule. *J Clin Invest* 1977; 59:1099–1104.

90. Schuster VL, Kokko JP, Jacobson HR. Interactions of lysyl-bradykinin and antidiuretic hormone in the rabbit cortical collecting tubule. *J Clin Invest* 1984; 73:1659–1667.

91. Balsano F. The kidney and essential hypertension. *Ann Ital Med Int* 1991; 6:93–106.

92. Katori M, Majima M. Role of the renal kallikrein-kinin system in the development of hypertension. *Immunopharmacology* 1997; 36:237–242.

93. Katori M, Majima M, Hayashi I, et al. Role of the renal kallikrein-kinin system in the development of salt-sensitive hypertension. *Biol Chem* 2001; 382:61–64.

94. Ardiles LG, Figueroa CD, Mezzano SA. Renal kallikrein-kinin system damage and salt sensitivity: insights from experimental models. *Kidney Int* 2003; suppl:S2–S8.

95. Bellini C, Ferri C, Piccoli A, et al. The influence of salt sensitivity on the blood pressure response to exogenous kallikrein in essential hypertensive patients. *Nephron* 1993; 65:28–35.

96. Chao J, Chao L. Kallikrein gene therapy: a new strategy for hypertensive diseases. *Immunopharmacology* 1997; 36:229–236.

97. Cervenka L, Harrison-Bernard LM, Dipp S, et al. Early onset salt-sensitive hypertension in bradykinin B2 receptor null mice. *Hypertension* 1999; 34:176–180.

98. Silva JA Jr, Araujo RC, Baltatu O, et al. Reduced cardiac hypertrophy and altered blood pressure control in transgenic rats with the human tissue kallikrein gene. *Faseb J* 2000; 14:1858–1860.

99. Weber H, Webb ML, Serafino R, et al. Endothelin-1 and angiotensin II stimulate delayed mitosis in cultures of rat aortic smooth muscle cells: evidence for common signalling mechanisms. *Mol Endocrinol* 1994; 8:148–158.

100. Yanagisawa M, Kurihara H, Kimura S, et al. A novel potent vasoconstrictor peptide produced by vascular endothelial cells. *Nature* 1988; 332:411–415.

101. Mortensen LH, Pawloski CM, Kanagy NL, Fink GD. Chronic hypertension produced by infusion of endothelin in rats. *Hypertension* 1990; 15:729–733.

102. Yokokawa K, Kohno M, Murakawa K, et al. Acute effects of endothelin on renal hemodynamics and blood pressure in anesthetized rats. *Am J Hypertens* 1989; 2:715–717.

103. Hishikawa K, Nakaki T, Marumo T, et al. Pressure enhances endothelin-1 released from cultured human endothelial cells. *Hypertension* 1995; 25:449–452.

104. Fujita K, Matsumura Y, Miyazaki Y, et al. Effects of the endothelin ETA-receptor antagonist FR139317 on development of hypertension and cardiovascular hypertrophy in deoxycorticosterone acetate-salt hypertensive rats. *Jpn J Pharmacol* 1996; 70:313–319.

105. Kohno M, Murakawa K, Horio T, et al. Plasma immunoreactive endothelin-1 in experimental malignant hypertension. *Hypertension* 1991; 18:93–100.

106. Whitworth CE, Veniant MM, Firth JD, et al. Endothelin in the kidney in malignant phase hypertension. *Hypertension* 1995; 26:925–931.

107. Gariepy CE, Ohuchi T, Williams SC, et al. Salt-sensitive hypertension in endothelin-B receptor-deficient rats. *J Clin Invest* 2000; 105:925–933.

108. Hansson JH, Nelson-Williams C, Suzuki H, et al. Hypertension caused by a truncated epithelial sodium channel gamma subunit: genetic heterogeneity of Liddle syndrome. *Nat Genet* 1995; 11:76–82.

109. Shimkets RA, Warnock DG, Bositis CM, et al. Liddle's syndrome: heritable human hypertension caused by mutations in the beta subunit of the epithelial sodium channel. *Cell* 1994; 79:407–414.

110. Matsumura Y, Kuro T, Kobayashi Y, et al. Exaggerated vascular and renal pathology in endothelin-B receptor-deficient rats with deoxycorticosterone acetate-salt hypertension. *Circulation* 2000; 102, 2765–2773.

111. Haneda M, Kikkawa R, Koya D, et al. Endothelin-1 stimulates tyrosine phosphorylation of p125 focal adhesion kinase in mesangial cells. *J Am Soc Nephrol* 1995; 6:1504–1510.

112. Busauschina A, Schnuelle P, van der Woude FJ. Cyclosporine nephrotoxicity. *Transplant Proc* 2004; 36:229S–233S.

113. Nassar GM, Badr KF. Endothelin in kidney disease. *Curr Opin Nephrol Hypertens* 1994; 3:86–91.

114. Hocher B, Liefeldt L, Thone-Reineke C, et al. Characterization of the renal phenotype of transgenic rats expressing the human endothelin-2 gene. *Hypertension* 1996; 28:196–201.

115. Liefeldt L, Schonfelder G, Bocker W, et al. Transgenic rats expressing the human ET-2 gene: a model for the study of endothelin actions in vivo. *J Mol Med* 1999; 77:565–574.

116. Herrera VL, Xie HX, Lopez LV, et al. The alpha1 Na,K-ATPase gene is a susceptibility hypertension gene in the Dahl salt-sensitive HSD rat. *J Clin Invest* 1998; 102:1102–1111.

117. Simonet L, St Lezin E, Kurtz TW. Sequence analysis of the alpha 1 Na+,(K+ATPase) gene in the Dahl salt-sensitive rat. *Hypertension* 1991; 18:689–693.

118. Ruiz-Opazo N, Barany F, Hirayama K, Herrera VL. Confirmation of mutant alpha 1 Na, K-ATPase gene and transcript in Dahl salt-sensitive/JR rats. *Hypertension* 1994; 24:260–270.

119. Michalkiewicz M, Michalkiewicz T, Ettinger RA, et al. Transgenic rescue demonstrates involvement of the Ian5 gene in T cell development in the rat. *Physiol Genomics* 2004; 19:228–232.

120. Buehr M, Nichols J, Stenhouse F, et al. Rapid loss of Oct-4 and pluripotency in cultured rodent blastocysts and derivative cell lines. *Biol Reprod* 2003; 68:222–229.

121. Vassilieva S, Guan K, Pich U, Wobus AM. Establishment of SSEA-1- and Oct-4-expressing rat embryonic stem-like cell lines and effects of cytokines of the IL-6 family on clonal growth. *Exp Cell Res* 2000; 258:361–373.

122. Roh S, Guo J, Malakooti N, et al. Birth of rats following nuclear exchange at the 2-cell stage. *Zygote* 2003; 11:317–321.

123. Mullins LJ, Wilmut I, Mullins JJ. Nuclear transfer in rodents. *J Physiol* 2004; 554:4–12.

124. Zan Y, Haag JD, Chen KS, et al. Production of knockout rats using ENU mutagenesis and a yeast-based screening assay. *Nat Biotechnol* 2003; 21:645–651.

125. Hasuwa H, Kaseda K, Einarsdottir T, Okabe M. Small interfering RNA and gene silencing in transgenic mice and rats. *FEBS Lett* 2002; 532:227–230.

126. Lewis DL, Hagstrom JE, Loomis AG, et al. Efficient delivery of siRNA for inhibition of gene expression in postnatal mice. *Nat Genet* 2002; 32:107–108.

127. McCaffrey AP, Meuse L, Pham TT, et al. RNA interference in adult mice. *Nature* 2002; 418:38–39.

128. Paddison PJ, Caudy AA, Hannon GJ. Stable suppression of gene expression by RNAi in mammalian cells. *Proc Natl Acad Sci U S A* 2002; 99:1443–1448.

129. Kubota H, Avarbock MR, Brinster RL. Growth factors essential for self-renewal and expansion of mouse spermatogonial stem cells. *Proc Natl Acad Sci U S A* 2004; 101:16489–16494.

130. Tesson L, Cozzi J, Menoret S, et al. Transgenic modifications of the rat genome. *Transgenic Res* 2005; 14:531–546.

131. Gibbs RA, Weinstock GM, Metzker ML, et al. Genome sequence of the Brown Norway rat yields insights into mammalian evolution. *Nature* 2004; 428:493–521.

132. Zimdahl H, Nyakatura G, Brandt P, et al. A SNP map of the rat genome generated from cDNA sequences. *Science* 2004; 303:807.

13 | Gene targeting in mice to study blood pressure regulation: role of the renin–angiotensin system

Willem J. de Lange and Curt D. Sigmund

INTRODUCTION

Over the last two decades, genetically modified mouse models have been used extensively in biomedical research. Mice are well suited for the generation of genetically modified animal models because of the relative ease with which we can modify their genome and obtain germline transmission of transgenes. There are two general classes of genetically modified mice: (1) those modified by gene addition, also known as additive transgenesis; and (2) those modified by gene ablation, also known as gene targeting. As the techniques needed to generate genetically manipulated mice have been described extensively elsewhere, we will give a brief overview of the basic strategies herein. Subsequently, we will provide selected examples of how we and others have used them to study blood-pressure regulation, focusing specifically on the renin–angiotensin system (RAS). Finally, we will discuss how mouse models have, and in the future might, contribute towards our understanding of how genetic variability contributes to the development of essential hypertension.

GENETIC MANIPULATION OF THE MOUSE

Transgenic expression of exogenous genes in mice

Transgenic animals are generated by microinjecting a construct consisting of exogenous DNA (transgene) directly into the male pronucleus of a fertilized one-cell mouse embryo (Fig. 13.1A, B).[1,2] Embryos are subsequently implanted into the oviduct of pseudopregnant females, resulting in the generation of transgenic offspring in which the transgene is physically integrated into all cells and transmitted through the germ line to subsequent generations (Fig. 13.1C). The strategy of expressing exogenous genes in mice has several advantages. First, transgenic mice are easy to generate in large numbers and provide an opportunity to examine the physiological consequences of overexpression of the target gene. The use of cell-specific and or inducible promoters also provides unique tools allowing investigators to control the spatial and temporal expression of

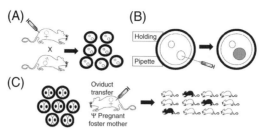

Fig. 13.1 Generation of transgenic mice via microinjection. (A) Female mice are hormonally superovulated by the injection of follicle stimulating hormone and luteinizing hormone. Eggs are fertilized by mating with male mice. One cell pronuclear stage embryos are obtained. (B) One-cell fertilized pronuclear-stage embryos are held in place with gentle suction through a holding pipette and the male pronucleus is injected with a solution of DNA. The pronucleus visibly grows in size due to the microinjection procedure. (C) The embryos divide to the two-cell stage embryos overnight and then are implanted into the oviduct of a hormonally (or pseudo-) pregnant female. Litters are born 18–19 days later, a fraction of which are transgenic (filled).

their target gene. The use of sensitive reporter genes also provides a mechanism with which to examine the expression pattern of specific genes that are endogenously expressed at levels that are not detectable using traditional methods such as Northern or Western blotting.

Of course, transgenic expression of an exogenous gene has a number of disadvantages as well. First, transgenic mice generated by pronuclear microinjection generally contain multiple copies of the transgene (between one and even several hundred). Although there is no strict copy-number proportional expression, multiple copy insertions could result in the transgene being overexpressed at supraphysiological levels, making their relevance questionable. Second, because the transgene is randomly inserted into the mouse genome, it is possible that it might insert into another gene, thus causing a mutation that might not be detected in the heterozygous state because one normal copy of the gene would remain. Additionally, expression of the transgene might be influenced by its position in the host genome, resulting in ectopic expression if integrated in close proximity to strong transcriptional enhancers, or it might insert into heterochromatin, thus causing its expression to be suppressed or absent.

It has now become clear that some of these disadvantages can be negated by using a construct design in which the transgene is embedded in a large segment of genomic DNA (i.e. 100–300 kb). Indeed, the generation of transgenic mice containing either PACs (P1 artificial chromosomes) or BACs (bacterial artificial chromosomes) has increased in popularity in recent years. Because the genomic segment is large, the approach maximizes the possibility that all the necessary regulatory sequences required for accurate and faithful tissue-specific, cell-specific and regulated expression are cotransferred along with the coding region of the target gene into the mouse genome. Additional advantages are the tendency for a lower copy number (not surprising given the size of BACs and PACs), expression of the inserted transgene that is predictably proportional to copy number and the presence of 'insulators', reducing the possibility that regulatory sequences in the vicinity of the insertion site would alter the expression of the transgene. The use of these large clones as transgenes was largely pioneered by studies on globin gene regulation[3] but has more recently been applied to study the regulation of the renin gene.[4]

Gene targeting through homologous recombination

Gene targeting strategies have classically been used to generate knockout mice deficient in a target gene of interest, but have more recently been exploited to create knockin mice in which an endogenous mouse gene is modified in some desirable way. Both approaches rely entirely on homologous recombination in embryonic stem (ES) cells, totipotent stem cells capable of being maintained in culture (for ease of genetic manipulation) yet retaining the ability to differentiate into all cells and tissues of a mouse (Fig. 13.2A).[5]

Gene ablation is generally achieved by generating a targeting construct homologous to the target gene, but where an essential part thereof (i.e. the exon containing the start codon, a critical domain for protein function, or an exon whose loss would result in a frame-shift) is replaced by a selectable marker (such as the neomycin resistance gene). Using strategies that have been described in detail elsewhere,[6] homologous recombinant clones are selected, expanded and microinjected into mouse blastocysts where they can join with the inner cell mass of the blastocyst and contribute to the genome of the resultant offspring (Fig. 13.2B). These offspring are called chimeras because their tissues are derived from a mix of normal cells derived from the blastocyst and altered cells derived from the genetically manipulated ES cells. Selection of chimeras is generally facilitated by using blastocysts and ES cells derived from mouse strains with different coat colors [i.e. blastocycts from strain C57/BL6 (black) and ES cells from strain 129 (agouti)]. Chimeras (F0 generation) are subsequently back crossed to the parental strain (e.g. C57BL/6 mice) to transmit the altered ES cell-derived genome to offspring (Fig. 13.2C). F1 mice heterozygous for the gene ablation are subsequently mated, resulting in the generation of offspring of which ~25% should be homozygous for the targeted allele (F2 generation). This approach has been used extensively and successfully to study the role of many genes in the development of hypertension, and some of these will be discussed in more detail in subsequent sections.

Despite the tremendous power of gene targeting, its greatest disadvantage is the ablation of the target gene in all cells and tissues of the organism. When the

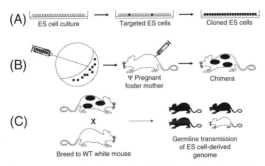

Fig. 13.2 Gene targeting in embryonic stem cells. (A) Embryonic stem (ES) cells in culture are manipulated by homologous recombination as described later in the text and illustrated in Figs 13.5 and 13.6. Targeted cells are obtained (black) and then are cloned into a pure population. (B) The target ES cells are microinjected onto the inner cell mass of a blastocyst-stage embryo and then implanted into the uterus of a pseudopregnant female. Chimeric mice are identified by the patchy coloration of the coat. (C) Germline transmission of the targeted genome is achieved by breeding the chimera with a wild-type mouse. Both gene target (black) and wild-type (white) are obtained from this cross.

target gene encodes an essential protein required during development or during early life, its ablation might result in a lethal phenotype. In recent years, investigators have developed strategies to avoid this problem by developing mouse models in which the target gene is only ablated in specific and investigator-selected cell types. One example has been the development of the Cre-LoxP Recombinase system, which provides a tool to ablate genes in a tissue- and cell-specific manner, or at specific developmental stages.[7] To accomplish this, LoxP sites – 34-bp palindromic sequences that recognize cre-recombinase – are inserted into the target gene through gene targeting in ES cells. In practice, as illustrated in Fig. 13.3, LoxP sites are inserted into introns surrounding a critical coding exon of the target gene. Each of these LoxP sites has the ability to bind two Cre-recombinase molecules, which in turn catalyze a recombination event between the sites, causing a deletion of the intervening DNA sequences. Several Cre-delivery systems have been developed to provide spatial and temporal control over the gene ablation. These include the use of tissue-specific targeting by adenoviral infection, or expression of Cre-recombinase transgenes under tissue-specific, inducible and temporally regulated promoters.[8–10] The development of Cre-recombinase molecules that are only induced in the presence of small ligands such as tamoxifen provides a means of temporal control over the deletion previously difficult to achieve by other means.[11]

THE RENIN–ANGIOTENSIN SYSTEM

The renin–angiotensin system (RAS) plays a critical role in regulating blood pressure and electrolyte homeostasis in mammals, and has been studied extensively for more than 100 years. This system is of particular importance in gaining an understanding of the genetic factors involved in the development of essential hypertension, as drug targets directed against two of its gene products [angiotensin-converting enzyme (ACE) and angiotensin II type 1 (AT_1) receptors] are among the most widely prescribed antihypertensive medications. Furthermore, the angiotensinogen (*hAGT*) gene remains one of only a handful of genes linked to hypertension in humans.[12] We will therefore give a brief overview of the basic components of this system and then provide selected examples of how we and others have used genetically modified mouse models to gain a better understanding of this system and its role in regulating blood pressure.

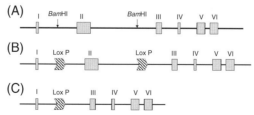

Fig. 13.3 Conditional knockout using Cre-Lox recombination. (A) Schematic representation of a hypothetical mouse gene containing six exons. (B) Schematic representation of the locus targeted to contain LoxP sites in introns A and B surrounding exon II. (C) Targeted mouse gene in which intervening sequences between LoxP sites have been deleted following Cre expression. Shaded boxes, exons of the mouse gene; hatched box arrows, LoxP sequences. Exon numbers are indicated by roman numerals above each exon.

According to classic dogma, renin – the rate limiting component of the RAS – is produced by the juxtaglomerular (JG) cells (modified smooth muscle cells lining the afferent arteriole near the glomerular hilus) in the kidney and is released into the bloodstream (Fig. 13.4). Here it cleaves AGT, produced by the liver, to form the decapeptide angiotensin I (Ang-I). Circulating Ang-I is subsequently further metabolized by ACE to produce the octapeptide angiotensin II (Ang-II). Ang-II is the primary active peptide of the RAS and interacts with Ang-II type 1 (AT_1) receptors throughout the body. Stimulation of AT_1 receptors results in arteriolar constriction, increased sodium reabsorption by directly stimulating the Na^+–H^+ exchanger in the proximal tubule and – indirectly – by enhancing sodium transport through the epithelial sodium channel via aldosterone. Ang-II also increases drinking response and increases vasopressin release and sympathetic outflow through its actions in the central nervous system. Ultimately, the effects of Ang-II result in increased arterial pressure and extracellular volume.

Ang-II is subsequently cleaved by aminopeptidases to form the heptapeptide angiotensin III (Ang-III) and the hexapeptide angiotensin IV (Ang-IV). Recent studies suggest that these peptides have important roles in cardiovascular regulation, in particular through their production in the brain.[13,14] The recent discovery of ACE-2, a carboxypeptidase that primarily hydrolyses Ang-II to form Ang-1-7, and a putative receptor for this peptide, provides support for the now long-held hypothesis that Ang-1-7 exerts actions that oppose those of Ang-II.[15,16]

MOUSE MODELS OF THE RAS

Systemic knockout of the RAS in mice

Using a gene knockout strategy, mice were generated in which the endogenous mouse angiotensinogen gene (*Agt*) was knocked out both heterozygously (*Agt$^{+/-}$*) or homozygously (*Agt$^{-/-}$*).[17,18] The Agt null genotype (*Agt$^{-/-}$*) was found to be compatible with survival until birth, but postnatal survival was markedly

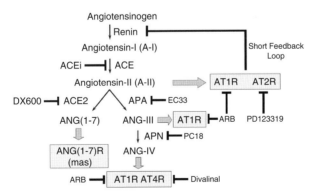

Fig. 13.4 The renin–angiotensin system. Extended pathway of the renin–angiotensin system is shown including receptors (shaded boxes) and the resultant peptides. Receptor blockers and enzyme inhibitors are also indicated. →, protien/peptide processing; ⇒, receptor binding; ⊤, inhibition; ACE, angiotensin converting enzyme; ACE2, angiotensin converting enzyme 2; ACEi, ACE inhibitors; ANG(1-7)R (mas), angiotensin 1-7 receptor; ANG-III, angiotensin III; ANG-IV, angiotensin IV; APA, aminopeptidase A; APN, aminopeptidase N; ARB, angiotensin II type 1 receptor blocker; AT1R, angiotensin II type 1 receptor; AT2R, angiotensin II type 2 receptor; AT4R, angiotensin type 4 receptor; DX600, ACE2 inhibitor; EC33, aminopeptidase A inhibitor; PC18, aminopeptidase N inhibitor; PD123319, angiotensin II type 2 receptor blocker.

reduced. Several renal abnormalities, including thinned cortices, medullary atrophy and medial thickening of arterial walls were present in $Agt^{-/-}$ mice, as well as imbalances in water and salt reabsorption. Additionally, $Agt^{-/-}$ mice were found to be hypotensive when compared to wild-type controls. Circulating mouse AGT was found to be reduced by about 65% in $Agt^{+/-}$ mice. $Agt^{+/-}$ were only moderately hypotensive, perhaps because circulating renin levels were elevated ~250% when compared to wild-type controls. One explanation suggests that a dynamic transcriptional feedback mechanism between various components of the RAS system exists, thereby ensuring physiologically regulated Ang-II production. Another explanation is an increase in the number of renin-expressing cells in states in which AGT (and Ang-II) are depleted, a hypothesis supported by physiological analysis of AGT-deficient mice and by recent gene-targeting experiments.[19,20]

Mice in which the *Ace* gene was knocked out ($Ace^{-/-}$) were severely hypotensive and showed renal abnormalities comparable to $Agt^{-/-}$ mice, strongly suggesting the renal abnormalities observed are due to either the absence of Ang-II, or the associated hypotension, rather than a lack of AGT *per se*.[21] Mice heterozygous for this knockout ($Ace^{+/-}$) had significantly reduced ACE levels but were normotensive. This finding indicates that ACE is unlikely to be the rate-limiting enzyme in the RAS cascade and supports previous findings of a positive feedback loop in the RAS in which a reduction in circulating ACE levels results in upregulation of renin transcription.

Most mammals, including humans, express two Ang-II receptor isoforms: type 1 (AT_1), expressed through the later stages of fetal development and throughout adult life, and type 2 (AT_2) expressed during early fetal development. Mice, however, express two AT_1 isoforms, each of which is encoded by distinct genes, termed AT_{1A} and AT_{1B}. These isoforms share 94% amino acid sequence homology and are both expressed throughout the cardiovascular system.[22,23] Studies of AT_{1A} knockout mice showed that expression of the AT_{1B} receptor was upregulated and that intracellular calcium signaling in renal vascular smooth muscle cells was comparable to that in cells obtained from wild-type animals.[24] These animals, however, had lower mean arterial pressure and an attenuated pressor response to Ang-II infusion when compared to wild-type animals, as well as impaired urinary concentrating ability.[25] Mice in which the AT_{1B} receptor was knocked out were, however, normotensive and responsiveness to Ang-II infusion did not differ from wild-type controls. Whereas mice containing either an AT_{1A} or AT_{1B} deficiency exhibited normal renal morphology, mice lacking both receptors exhibited renal lesions similar to those in *Agt*-deficient mice and the urinary concentrating defect was more severe in the double knockout mice than in mice lacking only the AT_{1A} receptor.[26] Taken together, these findings suggest that Ang-II signals primarily through the AT_{1A} receptor, but that there is a degree of redundancy allowing signaling through the AT_{1B} receptor in its absence.

The effect of AT_1 deficiency has also been studied in the brain. Central expression of AT_{1A} or AT_{1B} differentially responded to dehydration,[27] and an enhanced response to dehydration was observed in mice lacking the AT_{1A} receptor.[28] We were the first to report a potential divergence in the function of AT_{1A} or AT_{1B} receptors.[29] AT_{1A}-mediated signaling in the brain was essential for eliciting a pressor response to Ang-II, whereas stimulation of the AT_{1B} receptors was necessary for the dipsogenic response to Ang-II. As only one AT_1 receptor is found in humans, it has to be assumed that stimulation of this receptor would provoke both the pressor and drinking response.

The Mas receptor has been identified as the putative receptor for the vasodilatory peptide Ang-1-7.[16] In Mas receptor knockout mice, both the antidiuretic and vasodilatory effects of Ang-1-7 were abolished, indicating that Ang-1-7 is indeed an active peptide in the RAS and that its interaction with the Mas receptor results in both vasodilatation and antidiuresis.[16] Interestingly, however, Crackower et al reported that blood pressure remained normal in young mice lacking the *Ace2* gene but was reduced by 6 months of age.[30] This reduction was associated with hypoxia-induced cardiac hypocontractility (analogous to cardiac stunning and hibernation) and increased circulating Ang-II. This phenotype was completely abolished in mice in which both the *Ace* and *Ace2* genes were knocked out when compared to mice lacking only *Ace*.

Systemic overexpression of RAS in mice

In addition to generating Agt knockout mice, Smithies and coworkers also generated transgenic mice in which the endogenous mouse *Agt* gene was duplicated at the mouse *Agt* locus (using homologous recombination at the *Agt* locus).[17] Selective breeding between mice with the duplicated copy, $Agt^{+/-}$ mice and wild-type mice generated offspring in which the endogenous mouse *Agt* gene was either ablated ($Agt^{-/-}$), or present in one, two, three or four copies ($Agt^{+/-}$, $Agt^{+/+}$ (wt), $Agt^{++/+}$ or $Agt^{++/++}$). Studies on these animals revealed a nonlinear correlation between the *Agt* copy number and circulating AGT levels ($Agt^{-/-} = 0\%$; $Agt^{+/-} = 35\%$; $Agt^{+/+} = 100\%$, $Agt^{++/+} = 124\%$ and $Agt^{++/++} = 144\%$), but a linear relationship between *Agt* copy number and blood pressure (increase of about 8 mmHg per copy). This finding indicates that even though renin is generally accepted as the rate-limiting enzyme in the RAS, differences in *Agt* expression levels are sufficient to alter blood pressure (at least in mice). This could be relevant to human hypertension as altered expression levels of *hAGT* in humans have been reported to be associated with blood pressure and genetic variation of *hAGT*.[12] Moreover, some variants in the *hAGT* promoter might affect the level of AGT expression in tissues.[31,32] A number of models overexpressing *hAGT* using both its endogenous promoter and tissue-specific promoters have also been established.[33–35] These models will be discussed in detail below.

Numerous models overexpressing the human renin (*hREN*) gene have been reported, each differing in the extent of regulatory sequences employed in the construct. Transgenic mice containing relatively short extents of the *hREN* 5′ flanking region resulted in ectopic expression of the transgene, low JG cell transgene expression and poor regulation in response to physiological signals.[36] However, constructs with longer regulatory sequences were generally expressed in an appropriate tissue- and cell-specific manner and exhibited appropriate regulation.[4,37] For instance, we generated transgenic mice containing either 140 kb or 160 kb of human genomic DNA containing the *hREN* gene (designated PAC160 or PAC140 mice).[4] In these mice, *hREN* was spatially and temporally expressed, as was previously reported for endogenous renin expression, and it responded appropriately to physiological signals including plasma Ang-II, dietary sodium and blood pressure. We also recently reported that three genes neighboring renin in the human genome that are present on PAC160 are also coexpressed in the mice but exhibit very distinct tissue-specific expression profiles.[38]

Invariably, none of these models in which the *hREN* or *hAGT* transgene was overexpressed showed significant differences in arterial blood pressure as compared to nontransgenic controls. This observation supports the notion that there is a strict species-specific interaction between AGT and renin.[39] However, systemic infusion of human renin (hREN) into mice transgenically overexpressing *hATG* results in a transient elevation of arterial pressure.[33] In subsequent studies, mice overexpressing *hAGT* (A+ mice) were crossed with mice overexpressing either a poorly regulated *hREN* gene (termed R+) or a tightly regulated *hREN* transgene (PAC160) to generate double transgenic offspring. Baseline blood pressure in R+A+ and PAC160/A+ mice was found to be elevated by about 40 mmHg and 20 mmHg, respectively, when compared to either nontransgenic mice or single transgenic mice.[4,40] Blood pressure in these mice was normalized following administration of ACE inhibitors, indicative of the Ang-II dependence of the hypertensive phenotype in these mice. Subsequent studies have focused on some of the fundamental mechanisms controlling blood pressure in the R+A+ model. In short, hypertension in the R+A+ model is dependent on Ang-II action in the brain,[41] and the model exhibits severe endothelial dysfunction[42] and altered structure and function of cerebral arterioles.[43]

The functionality of the R+A+ model was confirmed by genetic complementation studies showing that the presence of both human genes can rescue defects observed in the AGT-deficient mice.[44] It is interesting to note that other complementation studies suggest that systemic or brain-specific RAS expression, but not kidney-specific expression is necessary for preventing the lethality associated with a defect in the RAS.[45,46]

Tissue-specific overexpression of RAS in mice: evidence for local RAS

That the RAS functions systemically as an endocrine system is unquestionable. However, the hypothesis that the system also has specific functions in individual tissues as a result of local Ang-II production continues to gain support. This notion of 'local RAS' was originally supported by the finding that many tissues, including brain, kidney, adrenal gland and the vasculature, all express essential components of a RAS. Mouse models have subsequently been used extensively and successfully to verify the existence of local RAS and have yielded invaluable information regarding their relative contribution in regulating blood pressure.

To establish whether extrarenal AGT is released into the circulating system, Stec et al[8] generated a transgenic mouse model in which the *hAGT* gene was specifically ablated in the liver in adult mice. Exon 2 of the *hAGT* transgene, containing the angiotensin precursor peptide and most of the angiotensinogen coding sequence, was flanked by LoxP sites ('floxed') (*hAGT(flox)*) and the liver-specific knockout was achieved through intravenous administration of an adenovirus containing Cre recombinase (Adcre). *hAGT* expression in the liver and systemic circulation were effectively ablated following Adcre infection, but there was no alteration in the expression of *hAGT* in other tissues. Circulating hAGT-levels 3-days post-Adcre infection were reduced to background levels, and intravenous hREN infusion 5-days post-Adcre infection failed to elicit a pressor response, effectively indicating the absence of hAGT in the circulation. Subsequently, hAGT(flox) mice were crossed with R+ mice to produce hypertensive double transgenic R+hAGT(flox) mice.[47] Adcre administration resulted in a significant reduction in blood pressure, which reached a peak at day 8 post-Adcre, after which blood pressure steadily increased back to the baseline. This increase in blood pressure correlated with a steady increase in circulating hAGT levels, presumably due to hepatocyte regeneration and a repopulation of the liver with hAGT-expressing cells. These findings indicate that most, if not all circulating AGT is liver-derived, and that extrahepatic AGT is unlikely to be secreted into the bloodstream.

Ding et al[34] generated a transgenic mouse model in which *hAGT* was expressed under control of the proximal convoluted tubule-specific kidney androgen-regulated promoter (KAP). This model is particularly useful for studying local kidney RAS, as AGT is endogenously expressed in proximal tubule cells and the level of transgene expression could be modulated in females by administering varying levels of androgen.[48] Mice in which *hAGT* expression was induced by testosterone, and which also expressed the *hREN* transgene systemically, exhibited hypertension.[49] The blood pressure was intermediate between wild-type mice and mice that express both the *hAGT* and *hREN* transgenes systemically. The finding that neither hAGT nor Ang-II level were elevated in the circulatory system clearly indicates that: (1) AGT synthesized in the kidney is not secreted into the circulatory system; and (2) a local kidney-specific RAS exists, which might be important in the regulation of blood pressure and, when unregulated, might cause hypertension. Mechanistically, it was speculated that proximal tubule AGT is secreted into the lumen of the proximal tubule through the apical membrane, and is converted to Ang-II that can then interact with luminal AT_1 receptors, resulting in activation of the Na^+–H^+ exchanger. Studies by a number of investigators support the regulated production of AGT[50] and the polarized secretion of AGT in proximal tubule cells.[51] Interestingly, the presence of renin has been reported in renal connecting tubule[52] and collecting duct,[53] and its targeted overexpression in proximal tubule causes a modest increase in blood pressure when bred with mice also expressing proximal tubule *hAGT*.[54]

Second to the kidney, the brain has received the greatest attention for its role in blood pressure regulation, the cardiovascular effects of direct administration of Ang-II, and the protective role of Ang-II receptor blockade in models of hypertension. Although there is no disputing the importance of Ang-II in the brain on blood pressure, its mechanism of synthesis remains controversial. It is well established that there is widespread expression of AGT in glial cells and recent evidence points to its focal expression in neurons.[55,56] Moreover, it has long been known that immunoreactive Ang-II can be detected in neuronal cell bodies and fibers throughout the CNS.[57] To further establish the identity of renin- and AGT-expressing cells in the brain, transgenic mouse models in which the *LacZ* and green fluorescent protein (*GFP*) reporter genes were driven by the *hAGT* and *hREN* promoters, respectively, were generated.[56,58] Expression of these reporter genes matched endogenous renin and AGT expression both spatially and temporally, and expression of GFP in the kidney was found to be responsive to physiological cues previously reported to alter renin expression, suggesting that these models could be successfully used to study renin and AGT expression in the CNS.[59] In subsequent experiments, mice expressing the *Ren-1-GFP* construct were crossed with mice expressing the *hAGT-LacZ* construct, thus generating double transgenic mice.[60] This study clearly showed the colocalization of GFP and β-gal (markers of renin and AGT expression, respectively) in adjacent cells in several brain regions, including rostral ventrolateral medulla (RVLM), subfornical organ (SFO), and the central nucleus of the amygdala. Additionally, it was found that individual neurons in the parabrachial nucleus (PB) and rostral ventrolateral medulla (RVLM) expressed both GFP and β-gal, implying that an intracellular RAS pathway may exist within this neural population. This possibility is further supported by the identification of a nonsecreted renin splice isoform in the brain.[61,62]

To establish whether 'local' brain RAS affects blood pressure, Morimoto and coworkers developed mouse models in which the *hAGT* and *hREN* genes were expressed under control of the astrocyte-specific glial fibrillary acidic protein (*GFAP*) promoter (GFAP-hAGT mice) and the neural-specific synapsin (*SYN*) promoter (SYN-hAGT mice), respectively.[35,63,64] Double transgenic models expressing both genes under *SYN* or *GFAP* promoter control exhibited a modest increase in blood pressure that was dependent on activation of central AT_1 receptors. They also exhibited a significant increase in baseline drinking and an increased appetite for salt.

STUDYING HUMAN GENETIC RISK FACTORS IN MICE

The genetics of angiotensinogen: a lesson in confusion

Over the last decade and a half, numerous studies have been undertaken to identify polymorphisms that convey a genetic predisposition to the development of essential hypertension in humans. Subsequent to their identification, many of these polymorphisms have been used in large-scale population-based case-control association studies. However, in nearly every case there are an equal number of studies refuting and supporting association with hypertension. A case in point is angiotensinogen.

Jeunemaitre et al[12] were the first to report linkage between the *hAGT* gene and hypertension in humans. An affected sibpair strategy was used to demonstrate linkage between a polymorphism of *hAGT* with elevated blood pressure in populations in Salt Lake City and Paris. Linkage was then independently verified in Caucasian European and African Caribbean populations.[65] Linkage between *hAGT* and pre-eclampsia was also reported,[66] however, linkage was *not* observed in a large European cohort.[67] A screen for variants in the *hAGT* gene revealed a number of polymorphisms in the 5′ flanking region, exons, and introns of the gene. Variant alleles of two of these (T174M and M235T) were found to be more prevalent in severely hypertensive cases than in controls and the 235T variant was more frequently identified in pre-eclamptic patients.[66] Over the past 10 years, the literature has become replete with contradictory reports arguing the importance of the 235T allele. Positive associations[68–72] and negative associations[65,73–76] have been reported for populations worldwide. The -6 polymorphism, which exists in strong linkage disequilibrium with the 235 polymorphism, was reported to play a minor role in blood pressure variation in the National Heart, Lung and Blood Institute (NHLBI) Family Blood Pressure Study.[77] Similarly, the frequency of the 235 TT genotype was more prevalent in some patients with diabetic nephropathy or IgA nephropathy than in others.[78–81] Positive and negative associations were reported in patients with coronary artery disease.[82,83] Therefore, like hypertension, there was no clear evidence supporting the importance of the 235T variant of *hAGT* in renal or coronary heart disease.

Nakajima et al identified 44 single nucleotide polymorphisms (SNPs) in the *hAGT* gene and assembled a comprehensive haplotype map of *hAGT* from both white and Japanese individuals.[84] Six major haplotypes of *hAGT* account for most of the variation in the *hAGT* gene, although the frequency of each differed substantially in the two populations. Chakravarti and colleagues generated a haplotype map of each gene in the RAS,[85] and then performed association studies with individual SNPs and haplotype blocks in African American and European American hypertensive populations.[86] Although a positive association was observed with several SNPs in *hAGT* (as with other genes in the RAS), there was no transmission distortion of any particular haplotype for *hAGT*, although positive results were obtained for haplotypes of the *hREN*, *ACE* and *AT₁* receptor genes.[86] Jeunemaitre identified five informative haplotypes of *hAGT* after stratification for the -6/T235 allele previously associated with hypertension.[87] Two of these haplotypes were associated with hypertension in Caucasian, but not Japanese, individuals.

Using mice to understand human genetic variation

The mice used for these types of studies are generated by one of two methods, both involving gene targeting. In the first, the endogenous mouse gene is 'humanized', i.e. modified to contain the analogs of the human polymorphism in question (Fig. 13.5). In the second, a human transgene is targeted to a specific locus in the mouse genome, such as the mouse hypoxantine phosphoribosyl transferase (*HPRT*) locus (Fig. 13.6). The major consideration to be taken into account when deciding which of these strategies to use is the degree of homology between the human and mouse genes and the number of variants and/or haplotypes to be tested.

The testing of a single SNP, or a set of SNPs, at a single position in a gene that is closely homologous across species would benefit from the first approach. Technically, the knockin approach is similar to the knockout approach described earlier in this chapter. In this case, however, instead of deleting an entire exon, the analog of the human polymorphism is introduced into the targeting construct by site-directed mutagenesis, and a floxed selectable marker is inserted into an adjacent intron (see Fig. 13.5). Chimeric mice are subsequently crossed

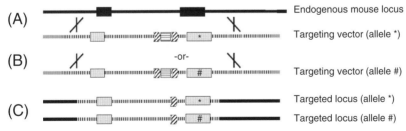

Fig. 13.5 Schematic illustration of gene targeting by knockin. (A) A simple two-exon mouse gene is shown as an example. Exons are in filled boxes. (B) Targeting vectors carry either the ˙ or # allele of interest. Homologous sequences are indicated by the vertically striped thick line and exons by the gray boxes. The positions of the ˙ or # allele in exon II are indicated. The selectable marker is indicated by a horizontal hatched box and LoxP sites by the crosshatched arrow. (C) The final targeted genome inserting either the ˙ or # allele is shown after Cre-mediated deletion of the selectable marker. The only difference between the final targeted genome and the starting genome is the insertion of the specific allele of interest and the presence of a single LoxP site in an intron.

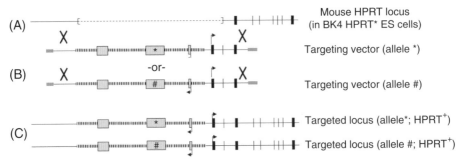

Fig. 13.6 Gene targeting at the hypoxantine phosphoribosyl transferase (HPRT) locus.
(A) Schematic representation of the HPRT locus in BK4 embryonic stem (ES) cells. The HPRT locus is disrupted and lacks several coding exons and the promoter region of the gene rendering the ES cells HPRT minus. This means they cannot grow on medium containing hypoxanthine, aminopterin, and thymidine (HAT). The disruption at HPRT is indicated by the [– – –]. (B) The targeting vectors have a number of important features. First, they carry the missing portion of the HPRT gene absent in BK4 ES cells along with homologous sequences necessary for homologous recombination. They also carry a hypothetical human gene carrying either the ˙ or # allele of interest. In this example, the human gene is oriented in the opposite direction (lower strand) than HPRT so that transcription of HPRT and the human gene will be in opposite directions. (C) Final targeted locus restoring the HPRT deficiency thus restoring growth of the targeted cells on HAT media. The human gene is inserted upstream and in the opposite orientation.

with mice expressing Cre-recombinase in the early embryo causing the deletion of the selectable marker, and thereby leaving only the analog of the human polymorphism and one intronic LoxP site as footprint. The major advantage of this approach is that the models generated closely resemble the human polymorphisms without having to introduce a foreign gene into the mouse genome, thereby maximizing the chances of small physiologically relevant changes being detected.

The second approach of inserting human gene variants into a known site of the mouse genome is best performed when the human and mouse genes are not particularly homologous or when multiple variants or haplotypes must be scored. As HPRT-targeting has been described in detail elsewhere,[88] we will only briefly describe the basic principles of this technique here. Like other gene targeting approaches, this method is also based on homologous recombination in ES cells. In this method, however, the human gene of interest is flanked by mouse DNA homologous to the mouse *HPRT* locus in a targeting construct (see Fig. 13.6). This construct is subsequently transformed into HPRT-deficient ES cells that are sensitive to growth in a special medium [hypoxanthine, aminopterin and thymidine (HAT) medium]. Successful homologous recombination results in both the insertion of the desired human gene at the *HPRT* locus and restoration of the mouse *HPRT* gene, allowing targeted ES cells to grow on the HAT medium. Transgenic mice are generated by blastocyst injection as previously described. The major advantages of this technique over traditional transgenic models are that: (1) only one copy of the transgene is inserted into the mouse genome; (2) all the insertions are targeted to the same location in the genome; and (3) direct comparisons can be made among constructs differing in haplotypes. The major disadvantages of HPRT-targeting are: (1) retention of the endogenous mouse gene, which could mask subtle allele-specific effects; (2) the sex-linked mode of inheritance caused by the presence of the *HPRT* locus on the X-chromosome; (3) random X-chromosome inactivation in females.

Human *AGT* polymorphisms

To investigate the functional significance of allelic variation in the *hAGT* gene, Chetkovic et al[89] used HPTR-targeting to introduce two of the most common human *AGT* haplotypes, namely -6a/235Thr (AT) and -6G/235Met (GM), into the mouse genome. In this study, HPRT-targeting – rather than a knockin approach – was followed because of a general lack of homology between the human and mouse *AGT* genes. There was no significant difference in the tissue- or cell-specific expression of the two haplotypes and no differences in circulating hAGT were detected. Mice expressing *hAGT*(AT) and *hAGT*(GM) were subsequently crossed with PAC160 mice expressing human renin to generate two PAC160/hAGT(AT) and PAC160/hAGT(GM) double transgenic mice.[90] Although phenotypic assessment revealed no alteration in blood pressure in females carrying either haplotype, there was a significant increase in blood pressure when double transgenic GM males were compared with their control littermates. A modest increase in heart rate was also noted in the GM males. It must, however, be noted that there was no significant difference in blood pressure between PAC160/hAGT(AT) and PAC160/hAGT(GM). Although these findings suggest that the AT and GM haplotypes are unlikely to result in hypertension in isolation, it is nevertheless possible that their phenotypic expression might become unmasked after exposure to certain environmental stressors, or in specific genetic backgrounds. Of course, it is possible that these polymorphisms might not have functional significance *per se*, but that they might be in linkage disequilibrium with other functional variants in *hAGT* or other closely linked genes.

CONCLUDING REMARKS

In this chapter we mention only a few selected examples in which gene targeting in mice has been used to study blood pressure regulation. There is no doubt that knockout and transgenic mouse models will remain an invaluable tool in delineating pathways involved in blood pressure regulation and their role in hypertension. Moreover, gene targeting might be a viable tool for understanding the physiological significance of genetic variation identified in humans and thus provide new insights into the complexities of the genetics of hypertension.

References

1. Gordon JW, Ruddle FH. Integration and stable germ line transmission of genes injected into mouse pronuclei. *Science* 1981; 214:1244–1246.
2. Sigmund CD. Manipulating genes to understand cardiovascular diseases: major approaches for introducing genes into cells. *Hypertension* 1993; 22:599–607.
3. Grosveld F, van Assendelft GB, Greaves DR, et al. Position-independent, high-level expression of the human beta-globin gene in transgenic mice. *Cell* 1987; 51:975–985.
4. Sinn PL, Davis DR, Sigmund CD. Highly regulated cell-type restricted expression of human renin in mice containing 140 kb or 160 kb P1 phage artificial chromosome transgenes. *J Biol Chem* 1999; 274:35785–35793.
5. Capecchi MR. Altering the genome by homologous recombination. *Science* 1989; 244:1288–1292.
6. Bronson SK, Smithies O. Altering mice by homologous recombination using embryonic stem cells. *J Biol Chem* 1994; 269:27155–27158.

7. Kilby NJ, Snaith MR, Murray JAH. Site-specific recombinases: tools for genome engineering. *Trends Genet* 1994; 9:413–421.

8. Stec DE, Davisson RL, Haskell RE, et al. Efficient liver-specific deletion of a floxed human angiotensinogen transgene by adenoviral delivery of cre-recombinase in vivo. *J Biol Chem* 1999; 274:21285–21290.

9. Sinnayah P, Lindley TE, Staber PD, et al. Targeted viral delivery of Cre recombinase induces conditional gene deletion in cardiovascular circuits of the mouse brain. *Physiol Genomics* 2004; 18:25–32.

10. Tsien JZ, Chen DF, Gerber D, et al. Subregion- and cell type-restricted gene knockout in mouse brain. *Cell* 1996; 87:1317–1326.

11. Feil R, Brocard J, Mascrez B, et al. Ligand-activated site-specific recombination in mice. *Proc Natl Acad Sci U S A* 1996; 93:10887–10890.

12. Jeunemaitre X, Soubrier F, Kotelevtsev YV, et al. Molecular basis of human hypertension: role of angiotensinogen. *Cell* 1992; 71:169–180.

13. Zini S, Fournie-Zaluski MC, Chauvel E, et al. Identification of metabolic pathways of brain angiotensin II and III using specific aminopeptidase inhibitors: Predominant role of angiotensin III in the control of vasopressin release. *Proc Nat Acad Sci U S A* 1996; 93:11968–11973.

14. Wright JW, Tamura-Myers E, Wilson WL, et al. Conversion of brain angiotensin II to angiotensin III is critical for pressor response in rats. *Am J Physiol Regul Integr Comp Physiol* 2003; 284:R725–R733.

15. Donoghue M, Hsieh F, Baronas E, et al. A novel angiotensin-converting enzyme-related carboxypeptidase (ACE2) converts angiotensin I to angiotensin 1-9. *Circ Res* 2000; 87:E1–E9.

16. Santos RA, Simoes e Silva AC, Maric C, et al. Angiotensin 1-7 is an endogenous ligand for the G protein-coupled receptor Mas. *Proc Natl Acad Sci U S A* 2003; 100:8258–8263.

17. Smithies O, Kim H-S. Targeted gene duplication and disruption for analyzing quantitative genetic traits in mice. *Proc Natl Acad Sci U S A* 1994; 91:3612–3615.

18. Kim HS, Krege JH, Kluckman KD, et al. Genetic control of blood pressure and the angiotensinogen locus. *Proc Natl Acad Sci U S A* 1995; 92:2735–2739.

19. Kim HS, Maeda N, Oh GT, et al. Homeostasis in mice with genetically decreased angiotensinogen is primarily by an increased number of renin-producing cells. *J Biol Chem* 1999; 274:14210–14217.

20. Sequeira Lopez ML, Pentz ES, Nomasa T, et al. Renin cells are precursors for multiple cell types that switch to the renin phenotype when homeostasis is threatened. *Dev Cell* 2004; 6:719–728.

21. Esther CR, Jr., Howard TE, Marino EM, et al. Mice lacking angiotensin-converting enzyme have low blood pressure, renal pathology, and reduced male fertility. *Lab Invest* 1996; 74:953–965.

22. Burson JM, Aguilera G, Gross KW, et al. Differential expression of angiotensin receptor 1A and 1B in mouse. *Am J Physiol* 1994; 267:E260–E267.

23. Johren O, Inagami T, Saavedra JM. AT1A, AT1B and AT2 angiotensin II receptor subtypes in rat brain. *Neuroreport* 1995; 6:2549–2552.

24. Zhu Z, Zhang SH, Wagner C, et al. Angiotensin AT1B receptor mediates calcium signaling in vascular smooth muscle cells of AT1A receptor-deficient mice. *Hypertension* 1998; 31:1171–1177.

25. Oliverio MI, Best CF, Kim H-S, et al. Angiotensin II responses in AT1A-receptor deficient mice: A role for AT1B receptors in blood pressure regulation. *Am J Physiol Renal Physiol* 1997; 272:F515–F520.

26. Oliverio MI, Kim HS, Ito M, et al. Reduced growth, abnormal kidney structure, and type 2 (AT2) angiotensin receptor-mediated blood pressure regulation in mice lacking both AT1A and AT1B receptors for angiotensin II. *Proc Natl Acad Sci U S A* 1998; 95:15496–15501.

27. Chen Y, Morris M. Differentiation of brain angiotensin type 1a and 1b receptor mRNAs: a specific effect of dehydration. *Hypertension* 2001; 37:692–697.

28. Morris M, Means S, Oliverio MI, et al. Enhanced central response to dehydration in mice lacking angiotensin AT(1a) receptors. *Am J Physiol Regul Integr Comp Physiol* 2001; 280:R1177–R1184.

29. Davisson RL, Oliverio MI, Coffman TM, et al. Divergent functions of angiotensin II receptor isoforms in brain. *J Clin Invest* 2000; 106:103–106.

30. Crackower MA, Sarao R, Oudit GY, et al. Angiotensin-converting enzyme 2 is an essential regulator of heart function. *Nature* 2002; 417:822–828.

31. Morgan T, Craven C, Nelson L, et al. Angiotensinogen T235 expression is elevated in decidual spiral arteries. *J Clin Invest* 1997; 100:1406–1415.

32. Inoue I, Nakajima T, Williams CS, et al. A nucleotide substitution in the promoter of human angiotensinogen is associated with essential hypertension and affects basal transcription in vitro. *J Clin Invest* 1997; 99:1786–1797.

33. Yang G, Merrill DC, Thompson MW, et al. Functional expression of the human angiotensinogen gene in transgenic mice. *J Biol Chem* 1994; 269:32497–32502.

34. Ding Y, Davisson RL, Hardy DO, et al. The kidney androgen-regulated protein (KAP) promoter confers renal proximal tubule cell-specific and highly androgen-responsive expression on the human angiotensinogen gene in transgenic mice. *J Biol Chem* 1997; 272:28142–28148.

35. Morimoto S, Cassell MD, Sigmund CD. Glial- and neuronal-specific expression of the renin-angiotensin system in brain alters blood pressure, water intake, and salt preference. *J Biol Chem* 2002; 277:33235–33241.

36. Sigmund CD, Jones CA, Kane CM, et al. Regulated tissue- and cell-specific expression of the human renin gene in transgenic mice. *Circ Res* 1992; 70:1070–1079.

37. Yan Y, Hu LF, Chen RP, et al. Appropriate regulation of human renin gene expression and secretion in 45-kb human renin transgenic mice. *Hypertension* 1998; 32:205–214.

38. Nistala R, Zhang X, Sigmund CD. Differential expression of the closely linked KISS1, REN, and FLJ10761 genes in transgenic mice. *Physiol Genomics* 2004; 17:4-10.

39. Hatae T, Takimoto E, Murakami K, et al. Comparative studies on species-specific reactivity between renin and angiotensinogen. *Mol Cell Biochem* 1994; 131:43–47.

40. Merrill DC, Thompson MW, Carney C, et al. Chronic hypertension and altered baroreflex responses in transgenic mice containing the human renin and human angiotensinogen genes. *J Clin Invest* 1996; 97:1047–1055.

41. Davisson RL, Yang G, Beltz TG, et al. The brain renin–angiotensin system contributes to the hypertension in mice containing both the human renin and human angiotensinogen transgenes. *Circ Res* 1998; 83:1047–1058.

42. Didion SP, Sigmund CD, Faraci FM. Impaired endothelial function in transgenic mice expressing both human renin and human angiotensinogen. *Stroke* 2000; 31:760–764.

43. Baumbach GL, Sigmund CD, Faraci FM. Cerebral arteriolar structure in mice overexpressing human renin and angiotensinogen. *Hypertension* 2003; 41:50–55.

44. Davisson RL, Kim HS, Krege JH, et al. Complementation of reduced survival, hypotension and renal abnormalities in angiotensinogen deficient mice by the human renin and human angiotensinogen genes. *J Clin Invest* 1997; 99:1258–1264.

45. Lochard N, Silversides DW, Van Kats JP, et al. Brain-specific restoration of angiotensin II corrects renal defects seen in angiotensinogen-deficient mice. *J Biol Chem* 2003; 278(4): 2184–2189.

46. Ding Y, Stec DE, Sigmund CD. Genetic evidence that lethality in angiotensinogen-deficient mice is due to loss of systemic but not renal angiotensinogen. *J Biol Chem* 2001; 276:7431–7436.

47. Stec DE, Keen HL, Sigmund CD. Lower blood pressure in floxed angiotensinogen mice after adenoviral delivery of cre-recombinase. *Hypertension* 2002; 39:629–633.

48. Ding Y, Sigmund CD. Androgen-dependent regulation of human angiotensinogen expression in KAP-hAGT transgenic mice. *Am J Physiol Renal Physiol* 2001; 280:F54–F60.

49. Davisson RL, Ding Y, Stec DE, et al. Novel mechanism of hypertension revealed by cell-specific targeting of human angiotensinogen in transgenic mice. *Physiol Genomics* 1999; 1:3–9.

50. Kobori H, Harrison-Bernard LM, Navar LG. Enhancement of angiotensinogen expression in angiotensin II-dependent hypertension. *Hypertension* 2001; 37:1329–1335.

51. Loghman-Adham M, Rohrwasser A, Helin C, et al. A conditionally immortalized cell line from murine proximal tubule. *Kidney Int* 1997; 52:229–239.

52. Rohrwasser A, Morgan T, Dillon HF, et al. Elements of a paracrine tubular renin-angiotensin system along the entire nephron. *Hypertension* 1999; 34:1265–1274.

53. Prieto-Carrasquero MC, Harrison-Bernard LM, Kobori H, et al. Enhancement of collecting duct renin in angiotensin II-dependent hypertensive rats. *Hypertension* 2004; 44:223–229.

54. Lavoie JL, Lake-Bruse KD, Sigmund CD. Increased blood pressure in transgenic mice expressing both human renin and angiotensinogen in the renal proximal tubule. *Am J Physiol Renal Physiol* 2004; 286(5):F965–F971.

55. Stornetta RL, Hawelu Johnson CL, Guyenet PG, et al. Astrocytes synthesize angiotensinogen in brain. *Science* 1988; 242:1444–1446.

56. Yang G, Gray TS, Sigmund CD, et al. The angiotensinogen gene is expressed in both astrocytes and neurons in murine central nervous system. *Brain Res* 1999; 817:123–131.

57. Lind RW, Swanson LW, Ganten D. Organization of angiotensin II immunoreactive cells and fibers in the rat central nervous system. An immunohistochemical study. *Neuroendocrinology* 1985; 40:2–24.

58. Jones CA, Hurley MI, Black TA, et al. Expression of a renin-green fluorescent protein transgene in mouse embryonic, extra-embryonic and adult tissues. *Physiol Genomics* 2000; 4:75–81.

59. Lavoie JL, Cassell MD, Gross KW, et al. Localization of rennin-expressing cells in the brain using a REN-eGFP transgenic model. *Physiol Genomics* 2004; 16:240–246.

60. Lavoie JL, Cassell MD, Gross KW, et al. Adjacent expression of renin and angiotensinogen in the rostral ventrolateral medulla using a dual-reporter transgenic model. *Hypertension* 2004; 43:1116–1119.

61. Sinn PL, Sigmund CD. Identification of three human renin mRNA isoforms resulting from alternative tissue-specific transcriptional initiation. *Physiol Genomics* 2000; 3:25–31.

62. Lee-Kirsch MA, Gaudet F, Cardoso MC, et al. Distinct renin isoforms generated by tissue-specific transcription initiation and alternative splicing. *Circ Res* 1999; 84:240–246.
63. Morimoto S, Cassell MD, Beltz TG, et al. Elevated blood pressure in transgenic mice with brain-specific expression of human angiotensinogen driven by the glial fibrillary acidic protein promoter. *Circ Res* 2001; 89:365–372.
64. Morimoto S, Cassell MD, Sigmund CD. Neuron-specific expression of human angiotensinogen in brain causes increased salt appetite. *Physiol Genomics* 2002; 9:113–120.
65. Caulfield M, Lavender P, Farrall M, et al. Linkage of the angiotensinogen gene to essential hypertension. *N Engl J Med* 1994; 330:1629-1633.
66. Ward K, Hata A, Jeunemaitre X, et al. A molecular variant of angiotensinogen associated with preeclampsia. *Nat Genet* 1993; 4:59–61.
67. Brand E, Chatelain N, Keavney B, et al. Evaluation of the angiotensinogen locus in human essential hypertension: a European study. *Hypertension* 1998; 31:725–729.
68. Jeunemaitre X, Inoue I, Williams C, et al. Haplotypes of angiotensinogen in essential hypertension. *Am J Hum Genet* 1997; 60:1448–1460.
69. Hegele RA, Brunt JH, Connelly PW. A polymorphism of the angiotensinogen gene associated with variation in blood pressure in a genetic isolate. *Circulation* 1994; 90:2207–2212.
70. Hegele RA, Harris SB, Hanley AJ, et al. Angiotensinogen gene variation associated with variation in blood pressure in aboriginal Canadians. *Hypertension* 1997; 29:1073–1077.
71. Hata A, Namikawa C, Sasaki M, et al. Angiotensinogen as a risk factor for essential hypertension in Japan. *J Clin Invest* 1994; 93:1285–1287.
72. Kamitani A, Rakugi H, Higaki J, et al. Association analysis of a polymorphism of the angiotensinogen gene with essential hypertension in Japanese. *J Hum Hypertens* 1994; 8:521–524.
73. Bloem LJ, Manatunga AK, Tewksbury DA, et al. The serum angiotensinogen concentration and variants of the angiotensinogen gene in white and black children. *J Clin Invest* 1995; 95:948–953.
74. Hingorani AD, Sharma P, Jia H, et al. Blood pressure and the M235T polymorphism of the angiotensinogen gene. *Hypertension* 1996; 28:907–911.
75. Fornage M, Turner ST, Sing CF, et al. Variation at the M235T locus of the angiotensinogen gene and essential hypertension: A population-based case-control study from Rochester, Minnesota. *Hum Genetics* 1995; 96:295–300.
76. Rotimi C, Morrison L, Cooper R, et al. Angiotensinogen gene in human hypertension: lack of an association of the 235T allele among African Americans. *Hypertension* 1994; 24:591–594.
77. Province MA, Boerwinkle E, Chakravarti A, et al. Lack of association of the angiotensinogen-6 polymorphism with blood pressure levels in the comprehensive NHLBI Family Blood Pressure Program. National Heart, Lung and Blood Institute. *J Hypertens* 2000; 18:867–876.
78. Fogarty DG, Harron JC, Hughes AE, et al. A molecular variant of angiotensinogen is associated with diabetic nephropathy in IDDM. *Diabetes* 1996; 45:1204–1208.
79. Pei Y, Scholey J, Thai K, et al. Association of angiotensinogen gene T235 variant with progression of immunoglobin A nephropathy in Caucasian patients. *J Clin Invest* 1997; 100:814–820.
80. Marre M, Jeunemaitre X, Gallois Y, et al. Contribution of genetic polymorphism in the renin-angiotensin system to the development of renal complications in insulin-dependent diabetes. *J Clin Invest* 1997; 99:1585–1595.
81. Tarnow L, Cambien F, Rossing P, et al. Angiotensinogen gene polymorphisms in IDDM patients with diabetic nephropathy. *Diabetes* 1996; 45:367–369.
82. Katsuya T, Koike G, Yee TW, et al. Association of angiotensinogen gene T235 variant with increased risk of coronary heart disease. *Lancet* 1995; 345:1600–1603.
83. Ichihara S, Yokota M, Fujimura T, et al. Lack of association between variants of the angiotensinogen gene and the risk of coronary artery disease in middle-aged Japanese men. *Am Heart J* 1997; 134:260–265.
84. Nakajima T, Jorde LB, Ishigami T, et al. Nucleotide diversity and haplotype structure of the human angiotensinogen gene in two populations. *Am J Hum Genet* 2002; 70:108–123.
85. Zhu X, Yan D, Cooper RS, et al. Linkage disequilibrium and haplotype diversity in the genes of the renin–angiotensin system: findings from the family blood pressure program. *Genome Res* 2003; 13:173–181.
86. Zhu X, Chang YP, Yan D, et al. Associations between hypertension and genes in the renin-angiotensin system. *Hypertension* 2003; 41:1027–1034.
87. Jeunemaitre X, Inoue I, Williams C, et al. Haplotypes of angiotensinogen in essential hypertension. *Am J Hum Genet* 1997; 60:1448–1460.
88. Bronson SK, Plaehn EG, Kluckman KD, et al. Single-copy transgenic mice with chosen-site integration. *Proc Natl Acad Sci U S A* 1996; 93:9067–9072.
89. Chetkovic B, Yang B, Williamson RA, et al. Appropriate tissue- and cell-specific expression of a single copy human angiotensinogen transgene specifically targeted upstream of the HPRT locus by homologous recombination. *J Biol Chem* 2000; 275:1073–1078.
90. Chetkovic B, Keen HL, Davis DR, et al. Physiological significance of two common haplotypes of human angiotensinogen using gene targeting in the mouse. *Physiol Genomics* 2002; 11:253–262.

14 | Gene therapy for hypertension: a promise waiting to be fulfilled

M. Ian Phillips and Y. Clare Zhang

INTRODUCTION

Despite decades of research on the physiological and molecular mechanisms regulating blood pressure, we do not know precisely the genes that cause hypertension. Numerous genomic studies using linkage and association analyses or family genetics have failed to correlate genes to hypertension except in those very rare cases of single gene mutations. Lifton et al have extensively studied hypertension due to single mutations.[1] However, because these occur in extremely rare forms of hypertension, they are not targets for treating hypertension at large. When we first proposed that hypertension could be treated with gene therapy,[2] a number of questions were raised, one of which was: 'How can we have a gene therapy when we don't know which genes are involved?' The short answer is that we target the genes that produce proteins that have been targeted by the drug industry for many years. Beta-blockers target beta-adrenergic receptors. Angiotensin-converting enzyme (ACE) inhibitors target angiotensin-converting enzyme. Angiotensin receptor blockers (ARBs) inhibit angiotensin type1 receptors. All of these drugs are very effective for drug treatment of hypertension, so these proteins and the DNA and RNA that produce them are among the first targets for gene therapy. Thanks to years of pharmaceutical use we have so much clinical experience with short-term inhibition of these proteins that a gene-therapy approach to these targets is appropriate even without knowing which genes cause hypertension. Gene therapy that provides highly specific, long-term inhibition of the same proteins should be even more efficacious and, because of the precise specificity, there should be fewer side effects. The currently available beta-blockers are small-molecule drugs that are either nonspecific or selective for beta-adrenergic receptors (AR). None is specific, yet it is the beta-1 receptor that needs to be inhibited to lower blood pressure. The crossover of blockade of beta-1 and beta-2 with beta-AR blockers leads to side effects and, as they cross the blood–brain barrier (BBB), they induce side effects such as sleep disturbance and sexual impotence. Antisense gene therapy with beta-1 antisense oligonucleotides is highly specific and inhibits only the beta-1 receptor, leaving the beta-2 receptor active.[3] Recently, we have also developed a highly specific, small interfering RNA (siRNA), which silences beta-1 ARs and does not inhibit beta-2 ARs The specific gene-based inhibitors – antisense or siRNA – reduce some of the side effects such as bradycardia. Further, as antisense oligos do not cross the BBB, they lack a central effect unless injected directly into the brain. Therefore, if beta 1 antisense therapy were developed, we would predict that there would not be the central side effects, such as impotence and intolerable dreams, that are contraindicated with current beta-blockers.

The gene therapy that we have proposed for hypertension is not a cure: it is a treatment aimed at producing far better rates of control of high blood pressure than are presently achieved by a daily regimen of drugs. Poor compliance with drug treatments is related to the fact that patients have to take antihypertensive pills daily and because they fail to maintain their prescription. Patients change their drug choice because of side effects. As a result of these and other factors, nearly three-quarters of people with hypertension do not have control of their high blood pressure. Gene therapy could not only provide long-lasting therapy, it could also avoid the peaks and troughs of high blood pressure control that occur with drugs. Even when compliant, hypertensive patients – some with a high risk for heart failure – generally take their pills at around 8 a.m. Because of the rising blood pressure in the waking hours, and because 24 hours after taking the pill the antihypertensive effect has worn off or is minimal, they are at their least protected from heart attacks at this time of day. Gene therapy could provide constant blood pressure control throughout weeks or months and we would therefore predict a decrease in heart attacks and stroke as a further benefit of gene therapy.

So why has gene therapy not taken off? Gene therapy is a promise still waiting to be fulfilled. Huge setbacks have come from deaths in early clinical trials of gene therapy applied to other diseases. The rush to test some gene therapies in patients who had not been thoroughly tested preclinically has tarnished all gene therapy approaches, even those with real possibilities of being viable treatments. There is, to date, no real gene therapy in practice. The case of 17-year-old Jesse Gelsinger is a tragic milestone that has been widely discussed.[4] Mr Gelsinger had volunteered to be in a Phase I trial at the University of Pennsylvania to test a gene delivered by the adenovirus vector. The vector killed him; the adenovirus produced numerous proteins, which activate the immune system, and Mr Gelsinger responded to the adenovirus with a multiple organ system inflammation and died. There are many implications of this failure – moral, ethical and scientific. Many feel that the trial should not have used adenovirus; others argue that Mr Gelsinger was prone to inflammatory response and should not have been included in the trial.

Another gene therapy trial, in France, with a retrovirus used to treat severe combined immunodeficiency disease (SCID) in children, has also resulted in deaths.[5] Three treated children were reported to develop leukemia and one died due to random integration of retrovirus in genome and consequent disruption of genes that control cell proliferation. Again, ethical questions have been raised. Were the benefits greater than the risks? In the case of SCID the outcome is death. Therefore when some children were cured of SCID but developed leukemia as a result of the therapy there was a basic ethical dilemma. However, despite the bad press, some gene therapy trials with vectors are progressing without such negative outcomes. Trials with adeno-associated virus (AAV) are proceeding for alpha trypsin 1 and cystic fibrosis.[6,7] AAV is the vector we have studied preclinically for long-term control of blood pressure.[8] Although we proposed using antisense by delivering DNA in the antisense orientation in AAV, trials with antisense inhibitors do not need to involve vectors. Antisense oligonucleotides (AS ODNs) have been tested in over 20 Phase II and III trials without serious side effects and one therapy based on antisense is Food and Drug Administration (FDA) approved and has been in use for several years. However, antisense inhibition, despite its early promise, has not been widely successful. Most of the 20 or more trials that have been completed failed to show large-enough statistical improvement to warrant adoption as an alternative therapy. In our view, a major reason for this is that antisense oligonucleotides have been targeting genes involved in cancer. Antisense is a competitive inhibitor of RNA and does not produce complete inhibition of mRNA. Therefore they are not a good choice for killing cancer cells. Indeed, some of the trials have sought only to make anticancer drugs more effective by combining antisense inhibition. The rise of RNA inhibition with siRNA as a gene silencer has boosted the hope that an RNA therapy is possible. However, for treating hypertension, AS ODNs do not have to silence mRNA; they have only to dampen the overproduction of gene targets mentioned above. Therefore we continue to have hope for a gene therapy that could be used to treat hypertension better than current drugs

The drugs available for the treatment of hypertension are very good if they are taken daily as prescribed .But many of the antihypertensive drugs are expensive, and therefore unavailable to poorer segments of all societies. Another problem is that hypertension is undetected in about 40% of the population of the United States, according to the NHANES III Report.[9] Of the 60% in whom hypertension has been detected, only about half receive treatment. The problem is further confounded because it is estimated that only 27% of those treated fully comply with their treatment and have their hypertension controlled.[9] Clearly, there is a need for rethinking our approach to the treatment of hypertension. Detection can be increased by education. Nonpharmacological treatment, such as exercise, weight loss and low-salt diets could provide inexpensive treatment but it has proved very difficult to achieve good compliance for these approaches. For treating hypertension on a world scale, we need something akin to an immunization against hypertension. As hypertension is polygenic and not a single-gene disease (except in very few cases[10]) immunization cannot be used. We need to develop ways that would improve hypertension control by providing longer-lasting effects with a single dose and reducing side effects that lead to poor compliance. To do this, we began developing a somatic gene therapy approach in 1993,[11,12] with the goal of producing prolonged control of hypertension. Two strategies have been taken. One by Chao and colleagues[13] to express genes for vasodilation, and the other by Phillips and colleagues to decrease genes for vasoconstriction.[12] They represent the two sides to transferring DNA into cells, one is the sense approach, i.e. the normal DNA sequence direction, and the other is the antisense approach, i.e. the opposite DNA sequence direction.

SENSE TO VASODILATION GENES

Chao et al have an extensive series of studies on gene transfer to genes that act to increase vasodilator proteins (Table 14.1). They have used genes such as kallikrein,[13] atrial natriuretic peptide,[14] adrenomedullin[15] and endothelial nitric

Table 14.1 Preclinical data of gene therapy for hypertension vasodilator genes

Target gene	Delivery	Model	Max Δ blood pressure (mmHg)	Duration of effect	Reference
Human tissue Kallikrein	Adenovirus	Dahl salt-sensitive		4 weeks	Chao et al 1997[13]
		5/6 renal mass	−37	5 weeks	Wolf et al 2000[42]
		SHR	−30	36 days	
	Adenovirus intramuscular	SHR		5 weeks	Zhang et al 1999[43]
		2K-1C	−26	24 days	
	Adenovirus iv	Doca-salt		23 days	Dobrzynski et al 1999[17]
Adreno-medullin	Adenovirus	Doca-salt	−41	9 days	Dobrzynski et al 2000[28]
	iv	SHR		4 weeks	Chao et al 1997[15]
	iv	Dahl salt-sensitive			Zhang et al 2000[43]
Atrial natriuretic peptide (ANP)	Adenovirus	Dahl salt-sensitive	−32	5 weeks	Lin et al 1977[14]
Nitric oxide	Plasmid	SHR	−21	5-6 weeks (lst injection) 10-12 weeks (2nd injection)	Lin et al 1997[16]

AAV, adeno-associated virus; ACE, angiotensin-converting enzyme; AGT, angiotensinogen; AS-ODN, antisense oligodeoxynucleotide; AT1-R, angiotensin type 1 receptor; CIH, cold-induced hypertension; iv, intravenous; LNSV, retrovirus; SHR, spontaneously hypertensive rat.

oxide synthase.[16] In different rat models of hypertension [spontaneously hypertensive rats (SHR), Dahl salt-sensitive, Doca-salt] they showed that they could achieve blood pressure lowering effects for 3–12 weeks with the overexpression of these genes. The fall in pressure resulting from these vasodilator proteins was from −21 to −41 mmHg. The results of this group are consistent and impressive. Even though the effects were not very prolonged, there were reductions in end-organ damage with these therapies.[17] However, the use of adenovirus limits the possibility of translating these strategies to humans. The use of plasmids, however, had very prolonged effects in their hands.

ANTISENSE TO VASOCONSTRICTOR GENES

To counter overexpression of a gene as a critical factor contributing to hypertension, we introduced antisense somatic gene therapy. Antisense provides a highly specific, biological approach to produce attenuation of the sense DNA expression that produces too much protein, e.g. angiotensin II (Ang II), which is responsible for increased vasoconstriction. Antisense gene therapy involves recombinant antisense DNA to express an antisense mRNA or antisense oligonucleotides to inhibit mRNA designed to specifically reduce an overexpressed protein that is critical to the disease. As hypertension is a multigene disease, how can we decide on the candidate genes for gene therapy? We have ignored the difficulties of defining all the candidate genes by concentrating on the genes that have already been shown to be successful targets by the experience with current drugs. These include beta-receptors,[10,11] ACE,[21,22] and angiotensin type 1 receptor (AT$_1$-R).[23] Other targets follow logically, including angiotensinogen (AGT).[21] Transfer of the antisense genes to somatic cells is achieved by an *in vivo* approach. It would be possible to try an *ex vivo* approach in which target cells are removed from the host, transduced *in vivo* and then reimplanted as genetically modified cells. However, this strategy has no obvious applicability to hypertension, where the cause of the disease lies in the reaction of blood vessels that are not in one specific tissue (although the heart, kidney and brain are obviously very important in hypertension). The *in vivo* approach is challenging. One challenge is to provide sufficient antisense DNA, either alone or in a vector, to produce a sufficient concentration for uptake in a large number of cells. To do this we have developed two different strategies for hypertension gene therapy based on antisense with: (1) antisense oligonucleotides (Table 14.2); and (2) viral vectors to deliver antisense DNA (Table 14.3).

NONVIRAL DELIVERY

Antisense oligonucleotides

Antisense oligonucleotides are short lengths of synthetically made nucleotides (DNA) designed to hybridize with a specific sequence of mRNA. The hybridization can have differing effects: it can stimulate RNAase H, or sterically inhibit the mRNA from translating its message in the readthrough process at the ribosome, or both.

Delivery of antisense oligodeoxynucleotides (AS-ODNs) can be carried out with direct injection of 'naked DNA'. We have found that direct injection is effective, but the efficiency of uptake is greatly increased by delivering the ODN in cationic liposomes, provided the correct ratio has been calculated.[18]

Beta-1-adrenoceptor antisense

Nonviral gene delivery, using cationic liposomes such as DOTAP and DOPE, has been successfully used by our group to deliver β_1 adrenoceptor antisense oligonucleotides (β_1-AR-AS-ODN) to act as novel beta-blockers with prolonged effects.[18,19] By optimizing the liposome : ODN ratio and the incubation procedure, we are able to produce antihypertensive effects with β_1-AS-ODN for 33–40 days with a single dose.[19] The beauty of the β_1-AS-ODN is its specificity. The β_1-AS-ODN reduces β_1-adrenoceptors but does not affect β_2-adrenoceptors. Also, the β_1-AS-ODN does not cross the BBB and therefore the novel β_1 blocker, based on antisense, will have no central nervous system side effects. The strongest uptake sites are in the heart and kidney, where the β_1-adrenoceptors play a significant role. In the heart they control the force of contraction and this is reduced by the β_1-adrenoceptor. However, the heart rate is not affected by the β_1-AS-ODN.[11] This is in contrast to the effects of currently available beta-blockers that have both β_1 and β_2 actions and which reduce heart rate as well as heart contractility. Therefore, the specificity offered by the ODN provides a more precise and accurate way of controlling the mechanisms contributing to high blood pressure without the side effects of bradycardia.[18] Furthermore, since the effect lasts for 30–40 days with a single injection, the antisense ODN is greatly superior

Table 14.2 Preclinical data of gene therapy for hypertension vasoconstrictor genes: antisense oligodeoxynucleotides

Target gene	Delivery	Model	Max Δ blood pressure (mmHg)	Duration of effect	Reference
AT1-R	AS-ODN icv	SHR	−30	Unknown	Gyurko et al 1993[11]
AGT	AS-ODN icv	SHR	−35	Unknown	Phillips et al 1994[12]
AT1-R	AS-ODN pvn microinjection	MRen2	−24	4 days	Li et al 1997[26]
Thyrotropin-releasing hormone	AS-ODN intrathecal	SHR	−38	Unknown	Suzuki et al 1994[41]
Angiotensin-gene activating elements	AS-ODN portal vein	SHR SHR	−20 −28	6 days 7 days	Morishita et al 1996[38]
Carboxy-peptidase Y	AS-ODN HJV liposome	Doca-salt	−15	4 days	Hyashi et al[47]
c-fos	AS-ODN microinjection in RVLM	WKY SD	−16 −17	4–6 hours Unknown	Suzuki et al 1994[41]
CYP4A1	AS-ODN continuous Infusion	SHR	16	Unknown	Wang et al 2001[44]
AGT	AS-ODN iv	SHR	−25	Unknown	Wielbo et al 1996[21]
AGT	AS-ODN hepatic vein HJV-liposome	SHR	−20	4 days	Tomita et al 1995[45]
AT1-R	AS-ODN icv	SHR	−30	7 days	Gyurko et al 1997[23]
AGT	AS-ODN with asialoglyco-protein iv	SHR	−30	7 days	Makino et al 1998[22]
AT1-R	AS-ODN iv	2K-1C acute	−30	> 7 days	Galli et al 2001[46]
AT1-R	AS-ODN icv	2K-1C 6 months	−30	> 5 days	Kagiyama et al 2001[24]
AT1-R	AS-ODN iv in liposomes	CIH	−38	Unknown	Peng et al 1998[25]
β1-AR	AS-ODN iv in liposomes	SHR	−35	30–40 days	Zhang et al 2000[3,19]

AGT, angiotensinogen; AS-ODN, antisense oligodeoxynucleotide; AT1-R, angiotensin type 1 receptor; CIH, cold-induced hypertension; HJV, Haemagglutinin Virus of Japan; ICV, intracerebroventricular; pvn, paraventricular nucleus; RVM, rostral ventral medulla; SHR, spontaneously hypertensive rat; unknown, recovery of pressure not recorded; WKY, Wistar Kyoto.

to any currently available drug, all of which have to be taken on a daily basis. Repeated injections at intervals of 3–4 weeks of intravenous β_1-AS-ODN produce prolonged control of high blood pressure without any toxic effects in the liver, blood or organs.

Angiotensinogen antisense ODN

We have also established that angiotensinogen AS-ODN is effective for antisense ODN for hypertension therapy. In human hypertension, the angiotensinogen

Table 14.3 Preclinical data of gene therapy for hypertension vasoconstrictor genes: viral vector delivery of antisense

Target gene	Delivery	Model	Max Δ blood pressure (mmHg)	Duration of effect	Reference
AGT	AAV-based plasmid	SHR	−22.5	8 Days	Tang et al 1999[30]
AT1-R	AAV ic	SHR adult	−40	9 weeks plus	Phillips 1997[33]
AGT	AAV ic	SHR adult	−40	10 weeks plus	Phillips 1997[8]
AT1-R	LNSV ic	SHR (neonates)	−40	90 days	Iyer et al 1996[35]
AT1-R	LNSV iv	SHR	−30	36 days	Wang et al[48]
ACE	LNSV ic	SHR (neonates)	−15		Tang et al 1999[30]
AGT	AAV ic	SHR (neonates)	−30	6 months	Kimura et al 2000[34]
AT1-R	AAV iv	Double transgenic mice (adult)	−40	6 months	Phillips et al (in press)[49]

AAV, adeno-associated virus; AGT, angiotensinogen; AT1-R, angiotensin type 1 receptor; ic, intracerebral; iv, intravenous; LNSV, retrovirus; SHR, spontaneously hypertensive rat.

gene has been shown to be linked and play a role in the disease.[20] However, there is no currently available drug to inhibit angiotensinogen. We have designed antisense, targeted to AGT mRNA and tested it *in vivo* and *in vitro*.[21] When given intravenously, the angiotensinogen AS-ODN reduces blood pressure significantly when delivered with a liposome. These studies have been confirmed by others independently, showing that AGT-AS-ODN reduces blood pressure for up to 7 days with a single systemic dose.[22]

AT₁-R antisense ODN

A similar story is true for the effects of AT$_1$-AS-ODN. This has been tested centrally with intracerebroventricular injections and with intravenous injections. It has been tested in SHR rats,[23] in 2-kidney-1 clip animals[24] and in environmentally induced hypertension.[25] In these three different models of hypertension – genetic, surgical and environmental – the antisense produces a decrease in blood pressure within 24 hours of administration. The effect lasts for up to 7 days and there is no effect on heart rate.[23] The distribution of antisense is in blood vessels, kidney, liver and heart.[25] The majority of uptake is in the kidney and liver.[17] A reduction in AT$_1$ receptors after treatment with the AT$_1$-AS-ODN reveals reductions in the protein in kidney, aorta and liver.[25]

In summary, AS-ODNs have proved to be useful in demonstrating in the preclinical setting and can target specific genes and reduce blood pressure for several days (or weeks) with a single administration. Laboratory data indicate that these effects are the result of rapid uptake of the antisense ODN into cells,[26] where they migrate to the nucleus and inhibit the production of protein, most likely through translational inhibition of messenger RNA.[26,27] This could occur by the hybridization of ODN with specific mRNA, preventing the passage of the mRNA through the ribosome. Alternatively, in some tissues, DNA hybridization to RNA will stimulate the production of RNAse-H for the specific sequence of mRNA bound to the ODN. RNAse-H destroys the RNA that is hybridized to

DNA and thereby releases the oligo for further hybridization. This recycling action induced by RNAse-H might account for the long action of AS-ODNs.

Other useful features that make oligos attractive for hypertension therapy are, first, that they can be produced relatively cheaply, rapidly and in large quantities. Second, the demand for oligos and primers has reduced the cost per base to a few cents. They do not cross the BBB and, therefore, when given peripherally, will not have central effects.[18] Third, they are most effective when delivered in the right combination of ODN to cationic liposome.[18,19] Treatment of rats with liposome ODN complexes has not shown any toxicity in our experience.

VIRAL VECTOR DELIVERY

To produce very prolonged effects (i.e. several months) with a single injection, we use antisense DNA delivery by viral vector. Several viral vectors are available but the adeno-associated virus (AAV) is both safe for use in humans and large enough to carry antisense genes with tissue specific promoters.[28] The AAV is not to be confused with the adenovirus. Adenoviruses, although easy to use in laboratory animals, have caused a human death during trials and are not, in their present form, acceptable vectors. AAV is a parvovirus that does not replicate and does not induce inflammatory reactions. The AAV can be stripped of its *rep* and *gag* genes to carry up to 4.5 kb and deliver it to the nuclei of cells where it integrates in the genome.[29] When antisense DNA is used, the AAV allows the continuous production of an RNA that is in the antisense direction. This antisense RNA hybridizes to specific mRNA and inhibits translation. Therefore, we are developing antisense therapy using the AAV as a vector. To construct a viral vector requires the design and production of plasmids and gene packaging into the vector.

DELIVERY BY PLASMIDS

Plasmids are effective vectors but last for a shorter time than the viral vector because they do not allow integration into the genome. This is illustrated with the adeno-associated-based vector for angiotensinogen antisense cDNA.[30] A plasmid containing AAV terminal repeats was prepared with a cassette, consisting of a cytomegalovirus (CMV) promoter, the rat AGT cDNA based on the sequence by Lynch et al.[31] The cDNA is oriented in the antisense direction. In addition, the cassette contains an internal ribosome entry site (IRES) and as a marker, the green fluorescent protein gene (GFP).[32] At 48 hours after transfection into pAAV-AGT-AS, there was clear dominant expression of GFP in the H-4 cells. There was a significant reduction of AGT (120 ± 14 versus 230 ± 20 ng/mg protein, $P < 0.01$). Transgene expression detected by RT-PCR in the H-4 cells started at 2 hours and continued for at least 72 hours.

The plasmid was then tested *in vivo* by injecting the S and AS plasmids intravenously into SHR rats.[30] AGT-AS expression was positive in heart and lung at 3 days and 7 days. Expression in the kidney was absent or weak. When injected with 3 mg/kg plasmid, pAAV-AGT-AS produced a significant drop in blood pressure ($P < 0.01$) for 6–8 days in SHRs. The drop in blood pressure correlated to a drop in plasma angiotensinogen levels that was significant at days 3 and 5 after injection. The decrease in blood pressure with injection of plasmid could be prolonged by injecting the plasmid with cationic liposome (DOTAP/DOPE).

Plasmids are useful for delivery of AS to produce an antihypertensive effect lasting about 1 week. They do not require the more complex packaging needed for recombinant AAV (rAAV).

DELIVERY BY RECOMBINANT AAV VECTOR

To produce long-term decreases in hypertension, we developed rAAV to deliver antisense to AT_1-R in SHR.[28,33] The results showed that single intracardiac injection of rAAV-AT_1-R-AS effectively reduced blood pressure by 30 mmHg for at least 5 weeks compared to controls.

To test whether an AAV delivery of an AT_1-R antisense would inhibit development of hypertension, we injected 5-day-old SHRs. Hypertension in SHR develops between the eighth and tenth weeks after birth. Therefore, injecting in 5-day-old SHRs allowed us to observe if the development of hypertension would be reduced. A single injection of AAV-AGT-AS in 5-day-old SHRs significantly attenuated the full development[34] and level of hypertension for up to 6 months. In 3-week-old SHRs, rAAV-AT_1-R-AS significantly reduced hypertension by about 30 mmHg for at least 5 weeks (the length of the study). However, contrary to the reports of the effect of retrovirus delivery of an AT_1-R-AS in 5-day-old SHRs 'curing' hypertension,[35] we did not find a complete inhibition of the rise in blood pressure.

In rAAV-AGT-AS-treated SHRs, measures of plasma AGT levels showed a corresponding lack of increase in AGT in the AS-treated groups, compared to the significant increase of AGT in the control animals.[34] Correlation of AGT versus blood pressure was significant ($P < 0.05$) in the control-treated animals and not significant in the AS-treated animals. This shows that angiotensinogen in the SHR is correlated with an increase in blood pressure. The AAV was expressed in kidney, heart and liver throughout the time of the reduction in blood pressure. Thus, we concluded that the early treatment with a single dose of rAAV-AGT-AS, given systemically, prevents the full development of hypertension in the adult SHR by a prolonged reduction in AGT levels. Similarly, the results with the rAAV-AT_1-AS showed a reduction in hypertension development correlated with a consistent reduction in AT_1 receptors in VSMC.[33] No toxicity was noted.[34] To prove the potential therapeutic value of rAAV, we recently used a mouse model of hypertension that clearly depends on an overactive renin–angiotenisn system. In this model, which has human renin and human AGT transgenes, rAAV-AS-AT_1-R reduced high blood pressure for up to 6 months with a single systemic injection.[36] These latest data with rAAV-AT_1-R-AS confirm the results in adult SHRs[28] and give an even clearer picture that the AAV as vector has many advantages for hypertension therapy.

OTHER VECTORS

Other vectors are being tested for hypertension gene therapy. As noted above, adenovirus vectors have been used with kallikrein gene insertion[13] and recently to deliver calcitonin gene-related peptide for hypoxia-induced pulmonary hypertension in mice.[37] However, the adenovirus synthesizes proteins that trigger the immune system and cause inflammation, which has limited use in human therapy so far. Raizada and colleagues have worked with LNSV, a retrovirus, with antisense AT_1 receptor injected into newborn SHRs to prevent the development of hypertension in the adults.[35,38] In a series of papers they have evidence that AT_1-R-AS normalizes blood pressure and prevents organ damage. Retroviruses are appropriate only for dividing cells and therefore are not suitable for hypertension therapy in adults. As a therapy, the idea of injecting infants with AT_1-R antisense on the chance they might have become hypertensive as adults is farfetched, but these studies offer a demonstration of the effectiveness of antisense. Retroviruses might be useful in treating cardiomyopathy, restenosis and vascular remodeling, where cells are actively dividing, but retroviruses integrate randomly into the genome and the risk of tumorgenesis is high. Lentivirus vectors, which can infect dividing cells, are just beginning to be explored for their therapeutic value. They offer large gene-carrying capacity, are stable, and are easily produced. Their disadvantage is the risk of uncontrolled infection and the potential for neoplastic changes. Other vectors, such as herpex simplex virus and Japan Sendai virus, are being tested as vectors but all vectors are as yet only in limited use by certain laboratories.

ENGINEERING VIRUSES

In addition to the choice of vectors, the control of transgene expression needs to be engineered and new promoters need to be explored before viral vectors can be used in humans.[38] The ideal promoter will be active for prolonged periods to maintain transgene expression and specific for a tissue cell type. However, there might be circumstances when the vectors will need mechanisms to switch them on or off as required. Various attempts are being made to develop gene switches, such as the tetracycline transactivator system (tTA), by which a transgene can be activated in the presence (or absence) of tetracycline. Ultimately, the promoters and transactivating factors will have to be so specific that the antisense can be turned on in a specific tissue when the need arises.

CONCLUSION

Both antisense oligonucleotides and antisense DNA delivered in a vector have advantages for gene therapy. Antisense ODNs can be used as long-lasting drugs. They have an action that lasts for days or weeks, depending how they are delivered. They are specific for a target protein, and reduce overactive production of proteins but, because the inhibition is never total, they permit normal physiology. Antisense oligos are not toxic at therapeutic doses. They can be produced in large quantities, relatively cheaply for humans. The challenge for antisense ODNs is to deliver them. They can be delivered systemically by injection with liposomes,[19] but a goal for therapy is either a skin patch or oral delivery.

The AAV vector with antisense DNA has very prolonged action (weeks/months) with a single dose,[34] and is safe, nonpathogenic and noninflammatory.[6,7] The AAV is extremely stable.[6,7] The challenge for clinical use is to increase production of large amounts at reasonable cost and to further engineer the control of the vector, as described above.

This brief review of some of the preclinical data suggests that gene therapy for hypertension is possible.[38] The question remains: will these strategies be tested at the clinical level? The rAAV antisense strategy appears to be effective for reducing high blood pressure in different models of hypertension. Its development could provide a new generation of antihypertensive agents that would be administered in a single dose for prolonged effects lasting several months. Alternatively, antisense oligonucleotides are effective and highly specific. They could be used like long-acting drugs to provide sustained control of hypertension with infrequent administration. It seems that of the two strategies, the antisense oligonucleotides will be clinically acceptable first, because of our familiarity with drug treatments. The viral vector approach might come much later, when all the basic science has been done to assure the patient that it is safe.

In addition to the gene targets we have discussed in this chapter there are others related to hypertension and vascular disease that as yet have no drug treatment, e.g. the gene encoding apolipoprotein B (apo B), which is essential to the formation of low-density lipoproteins (LDL) and stimulates LDL receptors. The heterozygous apo B knockout mice have a 20% decrease in cholesterol and do not develop hypercholesterolemia when fed a high-cholesterol diet.[39] RNAi delivered systemically silenced the apo B mRNA in the liver and jejuneum, resulting in decreased cholesterol and plasma levels of apo B.[40] The RNAi degraded mRNA, preventing it from translating the specific protein, apo B. This encouraging result may have two benefits. It renews interest in a gene therapy by inhibiting specific mRNA and focuses the therapeutic hope on a cardiovascular disease.

References

1. Lifton RP, Gharavi AG, Geller DS. Molecular mechanisms of human hypertension. *Cell* 2001; 104:445–456.
2. Phillips MI. Is gene therapy for hypertension possible? *Hypertension* 1999; 33:1–13.
3. Zhang YC, Bui JD, Shen L, Phillips MI. Antisense inhibition of (beta1adrenergic) receptor mRNA in a single dose produces a profound and prolonged reduction in high blood pressure in spontaneously hypertensive rats. *Circulation* 2000; 101:682–688.
4. Marshall E. Gene therapy death prompts review of adenovirus vector. *Science* 1999; 286(5448):244–245.
5. Check E. Gene therapy put on hold as third child develops cancer. *Nature* 2005; 433(7026):61.
6. Flotte TR, Brantly ML, Spencer LT, et al. Phase I trial of intramuscular injection of a recombinant adeno–associated virus alpha 1-antitrypsin (rAAV2-CB-hAAT) gene vector to AAT-deficient adults. *Hum Gene Ther* 2004; 15:13–128.
7. Moss RB, Rodman D, Spencer LT, et al. Repeated adeno-associated virus serotype 2 aerosol-mediated cystic fibrosis transmembrane regulator gene transfer to the lungs of patients with cystic fibrosis: a multicenter, double-blind, placebo-controlled trial. *Chest* 2004; 125:209–221.
8. Phillips MI. Antisense inhibition and adeno-associated viral vector delivery for reducing hypertension. *Hypertension* 1997; 29(1 Pt 2):177–187.
9. NM Kaplan. *Clinical hypertension.* Baltimore: Williams and Williams; 1998.
10. Lifton RP. Molecular genetics of human blood pressure variation. *Science* 1996; 272(5262):676–680.
11. Gyurko R, Wielbo D, Phillips MI. Antisense inhibition of AT1 receptor mRNA and angiotensinogen mRNA in the brain of spontaneously hypertensive rats reduces hypertension of neurogenic origin. *Regul Pept* 1993; 49:267–274.
12. Phillips MI, Wielbo D, Gyurko R. Antisense inhibition of hypertension: a new strategy for renin-angiotensin candidate genes. *Kidney Int* 1994; 46(6):1554–1556.
13. Chao J, Chao L. Kallikrein gene therapy: a new strategy for hypertensive diseases. *Immunopharmacology* 1997; 36(2–3):229–236.

14. Lin KF, Chao J, Chao L. Atrial natriuretic peptide gene delivery attenuates hypertension, cardiac hypertrophy, and renal injury in salt-sensitive rats. *Hum Gene Ther* 1998; 9(10):1429–1438.

15. Chao J, Jin L, Lin KF, Chao L. Adrenomedullin gene delivery reduces blood pressure in spontaneously hypertensive rats. *Hypertens Res* 1997; 20:469–477.

16. Lin KF, Chao L, Chao J. Prolonged reduction of high blood pressure with human nitric oxide synthase gene delivery. *Hypertension* 1997; 30(3 Pt 1):307–313.

17. Dobrzynski E, Yoshida H, Chao J, Chao L. Adenovirus-mediated kallikrein gene delivery attenuates hypertension and protects against renal injury in deoxycorticosterone-salt rats. *Immunopharmacology* 1999; 44(1–2):57–65.

18. Wang H, Katovich MJ, Gelband CH, et al. Sustained inhibition of angiotensin I-converting enzyme (ACE) expression and long-term antihypertensive action by virally mediated delivery of ACE antisense cDNA. *Circ Res* 1999; 85:714–722.

19. Zhang ClareY, Kimura B, Shen L, Phillips MI. New beta-blocker: prolonged reduction in high blood pressure with beta1 antisense oligodeoxynucleotides. *Hypertension* 2000; 35(1 Pt 2):219–224.

20. Jeunemaitre X, Soubrier F, Kotelevtsev YV, et al. Molecular basis of human hypertension: role of angiotensinogen. *Cell* 1992; 71:169–180.

21. Wielbo D, Simon A, Phillips MI, Toffolo S. Inhibition of hypertension by peripheral administration of antisense oligodeoxynucleotides. *Hypertension* 1996; 28:147–151.

22. Makino N, Sugano M, Ohtsuka S, Sawada S. Intravenous injection with antisense oligodeoxynucleotides against angiotensinogen decreases blood pressure in spontaneously hypertensive rats. *Hypertension* 1998; 31:5166–5170.

23. Gyurko R, Tran D, Phillips MI. Time course of inhibition of hypertension by antisense oligonucleotides targeted to AT1 angiotensin receptor mRNA in spontaneously hypertensive rats. *Am J Hypertens* 1997; 10(5 Pt 2):56S–62S.

24. Kagiyama S, Varela A, Phillips MI, Galli SM. Antisense inhibition of brain renin-angiotensin system decreased blood pressure in chronic 2-kidney, 1 clip hypertensive rats. *Hypertension* 2001; 37(2 Pt 2):371–375.

25. Peng JF, Kimura B, Fregly MJ, Phillips MI. Reduction of cold-induced hypertension by antisense oligodeoxynucleotides to angiotensinogen mRNA and AT1-receptor mRNA in brain and blood. *Hypertension* 1998; 31:6317–6323.

26. Li B, Hughes JA, Phillips MI. Uptake and efflux of intact antisense phosphorothioate deoxyoligonucleotide directed against angiotensin receptors in bovine adrenal cells. *Neurochem Int* 1997; 31:393–403.

27. Crooke ST. Progress in antisense technology: the end of the beginning. *Methods Enzymol* 2000; 313:3–45.

28. Dobrzynski E, Wang C, Chao J, Chao L. Adrenomedullin gene delivery attenuates hypertension, cardiac remodeling, and renal injury in deoxycorticosteroneacetate–salt hypertensive rats. *Hypertension* 2000; 36:695–1001.

29. Wu P, Phillips M I, Bui J, Terwilliger EF. Adeno-associated virus vector-mediated transgene integration into neurons and other nondividing cell targets. *J Virol* 1998; 72:7919–7926.

30. Tang X, Mohuczy D, Zhang YC, et al. Intravenous angiotensinogen antisense in AAV-based vector decreases hypertension. *Am J Physiol* 1999; 277(6 Pt 2):H2392–H2399.

31. Lynch KR, Simnad VI, Ben-Ari ET, Garrison JC. Localization of preangiotensinogen messenger RNA sequences in the rat brain. *Hypertension* 1986; 8:640–643.

32. Zolotukhin S, Potter M, Hauswirth WW, et al. A 'humanized' green fluorescent protein cDNA adapted for high-level expression in mammalian cells. *J Virol* 1996; 70:7646–7654.

33. Phillips MI, Mohuczy-Dominiak D, Coffey M, et al. Prolonged reduction of high blood pressure with an in vivo, nonpathogenic, adeno-associated viral vector delivery of AT1-R mRNA antisense. *Hypertension* 1997; 29(1 Pt 2):374–380.

34. Kimura B, Mohuczy D, Tang X, Phillips MI. Attenuation of hypertension and heart hypertrophy by adeno-associated virus delivering angiotensinogen antisense. *Hypertension* 2001; 37(2 Pt 2):376–380.

35. Iyer SN, Lu D, Katovich MJ, Raizada MK. Chronic control of high blood pressure in the spontaneously hypertensive rat by delivery of angiotensin type 1 receptor antisense. *Proc Natl Acad Sci U S A* 1996; 93(18):9960–9965.

36. Phillips MI. Gene therapy for hypertension: sense and antisense strategies. *Expert Opin Biol Ther* 2001; 1:455–462.

37. Champion HC, Bivalacqua TJ, Toyoda K, et al. In vivo gene transfer of prepro-calcitonin gene-related peptide to the lung attenuates chronic hypoxia-induced pulmonary hypertension in the mouse. *Circulation* 2000; 101:823–830.

38. Morishita R, Higaki J, Tomita N, et al. Role of transcriptional cis-elements, angiotensinogen gene-activating elements, of angiotensinogen gene in blood pressure regulation. *Hypertension* 1996; 27(3 Pt 2):502–507.

39. Farese RV Jr, Ruland SL, Flynn LM, et al. Knockout of the mouse apolipoprotein B gene results in embryonic lethality in homozygotes and protection against diet-induced hypercholesterolemia in heterozygotes. *Proc Natl Acad Sci U S A* 1995; 92:5774–5778.

40. Soutschek J, Akinc A, Bramlage B, et al. Therapeutic silencing of an endogenous gene by systemic administration of modified siRNAs. *Nature* 2004; 432(7014):173–178.

41. Suzuki S, Pilowsky P, Minson J, et al. c-fos antisense in rostral ventral medulla reduces arterial blood pressure. *Am J Physiol* 1994; 266(4 Pt 2):R1418–R1422.

42. Wolf WC, Evans DM, Chao L, Chao J. A synthetic tissue kallikrein inhibitor suppresses cancer cell invasiveness. *Am J Pathol* 2001 159; 1797–1805.

43. Zhang JJ, Wang C, Lin KF, et al. Human tissue kallikrein attenuates hypertension and secretes into circulation and urine after intramuscular gene delivery in hypertensive rats. *Clin Exp Hypertens* 1999; 21:7145–7160.

44. Wang MH, Zhang F, Marji J, et al. CYP4A1 antisense oligonucleotide reduces mesenteric vascular reactivity and blood pressure in SHR. *Am J Physiol Regul Integr Comp Physiol* 2001; 280:1255–1261.

45. Tomita N, Morishita R, Higaki J, et al. Transient decrease in high blood pressure by in vivo transfer of antisense oligodeoxynucleotides against rat angiotensinogen. *Hypertension* 1995; 26:131–136.

46. Galli SM, Phillips MI. Angiotensin II AT(1A) receptor antisense lowers blood pressure in acute 2-kidney, 1-clip hypertension. *Hypertension* 2001; 38(3 Pt 2):674–678.

47. Hayashi I, Majima M, Fujita T, et al. In vivo transfer of antisense oligonucleotide against urinary kininase blunts deoxycorticosterone acetate-salt hypertension in rats. *Br J Pharmacol* 2000; 131(4):820–826.

48. Wang H, Lu D, Reaves PY. Retrovirally mediated delivery of angiotensin II type 1 receptor antisense in vitro and in vivo. *Methods Enzymol* 2000; 314:581–590.

49. Phillips MI, Kimura B. Normalization of Hypertension with AAV delivery of AT1 receptor and ACE antisense DNA. (Presented at the *Amer J Hypert Ann meeting* 2003 New York).

Index